RENAL TRANSPLANTATION – UPDATES AND ADVANCES

Edited by **Layron Long**

Renal Transplantation – Updates and Advances
Edited by Layron Long

Published by InTech
Janeza Trdine 9, 51000 Rijeka, Croatia

Publishing Process Manager Adriana Pecar

Technical Editor Teodora Smiljanic

Cover Designer InTech Design Team

Additional hard copies can be obtained from orders@intechopen.com

Renal Transplantation – Updates and Advances, Edited by Layron Long
p. cm.
ISBN 978-953-51-0173-4

For EU product safety concerns:
IN TECH d.o.o., Prolaz Marije Krucifikse Kozulić 3, 51000 Rijeka, Croatia,
info@intechopen.com or visit our website at intechopen.com.

Meet the editor

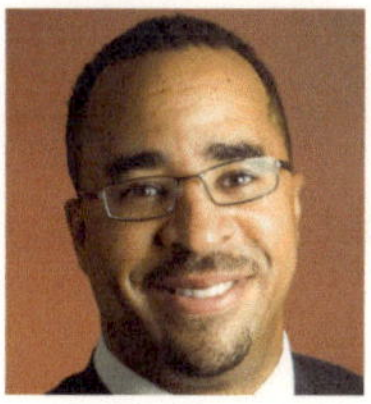

Dr Layron Long (Samaritan Urology, Good Samaritan Regional Medical Center, Corvallis, OR, USA) is a board-certified urologist who earned a medical degree from Meharry Medical College in Nashville, Tenn. He completed an internship in general surgery at Vanderbilt University Medical Center in Nashville and a fellowship in molecular genetics at Howard University/Johns Hopkins University in Washington, D.C. Dr Long trained in urological surgery at TUFTS New England Medical Center in Boston and finished his training as a senior and chief resident at the University of Washington Medical Center in Seattle. After completing residency training, Dr Long was an acting instructor and completed an Endourological Society fellowship in robotic surgery, laparoscopy and endo-urology at the University of Washington. He is a member of the American Urological Association, American Association of Clinical Urologists, Society of Endourology, Society of Laparoendoscopic Surgeons and the American College of Surgeons.

Contents

Preface

Due to the advances in renal transplantation, the treatment of end stage renal disease has been revolutionized. The modern progression of transplant surgery, molecular genetics, and pharmacogenetics has led to a reduction in surgical complications, prolonged survival, and improvements in the coset effectiveness of renal transplants. This text offers a medley of international papers that address the most recent advances in the field. "Renal Transplantation - Updates and Advances" provides a comprehensive , concise, evidence based codification of the current state of surgical techniques, immunology, pharmacology, and molecular science regarding the treatment and management of renal transplantation for end stage renal disease. This book is a treasure – trop of data, providing access to vital information, providing a great reference to state of the art perspectives on the subject at hand.

Dr. Layron Long
Samaritan Urology
Good Samaritan Regional Medical Center
Corvallis, OR
USA

1

Preservation of Renal Allografts for Transplantation

Marco Antonio Ayala-García[1,2], Miguel Ángel Pantoja Hernández[3], Éctor Jaime Ramírez-Barba[4,5,6], Joel Máximo Soel Encalada[1] and Beatriz González Yebra[1,6]

[1]*Hospital Regional de Alta Especialidad del Bajío*
[2]*HGSZ No. 10 del Instituto Mexicano del Seguro Social, Delegación Guanajuato*
[3]*Universidad de Celaya*
[4]*Instituto de Salud Pública del Estado de Guanajuato*
[5]*Secretaria de Salud del Estado de Guanajuato*
[6]*Universidad de Guanajuato*
México

1. Introduction

Kidney transplantation requires the availability of allografts obtained from diverse types of donors. Once the kidney is outside of the donor's body, it must be preserved in a state in which, after being transplanted, its normal operation can be quickly restored. Proper preservation of the renal graft is crucial, because it extends the viability of the organ, thus providing time for the complex preparation steps that are required for the transplantation procedure. These preparatory steps include the selection of the recipient, histocompatibility testing, transportation of the organ over long distances, and preparation of the recipient in the operating room.

The first documented case of perfusion and preservation of an isolated organ was performed by Loebel in 1849. Other pioneers have subsequently contributed to this area: Langendorf in 1845 used a siphoning tube connected to the organ, while Martin created a method to perfuse the coronary artery *in vitro* in the early 1900's. In 1905 Carrel published "Anastomosis and Transplant of Blood Vessels". Around 1930, Heinz Rosenberg built a perfusion machine, and in 1935 Lindbergh built a pulsatory perfusion machine.

In the early 1960's, the only known preservation method was simple organ cooling. Lapchinsky in the former Soviet Union started transplanting extremities and kidneys that were preserved at +2°C and +4°C, preserving them for up to 28 hours. In 1963 Calne and Pegg demonstrated that perfusion of cold blood to an ischemic kidney could prolong its preservation up to 12 hours. In 1967, Belzer preserved kidneys for up to 72 hours, using a method of continuous perfusion "*ex situ*". In 1969 Collins described the use of a preservation solution that resembled the composition of the intracellular fluid, and was used for perfusion/rinsing of the organ in cold temperature "*in situ*", and also for its further hypothermic storage, achieving kidney preservation for up to 30 hours. In the 1980's Belzer,

Southard and many other investigators started to lay the foundations for understanding the metabolic changes that occur in the extracted organs after explantation.

In this chapter the techniques for kidney allograft preservation will be briefly reviewed, and the pathophysiological changes that occur during preservation and reperfusion of the allograft will be discussed. Finally, the currently used preservation solutions will be described.

2. Techniques for preservation of the renal allograft

2.1 Hypothermic perfusion techniques

The combination of continuous perfusion and hypothermic storage used by Belzer *et al.* in 1967 represented a new paradigm in regards to organ preservation, achieving successful canine kidney preservation for 72 hours. In this technique, after the initial washes performed during perfusion in the operating room, the organ is introduced in a device that keeps a controlled flow (continuous or pulsatory) with cold preservation solution (0-4°C). This flow allows complete perfusion of the organ and clearing of any micro thrombi in the blood stream, while facilitating the elimination of final metabolic products. Its beneficial effects include a lower incidence of delay in the initial functioning of the graft, the possibility to assess its viability in real time, and the possibility of providing metabolic (oxygen or substrates) or pharmacologic support during the perfusion. The hypothermic perfusion machine (HPM) with continuous flow has not shown advantages with respect to the pulsatory flow machine. Figures; 1 and 2, shows some of the perfusion machines currently being used.

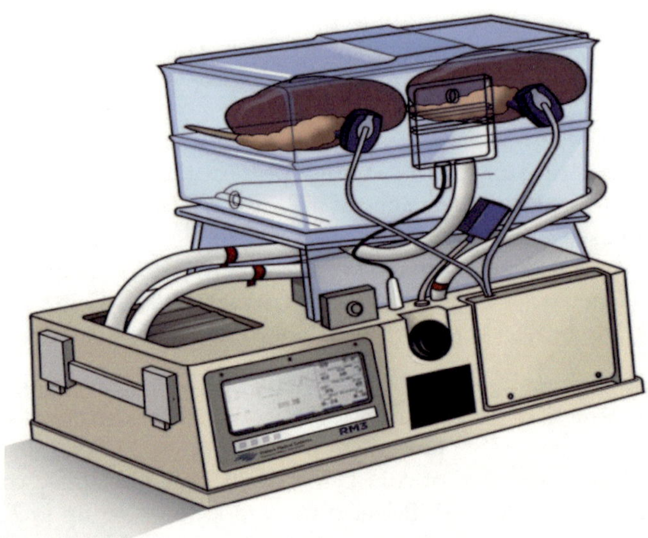

Fig. 1. Hypothermic perfusion machine: Waters RM3® Renal Preservation System from Waters Medical System®.

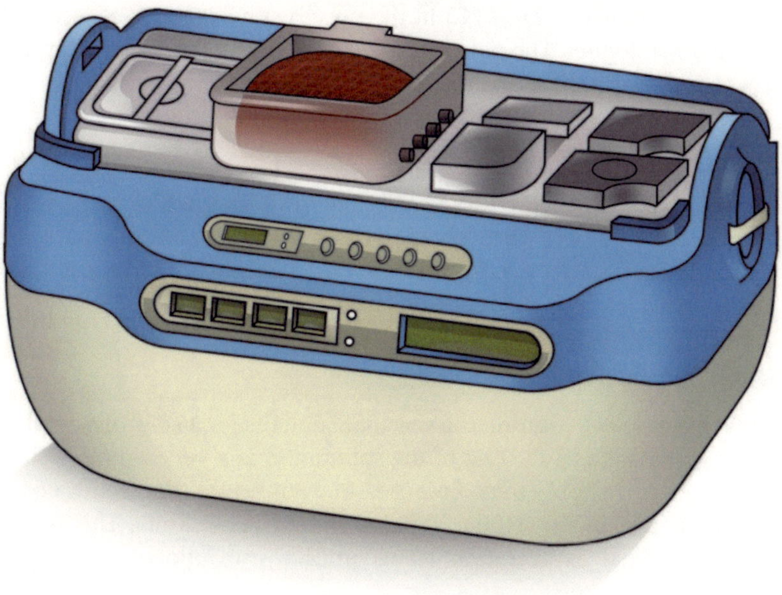

Fig. 2. Hypothermic perfusion machine: Life Port Kidney Transporter® from Organ Recovery Systems®.

To date, hypothermic perfusion is the approach that provides the longest possible preservation time for renal allografts. However, due to its complexity, high cost, and the need for abundant equipment, these techniques are only suitable for use in facilities highly specialized in renal preservation. Additionally, they require well prepared personnel with vast experience in the field of allograft preservation.

The use of HPM has the following advantages and disadvantages:

Advantages:

1. Less incidence of delay in the re-initiation of kidney allograft function.
2. Better preservation for longer periods of time (especially greater than 24 hours)
3. Ability to control flow and pressure, therefore ability to monitor intrarenal resistance during perfusion.
4. Decreased renal vasospasm.
5. Ability to provide metabolic support during perfusion.
6. Potential for pharmacological manipulation during perfusion.

Disadvantages:

1. Increased cost.
2. Endothelial injury.
3. Possibility of mechanical failure.

2.2 Normothermic preservation techniques

Just recently, interest has been arising on the beneficial effects of continuous normothermic or subnormothermic perfusion (25-37 °C) in the preservation process, especially of kidneys from non-beating heart donors. The potential benefits of normothermia during perfusion are the decrease of vascular resistance and the increase in oxygen release.

2.3 Oxygen insufflation technique

This technique was first described by Isselhard *et al.* in 1972, in which oxygen is insufflated through the kidney vessels and then escapes through small perforations on the organ's surface. This technique was attempted for the first time in canine kidneys, and has been the subject of a pilot clinical study.

2.4 Preservation by cold storage

This technique consists in substituting the vascular contents for a cold preservation solution, replacing the intracellular fluid for that of the solution. It is a very simple technique, but it only partially achieves its objective, because, in contrast to the continuous perfusion techniques, it does not maintain cellular metabolism in hypothermia. This is the technique that the majority of renal explantation teams utilize. The following is required for its application:

1. Preservation solution.
2. The temperature of the preservation solution should be 4°C.
3. The perfusion fluid should be infused at a pressure greater than 60 torr, ensuring the complete elimination of the graft's vascular contents. In practice, this is achieved by placing the perfusion fluids at 100-150 cm above the organs to be perfused.
4. The amount of solution necessary to preserve the kidney is 1 liter, but it is standard practice to stop perfusion only after the effluent fluid from the graft does not contain any blood.

3. Pathophysiology and basis for the preservation of a renal allograft

The extraction, storage, and transplantation of a renal allograft from a donor significantly alter the kidney's internal homeostasis. The extent of these changes influences the extent to which kidney function will be recovered after transplantation. Kidney injury mainly occurs as a result of ischemia, and the different preservation techniques serve to minimize this injury and improve the allograft's function and survival.

3.1 Basis for the preservation of the renal allograft

Any kidney that has been extracted from the body suffers a process known as ischemia. The graft does not receive oxygen or nutritional support, and at the same time, products of its own metabolism accumulate, resulting in injury. The injury to the tissue is initially reversible, but after a certain interval it becomes irreversible. This phenomenon is known as "hot ischemia", and under these conditions the time limit for organ viability is between 30 and 60 minutes.

The deterioration caused by ischemia is mediated by chemical reactions that happen more or less rapidly depending on the temperature. During hypothermia, reversible ischemic injury also appears early on ("cold ischemia"), but differs from hot ischemia in several ways.

The fundamental cause of ischemic injury resides in the molecular changes suffered by cellular membranes. Initially, the cells swell and become turgid due to the alterations in the functionality of the cell membrane. After 60 minutes of hot ischemia, rupture of renal cell membranes is observed, followed by cellular necrosis.

Another phenomenon also observed in hot ischemia is called "absence of reflux", which comprises the lack of blood flow when circulation is restored to the organ. This occurs when erythrocytes accumulate in the vessels. Therefore, completely eliminating erythrocytes in the vessels through rinsing during the ischemic period is essential.

3.2 Effects of hypothermia (cold ischemia)

The key to successful organ preservation is hypothermia. Cooling reduces the rate at which intracellular enzymes degrade the components that are essential for cellular viability. Hypothermia does not completely stop cellular metabolism, it only slows it down for a limited time, after which function ceases completely and viability is lost (cellular death). The length of this period is organ-specific.

The majority of enzymes in normothermic animal cells show a decrease in their activity from 1.5- 2 times for each 10°C decrease in temperature, following the Van Hoff rule:

$$Q_{10}= (K_2/K_1)^{10/(t2-t1)}$$

Where Q_{10} is the coefficient for a change of 10°C in temperature, and K_1 and K_2 are the rates of the enzymatic reactions at temperatures t_1 and t_2, respectively. In a renal cell with a Q_{10} of 2, a change in temperature from 37°C to 0°C decreases the rate of the metabolic reactions by a factor of 12 to 13.

The majority of organs tolerate between 30 to 60 minutes of hot ischemia, without completely losing their function. Thus, the simple cooling of a kidney increases its preservation time up to 12 to 13 hours, as shown by Calne and Pegg in 1963. After 13 hours, ultrastructural changes can be observed in the proximal tubules and, to a lesser extent, in the distal tubules.

The only methods that could in theory maintain a kidney viable for months or years are freezing of the organ, or its continuous aerobic perfusion. Temperatures below 0°C have been used to successfully preserve isolated cells and some simple tissues, but not kidneys. Cryopreservation is still an exciting and complex field of research. The method of continuous aerobic perfusion is complex, expensive and requires trained personnel with vast experience in organ preservation, and thus this technique is not routinely used in clinical practice.

The ideal preservation temperature for kidney allografts is between 0°C and 5°C (4°C seems to be the ideal temperature). Higher temperatures would accelerate cellular metabolism, making it necessary to provide nutrients to support its metabolic requirements through continuous perfusion during the preservation period.

As previously mentioned, in cold ischemia, besides hypothermia, perfusion fluids are also needed. Therefore, the renal allograft is subjected to ischemia in anaerobic hypothermia, which is accompanied by the events described below.

3.2.1 Cellular edema induced by ischemia and hypothermia

Under normal conditions, the cells are in an extracellular environment rich in sodium and low in potassium, while the intracellular environment is poor in sodium and rich in potassium. This equilibrium against a gradient between both sides of the plasma membrane is maintained by the Na+/K+ pump which requires energy (ATP) obtained from oxidative phosphorylation. The pump keeps this balance by avoiding the entrance of sodium into the cell and counteracting the colloidal osmotic pressure derived from proteins and other intracellular anions. Under normal conditions, the intracellular osmotic force is 110-140 mOsm/Kg.

Anaerobic hypothermia (such as in the kidney stored in the cold) decreases the activity of the Na+/K+ pump and reduces the plasma membrane potential. Sodium and chloride enter the cell following a concentration gradient, dragging with them water, which causes the cell to swell, causing cellular edema (Fig 3). This edema could be counteracted by adding to the preservation solution 110-140 mmol/l of substances that are impermeable to the cell (i.e. they cannot pass the plasma membrane due to their elevated molecular weight). We will refer to these substances as "waterproofing agents".

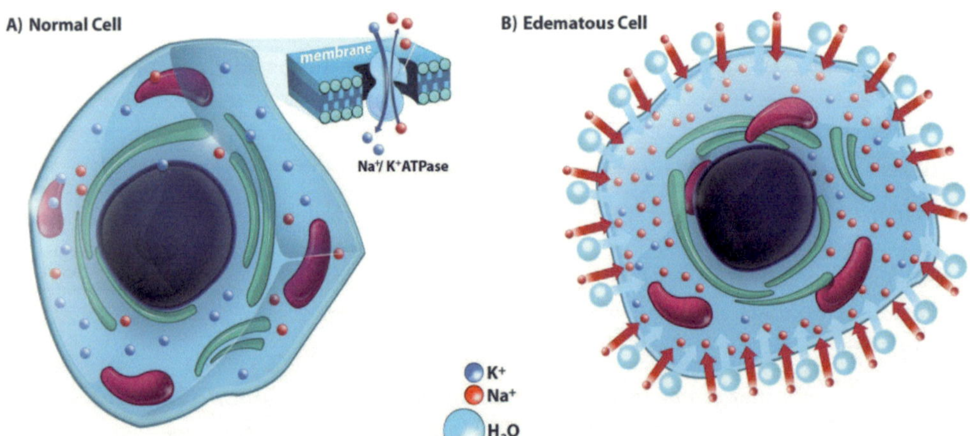

Fig. 3. Cellular edema.

The problem posed by waterproofing agents is that, even though they diffuse poorly across the membrane, they will eventually enter the cell over time. Therefore, when implanting the kidney in its new environment, the cells will suddenly be exposed to a relatively hypotonic extracellular osmolarity. Because the Na+/K+ pump is unable to start functioning quickly enough, potassium cannot be easily expelled to counteract this effect. One example of such agents is mannitol, which can be used as a waterproofing agent in preservation solutions.

Mannitol accumulates intracellularly, cannot be metabolized, and is only slowly eliminated from the cytosol, leading to cellular edema not directly related to hypothermia. Edema in endothelial cells can interfere with the reestablishment of normal blood flow, which by itself results in hot ischemia. Edema of parenchymal cells will also involve the mitochondria, with subsequent structural and functional deterioration of the tissue. The majority of preservation solutions contain waterproofing agents at a concentration close to 110 mmol/l. It seems that obtaining an adequate concentration of waterproofing agents in these solutions is essential to achieve adequate preservation by storage in cold.

3.2.2 Cellular acidosis

The cells of the organs stored in cold are under anaerobic conditions. To maintain their energy needs (ATP), they use anaerobic glycolysis which increases the concentration of lactate and hydrogen ions intracellularly. This causes acidosis that leads to lysosomal instability, activates lysosomal enzymes, and alters mitochondrial properties, which causes cell injury and death. (Fig 4).

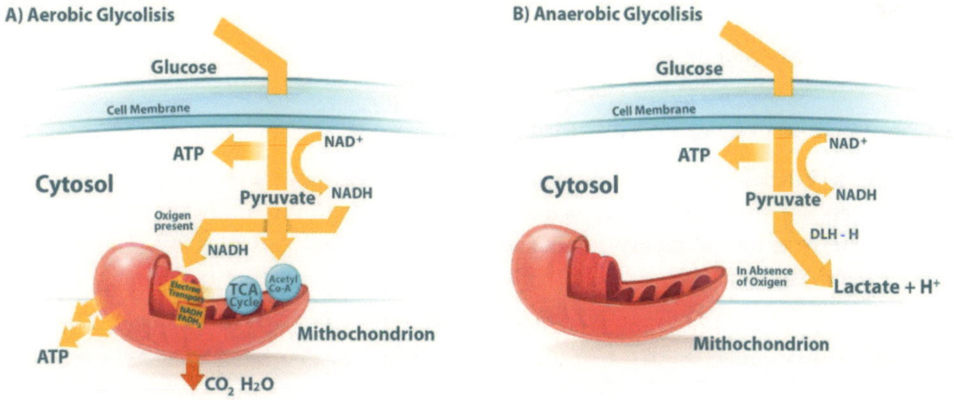

Fig. 4. Glycolysis.

To prevent intracellular acidosis, preservation solutions that contain substances that counteract acidosis (buffers) are used. Substances such as phosphate or histidine are used for this purpose. On the other hand, it seems advisable to have a slightly alkaline pH (7.6 - 8.0 at 37°C) in the solution destined for cold rinsing.

3.2.3 Expansion of the interstitial space

When an organ is perfused, and also later during its storage, there is an expansion of the interstitial space. This compresses the capillary system, causing the inadequate distribution of the preservation fluid across the tissue. Solutions that do not contain oncotic substances (such as albumin and other colloids) quickly diffuse to the interstitial space and cause edema when perfused. The preservation solution needs to contain substances that will create enough osmotic colloidal pressure to allow the free exchange of essential substances with the preserving solution, without expanding the interstitial space (Fig 5).

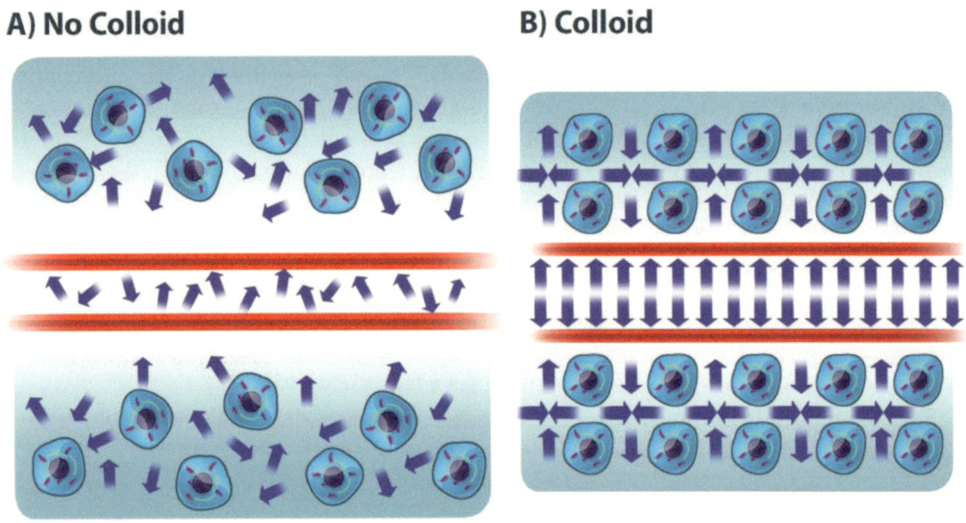

Fig. 5. Osmotic colloidal pressure.

3.2.4 Decrease of cellular energy output

Hypothermia blocks the production of energy at various levels, with cold-resistant enzymatic reactions remaining active, and with a limited supply of glycolytic intermediates and energetic reserves necessary for the maintenance of cellular integrity. These reactions stimulate synthesis of triglycerides from glucose.

The main source of energy in the renal cortex during hypothermia is the metabolism of free fatty acids. The octanoic acids (especially caprilic acid) are degraded to acetyl-coenzyme A and enter the Krebs cycle. In contrast, long-chain free fatty acids, such as palmitic and miristic acids, cannot be degraded in energy-producing cycles but are incorporated to tissue triglycerides through an energy-consuming process. Furthermore, phosphorylation is suppressed during hypothermia due to the inability of adenosine diphosphate to penetrate the mitochondrial inner membrane after hypothermic inactivation of adenosine diphosphate translocase. The adenosine diphosphate stays in the cytosol and degrades to adenosine monophosphate, and finally to hypoxanthine, which easily diffuses outside of the cell. Recovery of the depleted adenosine diphosphate occurs through *de novo* synthesis, and could require several hours after reestablishment of normal temperatures and appropriate oxygen levels. Thus, the preservation solution needs to contain substances that will maintain or replenish ATP (for example adenosine and glutamate).

3.2.5 Intracellular accumulation of calcium

The calcium-calmodulin complex plays a central role in the regulation of multiple enzymes responsible for mitochondrial respiration, adenosine triphosphate transport and regulation of the ion transport and membrane potentials. These effects increase the chances that the control of cytosolic calcium could help restore or preserve the enzymatic reactions necessary to maintain the integrity of cells subjected to hypothermic ischemia. Some calcium-mediated cellular reactions require maintenance of low levels of cytosolic calcium, together with an ability to rapidly fluctuate these levels along large ranges of concentration, in such a way that specific intracellular targets can be alternatively activated and deactivated.

During hypothermic ischemia, the enzymatic systems primarily responsible for calcium efflux are deactivated at the plasma membrane (calcium-specific adenosine triphosphatase and calcium-sodium exchange system). The rapid depletion of the energy reserves during hypothermic ischemia results in deactivation of calcium-specific adenosine-triphosphatase, which causes a massive influx of sodium into the cytosol; as a consequence, there is failure of the calcium-sodium exchange system. There is also a massive influx of calcium, which adversely affects numerous cellular enzymes, producing deterioration of cellular function and eventually cellular death.

The changes in the calcium-calmodulin complex can also generate mitochondrial and membrane dysfunction, damaging the phospholipid nature of these structures by activating the phospholipase pathway with subsequent production of prostaglandin derivatives. This damage primarily affects endothelial cells, and is observed prior to the damage to the parenchymal cells. Endothelial separation, due to cytoskeletal damage, could result in collagen exposure, which in turn produces platelet aggregation and intravascular coagulation. Although an organ in which the parenchymal cells have been damaged can be recovered, this is not feasible when the damage affects the endothelial cells.

4. Pathophysiology of renal allograft reperfusion upon implantation

Much of the injury to transplanted kidneys does not occur during ischemia, but instead during reperfusion at the time of implantation. This damage is a consequence of the following events:

4.1 Release of accumulated toxic metabolites

Re-establishment of blood flow allows the recovery of the oxygen supply and the elimination of accumulated toxic metabolites. Although reperfusion is necessary to recover the organ after the ischemic injury, the systemic release of these toxic metabolites into circulation could have metabolic consequences in distant sites, as well as produce local tissue damage. Additionally, some of these events can trigger inflammatory processes which are a direct stimulus to the immune system, significantly contributing to the risk of acute graft rejection.

4.2 Reactive oxygen species

Damage due to free radicals is less significant in the kidneys than other organs. The greatest source of oxygen radicals comes from the activation of the enzyme xanthine oxidase, although leukocyte and macrophage activation can also be involved. The end products of the degradation of ATP are frequently metabolized to urea by the action of xanthine dehydrogenase. However, in an acidic environment, xanthine dehydrogenase becomes xanthine oxidase. When oxygen is supplied to the cellular environment during reperfusion, xanthine oxidase converts accumulated extracellular waste into xanthine and superoxide anion (a reactive oxygen species). This anion rapidly reacts with itself to form hydrogen peroxide, a potent oxidizing agent capable of injuring the cell by oxidizing lipid membranes and cellular proteins. Hydrogen peroxide also triggers the production of other potent reactive oxygen species, including hydroxyl radical and singlet oxygen. Finally, these events lead to alteration of mitochondrial respiration and to lipid peroxidation with subsequent cellular destruction. The production of reactive oxygen species also initiates production of prostaglandins (by direct activation of phospholipase), including Leukotriene B4 and Platelet Activating Factor. These substances increase leukocyte adhesion to the vascular endothelium. Neutrophils could contribute to local injury by blocking microcirculation and by degranulation, which results in proteolytic damage to the kidney. It is therefore advisable to add substances to the preservation solution that protect against the formation of reactive oxygen species (for example, allopurinol), or "radical cleansers" (superoxide dismutase, iron chelating agents, mannitol, dimethylnitrosamine). However, it should be noted that the potential benefits of these components are the subject of debate.

4.3 Release of cytokines

Ischemia-reperfusion is associated with strong release of Tumor Necrosis Factor alpha, Interferon gamma, Interleukin 1 and Interleukin 8. These cytokines cause an up-regulation of adhesive molecules which produce leukocyte adherence and platelet plugs after revascularization, resulting in graft failure and kidney rejection.

The vascular endothelium modulates smooth muscle tone in the vessel by releasing various local hormones or autacoids. The production of one of them, nitric oxide, which is induced by inflammatory cytokines, correlates with acute rejection.

5. Available preservation solutions

For kidney preservation by cold storage, the Euro-Collins (EC) solution, University of Wisconsin (UW) solution, Histidine-Tryptophan-Ketoglutarate (HTK) solution, or Celsior solution can be used. The components are described in table 1.

The UW solution seems to be associated with better results when compared to the EC solution, showing better initial graft function and a 10% reduction in the need for dialysis after transplantation (the mean need for dialysis with preservation by storage in cold is between 20 and 50%). Both solutions guarantee preservation of up to 30 hours, so the kidney implantation surgery is completely elective (programmed).

Continuous hypothermic perfusion reduces the incidence of initial graft failure (need for postransplant dialysis) to 10%.

5.1 Euro-Collins solution

This solution is nowadays used as a preservation solution in isolated renal explantation, yielding preservation times of up to 30 hours with less cost than UW solution. However, muticentric studies show a better initial graft function with less need for dialysis in grafts preserved in UW solution.

COMPONENT	EC (mmol/l)	UW (mmol/l)	HTK (mmol/l)	Celsior (mmol/l)	Function
Sodium	10	30	15	100	Electrolyte
Potassium	115	120	10	15	Electrolyte
Magnesium	-	5	4	13	Electrolyte y cytoprotector
Chloride	15	-	50	-	Electrolyte
Calcium	-	-	0,015	0,25	Electrolyte
Phosphate	50	25	-	-	Buffer
Sulphate	-	5	-	-	Buffer
Bicarbonate	10	-	-	-	Buffer
Histidine	-	-	180	30	Buffer and waterproofing
Histidine CIH	-	-	18	-	Buffer
Glucose	195	-	-	-	Waterproofing
Mannitol	-	-	30	60	Waterproofing
Raffinose	-	30	-	-	Waterproofing
Lactobionate	-	100	-	80	Waterproofing and chelating Fe and Ca
Adenosine	-	5	-	-	Energy
Ketoglutarate	-	-	1	-	Energy
Glutamate	-	-	-	20	Energy
Glutathione	-	3	-	3, reduction	Anti-free radicals
Allopurinol	-	1	-	-	Anti-free radicals (inhibits xhantine-oxidase)
Tryptophan	-	-	2	-	Membrane stabilizer
Dexamethasone	-	8	-	-	Membrane stabilizer
Insulin	-	100 U/l	-	-	Membrane stabilizer
HES (Hydrox-Ethyl-Starch), a synthetic starch	-	50 g/l	-	-	Synthetic colloid
pH	7	7,4	7,2	7,3	
Osmolarity	355	320	310	340	
Viscosity	Low	High	Low	Low	

Table 1. Preservation solutions and their components. EC=Euro-Collins, UW=Universtiy of Wisconsin, HTK= Histidine-Tryptophan-Ketoglutarate.

5.2 Belzer or University of Wisconsin solution

Currently, this is the solution used for preservation of all abdominal organs, including the kidneys. Basically, it is composed of lactobionate and raffinose as waterproofing agents, hydroxyl-ethyl-starch (colloid), phosphate (buffer), adenosine (precursor of ATP synthesis), and glutathione and allopurinol (to counteract oxygen radicals). It does not contain glucose and it is an "intracellular" solution (rich in potassium and low in sodium), similar to the EC solution.

The disadvantages of UW are the following:

1. High cost
2. It has to be kept refrigerated until its use.
3. Supplements need to be added immediately before its use (insulin, penicillin and dexamethasone), although this can be excluded without adverse effects.
4. The glutathione losses efficacy with time (unstable).
5. The solution can precipitate, requiring filtering during kidney perfusion and rinsing.

5.3 HTK-bretschneider (Custodiol)

It is named HTK because of its components (Hisitidine-Tryptophan-Ketoglutarate) It is an "extracellular solution" (low in potassium) and its components include histidine (buffer and osmotic effect), mannitol (waterproofing agent, osmotic effect and anti-reactive oxygen species), tryptophan (membrane stabilizer) and ketoglutarate (substrate for cellular metabolism). Its osmolarity is similar to that of the UW solution (310 *vs.* 320) and has a lower osmotic pressure (15-25 mmHg *vs.* 0 mmHg). It has lower viscosity, which is why a smaller volume of solution is used during perfusion.

Regarding cost, HKT is comparable to the UW solution, when the specific requirements for the use of either solution are taken into account. HKT remains stable at room temperature, so it does not need to be refrigerated (unlike UW, although cooling to 4°C should be performed at least 2 to 3 hours before its use). HKT also does not precipitate and does not require filtering during perfusion. Being a low potassium solution, HKT also has the (theoretical) advantage of minimizing vascular injury.

5.4 Celsior

This is an "extracellular solution" (low in potassium). Its composition includes waterproofing agents like lactobionate and mannitol, antioxidants like reduced glutathione, metabolic substrates like glutamate, and a buffer (histidine). The solution is stable, it does not need refrigeration or filtering during perfusion. The volume needed to perfuse and its cost are similar to those of the UW solution.

6. Conclusions

Despite evidence that preservation techniques with perfusion machines provide better graft quality and longer periods of preservation, perfusion and subsequent storage at 4°C (for the shortest period possible) is still the standard procedure for preservation of renal grafts. A valid argument in favor of this practice is that it provides acceptable results with a simpler and cheaper method than the use of perfusion machines, which requires expensive and cumbersome equipment, as well as additional personnel. An important limitation of the preservation of organs by storage in cold is the impossibility of assessing whether the organ will adequately function after implantation. In this sense, machine perfusion offers a series of added advantages with respect to the preservation by simple cooling: a) it reduces the vascular resistance induced by ischemia and facilitates the elimination of erythrocyte remnants from the microcirculation, which allows better reperfusion after implantation, and b) it allows testing of the viability or quality of the organ before implantation, by monitoring the flow and pressure, or by determination of biochemical markers related to organ viability released into the preservation solution (alpha glutathione-S-transferase, pi-glutathione-S-transferase, alanineaminopeptidase, among others).

Preservation with HPM is routinely used in only few centers around the world. In Europe its use is not extensive, but in the United States it is used in about 20% of kidney transplant centers.

The most frequently used preservation fluids are Euro-Collins, University of Wisconsin and HTK-Custodiol, which yield preservation times between 18 and 36 hours.

7. Acknowledgment

We would like to thank Luis Felipe Alemón Soto and Gabriela Ramirez Tavares to help carry out this chapter.

8. References

Anaya Prado R; Rodríguez-Quilantan FJ & Toledo-Pereyra LH. (1999). Preservación de órganos, In: *Introducción al trasplante de órganos y tejidos*, Cuervas-Mons V & del Castillo-Olivares JL (Ed.), pp. 107-134, Arán Ediciones S.A., ISBN 84-86725-49-6, Madrid, España.

Baicu, S.; Taylor, M. & Brockbank, K. (1986). The role of perfusion solution on acid base regulation during machine perfusion of kidneys. *Clinical Transplantation*, Vol.20, No.1, (January 2006), pp. 113-121 ISSN 1399-0012

Balupuri, S.; Hoernich, N.; Manas, D.; Mohamed, M.; Snowden, C.; Strong, A. & Kirby, J. (1988). Machine perfusion for kidneys: how to do it a minimal cost. *Transplant International*, Vol.14, No.2, (March 2001), pp.103–107, ISSN 1432-2277

Belzer, F.; Ashby, B. & Dunphy, J. (1823). 24-hour and 72 hour preservation of canine kidneys. *Lancet*, Vol.290, No.7515, (September 1967), pp. 536-538, ISSN 0140-6736

Belzer, F. & Southard, J. (1969). Principles of solid organ preservation by cold storage. *Transplantation*, Vol.45, No.4, (April 1988), pp. 673-676, ISSN 0041-1337

Belzer, F. (1969). Evaluation of preservation of the intra abdominal organs. *Transplantation Proceedings*, Vol.25, No.4, (August 1993), pp. 2527-2530, ISSN 0041-1345

Boggi, U.; Vistoli, F.; Del Chiaro, M.; Signori, S.; Croce, C. & Pietrabissa, A. (1969). Pancreas preservation with University of Wisconsin and Celsior solutions: a single-center, prospective, randomized pilot study. *Transplantation*, Vol.77, No.8, (April 2004), pp. 1186-1190, ISSN 0041-1337

Booster, M.; Bonke, H.; Buurman, W.; Heineman, E.; Kurvers, H.; Maessen, J.; Stubenitsky, B.; Tiebosch, A.; Wijnen, R. & Yin, M.(1969). Enhanced resistance to the effect of normo thermic isquemia in kidneys using pulsatile machine perfusion. *Transplantation Proceedings*, Vol.25, No.6, (December 1993), pp. 3006-3011, ISSN 0041-1345

Calne R.; Pegg, D.; Pryse, D. & Brown, F. (1840). Renal preservation by ice cooling : an experimental study relating to kidney trnsplantation from cadavers. *British medical journal*, Vol.2, No.5358, (September 1963), pp.651-655, ISSN 0959-8138

Carrel, A. & Guthrie, C. (1880). Functions of a trasnplanted kidney. *Science*, Vol.22, No.563, (October1905), pp. 473, ISSN 1095-9203

Collins, G.; Bravo, M. & Terasaki, P. (1823). Kidney preservation for transportation. Initial perfusion and 30 hours' ice storage. *Lancet*, Vol.294, No.7632, (December 1969), pp. 1219-1222, ISSN 0140-6736

Clavien, P.; Sanabria, J.; Aravinda, U.; Harvey, P. & Strasberg, S. (1969). Evidence of the existence of a soluble mediator of cold preservation injury. *Transplantation*, Vol.56, No.1, (July 1993), pp. 44-53, ISSN 0041-1337

Daemen, J.; De Vries, B. & Kootstra, G. (1969). The effect of machine perfusion preservation on early function of non-heart-beating donors. *Transplantation Proceedings*, Vol.29, No.8, (December 1997), pp. 3489, ISSN 0041-1345

Escalante, J. & Rios, F. (2005). Preservación de órganos. *Medicina intensiva*, Vol.33, No.6, (June 2009), pp. 282-292, ISSN 0210-5691

Eugène, M.; Hauet, T. & Barrou, B. (1990). The use of preservation solutions in renal transplantation. *Progres en urologie journal del Association francaise durologie et de la Societe francaise durologie*. Vol.16, No.1, (February 2006), pp. 25-31, ISSN 1166-7087

Haloran, P. & Aprile, M. (1969). Randomized prospective trial of cold storage versus pulsatile perfusion for cadaver kidney preservation. *Transplantation*, Vol.43, No.6, (June 1987), pp. 827-832, ISSN 0041-1337

Henry, M. (1969). Pulsatile preservation in renal transplantation. *Transplantation Proceedings*, Vol.29, No.8, pp. 3575-3576, (December. 1997), ISSN 0041-1345

Isselhard, W.; Berger, M.; Denecke, H.; Witte, J.; Fischer, J.; Molzberger, H.; Freiberg, C. & Ammermann, D. (1868). Metabolism of canine kidneys in anaerobic ischemia and in aerobic ischemia by persufflation with gaseous oxygen. *Pflügers Archiv - European Journal of Physiology* ,Vol.337, No.2, (June 1972), pp. 87-106, ISSN 1432-2013

Koyama, I.; Bulkley, G.; Williams, G. & Im, M. (1969). The role of oxygen free radicals in mediating the reperfusion injury of cold-preserved ischemic kidneys. *Transplantation*, Vol.40, No.6, pp. 590-595 (December 1985), ISSN 0041-1337

Kozaki, K.; Kozaki, M.; Sakurai, E.; Tamaki, I.; Matsuno, N.; Saito, A.; Furuhaski, K.; Uchiyama, M.; Zhang, S. (1969). Usefulness of continuous hypothemic perfusion preservation for cadaveric renal grafts in poor condition. *Transplantation Proceedings*, Vol.27, No.1, (February 2005), pp.757-758, ISSN 0041-1345

Lapchinsky, A. (1823). Recent Results of experimental Transplantaion of Preserved Limbs and Kidneys and Possible use of this Technique in Clinical Practice. *Annals Of The New York Academy Of Sciences*, Vol.87, pp. 539-571, (May 1960), ISSN 1749-6632

Lee, C. & Mangino, M. (2004). Preservation methods for kidney and liver. *Organogenesis*, Vol.5, No.3, (September 2009), pp. 105-112, ISSN 1555-8592

Lillehei, R.; Manax, W. & Bloch, J. and Longerbeam, J.K. (1935). Successful 24 hour in vitro preservation of canine kidneys by the combined use of hyperbaric oxygenation and hypothermia. *Surgery*, Vol.56, (July 1964), pp. 275-282. ISSN 0039-6060

Lillehei, R.; Manax, W.; Bloch, J.; Lyons, G.; Eyal, Z. & Largiader, F. (1935). Organ Perfusion before transplantation, Minneapolis, MN with particular reference to the kidney Transplantation. *Surgery*, Vol.57,(April 1965), pp. 528-534, ISSN 0039-6060

Lindbergh, C.(1905). An apparatus for the culture of whole organs. *The Journal of Experimental Medicine*, Vol.62, No.3, (August 1935), pp.409-431, ISSN 0022 1007

Opelz, G. & Döhler, B. (2001). Comparison of Histidine-Triptophan-Ketoglutarate and University of Wisconsin Preservation in Renal Transplantation. *American Journal of Transplantation*, Vol. 8, No.3, (Sep 2008), pp. 567-573, ISSN 1600-6143

Maathuis, M.; Leuvenink, H. & Ploeg, R. (1969). Perspectives in organ preservation. *Transplantation*, Vol.83, No.10, (May 2007), pp. 1289-1298, ISSN 0041-1337

Matsumo, N.; Sakurai, E.; Tamaki, I.; Uchiyama, M.; Kozaki, K. & Kozaki, M. (1969). The effect of machine perfusion preservation versus cold storage on the function of kidneys from non-heart-beating-donors. *Transplantation*, Vol.57, No.2, pp. 293-294, (January 1994), ISSN 0041-1337

Matsumo, N.; Sakurai, E.; Uchiyama, M.; Kozaki, K.; Miyamoto, K. & Kozaki, M. (1969). Usefulnes of machine perfusion preservation for non-heart-beating-donors in kidney transplantation. *Transplantation Proceedings*, Vol.28, No.3, (June 1996), pp. 1551-1552, ISSN 0041-1345

Matsumo, N.; Konno, O.; Mejit, A.; Jyojima, Y.; Akashi, I.; Nakamura, Y.; Iwamoto, H.; Hama, K.; Iwahori, T.; Ashizawa, T. & Nagao, T. (1969). Application of machine perfusión preservation as a viability test for marginal kidney graft. *Transplantation*, Vol.82, No.11, (December 2006), pp.1425-1428, ISSN 0041-1337

McAnulty, J.; Vreugdenhil, P.; Southard, J. & Belzer, F. (1969). Use of UW cold storage solution for machine perfusion of kidneys. *Transplantation Proceedings*, Vol. 22, No.2, (April 1990), pp. 458-459, ISSN 0041-1345

Mozes, M.; Finch, W.; Reckard, F.; Merkel, & Cohen, C. (1969). Comparison of cold storage and machine perfusion in the preservation of cadaver kidneys: a prospective randomized study. *Transplantation Proceedings*, Vol.17, No.1, (Junuary 1985), pp. 1474-1477, ISSN 0041-1345

Nyberg, S.; Baskin, E.; Kremers, W.; Prieto, M.; Henry, M. & Stegall, M. (1969) improving the prediction of donor kidney quality: deceased donor score and resistive indices. *Transplantation*, Vol.80, No.7, (July 2005), pp. 925-929, ISSN 0041-1337

Opelz, G. & Terasaki, P. (1969). Advantage of cold storage over machine perfusion for preservation of cadaver kidneys. *Transplantation*, Vol.33, No.1, (January 1982), pp. 64-68, ISSN 0041-1337

Palmer, R. (June 2011). The History of Organ Perfusion and Preservation, In: *International Society for Organ Preservation*, 24.06.2011, Available from http://www.organpreservation.org/pages/about/history.aspx

Pedotti, P.; Cardillo, M .; Rigotti, P.; Gerunda, G.; Merenda, R.; Cillo, U.; Zanus, G.; Baccarani, U.; Berardinelli, M.; Boschiero, L.; Caccamo, L.; Calconi, G.; Chiaramonte, S.; Dal canton, A.; De carlis, L.; Di carlo, V.; Donati, D.; Pulvirenti, A.; Remuzzi, G.; Sandrini, S.; Valente, U. & Scalamogna, M. (1969). Comparative prospective study of two available solutions for kidney and liver preservation. *Transplantation*, Vol.77, No.10, (October 2004), pp. 1540-1545, ISSN 0041-1337

Polyak, M.; Arrington, B.; Stubenbord, W.; Boykin, J.; Brown, T.; Jean, M.; Kapur, S. & Kinkhabwala, M. (1969). The influence of pulsatile preservation on renal transplantation in the 1990s. *Transplantation*, Vol.69, No.2, (February 2000), pp. 249-258, ISSN 0041-1337

Sánchez, A.; Marques, M.; Del Río, F .; Núñez, J.; Barrientos, A.; Prats, D.; Conesa, J.; Calvo, N.; Pérez, M.; Blazquez, J.; Fernández, C. & Corral. (1927). Victims of cardiac arrest occurring outside the hospital: a source of transplantable kidney. *Annals of Internal Medicine*, Vol.145, No.3, (March 2006), pp. 157-164, ISSN 1539-3704

Szajer, M.; Shah, G.; Kittur, D.; Searles, B.; Li, L.; Bruch, D. & Darling, E. (1996). Novel extracorporal kidney perfusion system : a concept model. *Perfusion*, Vol.19, No.5, (September 2004), pp. 305-310, ISSN 1477-111X

St Peter, S.; Imber, C. & Friend, J. (1823). Liver and kidney preservation by perfusion. *Lancet*, Vol.359, No.9306, (February 2002), pp. 604-613, ISSN 0140-6736

Southard, J.; Senzig, K. & Belzer, F. (1964). Effects of hypothermia on canine kidney mitochondria. *Cryobiology*, Vol.17, No.2, (February 1980), pp. 148-153, ISSN 1090-2392

Southard, J. (1975). Advances in organ preservation. *Transplantation Proceedings*, Vol.21, No.1, (January 1989), pp: 1195-1196, ISSN 0041-1345

Tanabe, K.; Oshima, T.; Tokumoto, T.; Ishikawa, N.; Kanematsu, A.; Shinmura, H.; Koga, S.; Fuchinoue, S.; Takahashi, K. & Toma, H. (1969). Long term renal function in non-heart-beating donor hidney transplantation: a single center experience. *Transplantation*, Vol.66, No.12, (December 1998), pp. 1708-13, ISSN 0041-1337

Toledo, L. & Palma, J. (1992). Advances in organ preservation. *Transplantology*, Vol.7, No.2 (May 1996), pp. 67-75, ISSN 1134-315X

Valero, R.; Cabrer, C.; Oppenheimer, F.; Trias, E.; Sanchez, J.; ., De Cabo, F.; Navarro, A.; Paredes, D.; Alcaraz, A.; Gutiérrez, R. & Manyalich, M. (1988). Normothermic recirculation reduces primary graft dysfunction of kidneys obtained from non heart-beating donors. *Transplant International*, Vol.13, No.4, (August 2000), pp. 303-10, ISSN 1432-2277

Van, B.; Janssen, M. & Koostra, G. (1988). Functional relationship of alpha-glutatione-S-transferasa and glutathione-S-transferasa activity in machine-preserved non heart beating donor kidneys. *Transplant International*, Vol.15, No.11, (November 2002), pp. 546-549, ISSN 1432-2277

Van der Viet, J.; Vroemen, A. & Koostra, G. (1969). Comparison of cadaver kidney preservation methods in Eurotransplant. *Transplantation Proceeding*, Vol.16, No.1 (1984), pp. 180-181, ISSN 0041-1345

Wight, J.; Chilcott, J.; Holmes, M. & Brewer N. (1986). Pulsatile machine perfusion vs cold storage of kidneys for transplantation: a rapid systematic review. *Clinical Transplantation*, Vol.17, No.4, (August, 2003), pp. 293-307, ISSN 1399-0012

2

Renal Transplantation from Expanded Criteria Donors

Pooja Binnani, Madan Mohan Bahadur and Bhupendra Gandhi
Jaslok Hospital and Research Centre, Mumbai
India

1. Introduction

The 21st century has come as an era of chronic diseases including chronic kidney diseases. Treatment at the end stage of kidney failure involves replacing the lost functions of kidneys by dialysis or by a kidney transplant. The end stage renal disease (ESRD) population is increasing worldwide. The National Kidney Foundation says that "rates of chronic kidney disease (CKD) in the United States have increased by more than 20% over the past decade, causing dramatic loss of life and sky-rocketing health care costs, according to the 2008 annual report by the US Renal Data System"(National Kidney Foundation ,2009).

Kidney transplantation was proven unquestionably the preferred therapy for most patients with ESRD. Survival, cardiovascular stability and quality of life were found superior in allograft recipients compared to similar patients who remained on dialysis (Wolfe et al, 1999; Nathan et al, 2003).

There was a large gap between the number of patients waiting for a transplant and the number receiving a transplant. This gap has widened over the decade, according to 2009 OPTN/SRTR Annual report. The waiting list for a donor kidney has grown from slightly more than 40,000 people in 1998 to about 110,466 in 2011, as per UNOS (United Network for Organ Sharing) data base. Sometimes the wait is two or three years, but often it stretches to five or 10 years or longer. Some die while waiting. During the past few years, there has been renewed interest in the use of expanded criteria donors (ECD) for kidney transplantation to increase the numbers of deceased donor kidneys available. More kidney transplants would result in shorter waiting times and limit the morbidity and mortality associated with long-term dialysis therapy.

Performing renal transplant with a perfectly healthy kidney to all the patients with ESRD is an ideal scenario. But growing waiting lists and shortage of kidneys makes it necessary to make some compromises. Use of so-called, marginal or borderline donors can increase donor pool by almost 20 to 25%.

Terms- expanded criteria donor or marginal donor simply means accepting suboptimal quality grafts, either from a living donor or a cadaver donor with some acceptable medical risks. Scientific Registry of Transplant Recipients (SRTR)/Organ Procurement and Transplantation Network (OPTN) data showed 41% discard rate for ECD kidneys. Common reasons for discard of these donor kidneys were older donors, glomerulosclerosis on biopsy and poor renal perfusion (Sunga et al, 2008). Current utilization is 15% of all transplanted kidneys.

2. Marginal versus expanded criteria donor

Some authors believe that the term 'expanded' be used instead of "marginal" because the term 'marginal' may be considered pejorative by the patients who receive them, as well as by the programs that transplant them (Kauffman, 1997).

3. Standard donor versus expanded criteria donors

Graft and patient survival after ECD kidney transplantation are inferior to survival rates with SCD kidney transplantation. The differences are initially insignificant, but increase over time. The half-lives of deceased-donor kidneys (ECD or SCD) are shorter than the half-life of a living-donor kidney (Metzger, 2003). Many large retrospective database analysis compared outcomes of standard-criteria donor (SCD) kidney transplants with ECD kidney transplants. Overall, mortality in the perioperative period was greater in ECD kidney recipients (Merion et al, 2005; Remuzzi et al, 2006). Kidneys transplanted from expanded criteria donors have a higher rate of delayed graft function, more acute rejection episodes, and decreased long-term graft function. Several factors, including prolonged cold ischemia time (CIT), increased immunogenicity, impaired ability to repair tissue, and impaired function with decreased nephron mass may contribute to this (De Fijter et al, 2001). Despite these inferior results, these transplants had definitely survival advantage over patients still receiving dialysis (Ojo et al, 2001; Merion et al, 2005). It was also observed that, despite an increased mortality risk during the initial post-transplant period, the long-term mortality risk was > 50% lower for patients who were 60 to 74 years of age at the time of waiting list registration compared with those who remained on dialysis (Wolfe et al, 1999).

4. Optimised allocation

The strategy proposed by Bryce Kiberd et al was to retrieve all kidneys; but visibly scarred kidneys should be discarded. He also proposed performing biopsy in some deceased donors kidneys > age 65, > age 55 and donor Creatinine clearance<60 - 70 ml/min, discarding advanced arteriolar sclerosis or interstitial fibrosis. Allocating these grafts to Older (>59) or diabetic, avoid the sensitized, minimize cold ischemic time and avoid large weight or age mismatches (Bryce Kiberd, 2011). Schnitzler and colleagues used a Markov model to determine the best timing for an individual patient to accept an offer of an ECD kidney, based on registry data from the United States Renal Data System (USRDS) and expected quality-adjusted life years (Schnitzer et al, 2003). Common practice in the United States as well as Europe is to place older donor kidneys in older patients (Voiculescu et al, 2002; Smits et al, 2002; Kasiske et al, 2002; Lee et al, 1999).

5. Types of marginal donors

5.1 Living marginal donor

Living-related kidney donation is a way out of the current dilemma of insufficient supply of renal allografts. The risk to the donor is minimal, but not zero. Apart from these peri-operative risks, are there potential long-term risks with respect to renal function, proteinuria and hypertension. Potential risks must be excluded by careful work-up of the donor (Duraj et al, 1995; Natarajan et al, 1992; Foster et al, 1991). There is enough evidence to suggest that, standard living donors do not face risks for ESRD any higher than those of age- matched peers (Fehrman-Ekholm et al, 2001). But this doesn't hold true for marginal living donors. In fact, emphasis should be given to ascertain the risk of developing CKD as well as ESRD in these donors.

Marginal Donors - Inclusion

- Elderly donors
- GFR - 60 to 70 ml/ min
- Mild Hypertension
- Donor with Stone Disease
- Donors with Renal cysts
- Donors with BMI>30
- Other issues like tuberculosis, DM, proteinuria, hematuria, malignancy, family history of ESRD and CMV Infections

5.1.1 Aged kidney donors

Glomerulosclerosis increases with age. There is decrease in GFR of approx 1 ml/min per 1.73 m^2 per year after age 40. There is a documented acute decrease in GFR of approximately 30% after unilateral nephrectomy; however, the impact of unilateral nephrectomy on this rate of decline in GFR is unknown.

Twenty per cent glomerulosclerosis is usually considered the upper limit for accepting kidneys from a donor. There is higher incidence of delayed graft function with such kidneys. Further, there may be associated increased rate of acute rejection. Advancing age is associated with higher incidence of hypertension (Moreso et al, 1999). The influence of donor age on the outcome of living donor kidney transplantation is not very clear. Gill et al in their observational cohort study of 23,754 kidney transplantations performed in recipients 60 years and older, found that old living donor transplants were associated with inferior 3-year graft survival rates, but similar 3-year patient survival rates compared with young living donor transplants. Elderly deceased criteria donor transplantations were associated with a greater risk of graft loss. He proposed old living donors an important option for elderly transplantation (Gill et al, 2008). There are other few studies in the literature that found encouraging results with elderly living donor transplants (Kumar et al, 2000; De La Vega, 2004). Graft survival, patient survival, degree of hypertension and renal function were similar in elderly and young living donor transplant groups. Contrary to these encouraging results, others noted poor patient and graft survival in elderly donor transplants (Toma et al, 2001; Prommool et al, 2000). Long term outcome of this group is not known.

5.1.2 Hypertensive donors

There are no precise guidelines regarding donation from patients with arterial hypertension. It is now accepted that systolic blood pressure greater than 140 mmHg is a much more important cardiovascular risk factor than raised diastolic blood pressure. In fact, there is little evidence that well-controlled hypertension may lead to kidney damage in an otherwise healthy subject. According to a Consensus Conference held in Amsterdam (Delmonico, 2005), there is no reason to reject as a kidney donor a subject more than 50 years of age who has a normal blood pressure on therapy with a GFR > 80 ml/min and proteinuria < 300 mg per day(Delmonico et al, 2005). Ambulatory blood pressure monitoring has been proposed as a more sensitive method than office blood pressure measurements in identifying hypertension in living donors (Ozdemir et al, 2000).

5.1.3 Diabetic donors

Diabetics are generally excluded because of the increased risk of postoperative complications in the short term and because of the potential risk of developing diabetic nephropathy in the long term (Delmonico et al, 2005; Kasiske et al, 1995). Diabetic nephropathy occurs in familial clusters and heredity helps to determine susceptibility to diabetic nephropathy (Sequist et al, 1989). It was clearly stated in Consensus Conference held in Amsterdam, that individuals with a history of diabetes or fasting blood glucose of ≥ 126mg/dl (7.0mmol/L) on at least two occasions (or 2-h glucose with OGTT ≥ 200mg/dl (11.1mmol/L)) should not donate(Delmonico et al, 2005).

5.1.4 Patients with nephrolithiasis

It seems reasonable to accept as donors only those subjects without stones at the time of evaluation and with normal values within a 24-hour urine collection of calcium, urate, and oxalate. According to a Consensus Conference, patients with stones caused by inherited disorders, inflammatory bowel disease, or systemic disease are at high risk of recurrence and should not be considered for donation (Delmonico et al, 2005). In the series a cohort of 710 renal transplant recipients from mayo clinic, evaluation was done for the risk transplant graft renal calculus formation over duration of 4 years. 44 donor kidneys had calculi, majority being <2mm. Stable stone size was seen in four patients, increase in stone size averaging 2.9 millimeters in four patients. No loss of the transplanted kidneys occurred due to stone obstruction in the patients studied (Ho et al, 2005). Whether or not kidney stone formers should donate a kidney is controversial. The American Society of Transplantation (AST) position paper proposes guidelines that a kidney stone former may donate a kidney if: only one stone has ever formed; stones have been multiple, but none have formed for >10 years and none are seen on radiograph; and the donor is screened for metabolic abnormalities and is offered life-long follow-up that includes periodic risk reassessment, medical treatment, and hydration (Michelle et al, 2006).

5.1.5 Obese donors

There is little information on the long-term follow-up of obese donors. Of some concern, in patients submitted to unilateral nephrectomy for various reasons, those with a BMI > 30 had a significantly higher risk of developing proteinuria or renal dysfunction in the long term than did those with a BMI < 30 (Praga et al, 2000). The Consensus Conference held in Amsterdam discouraged donation from persons with a BMI higher than 35(Delmonico et al, 2005). Dyslipidemia are associated with decreased kidney function in the general population and have faster rates of progression in patients who have chronic kidney disease. However, isolated dyslipidemia is not a contraindication for donation.

5.1.6 Other issues

- Adult relatives of patients with polycystic kidney disease can be accepted for donation if they have a normal CT or renal ultrasound scan.
- Donors with malignancy- a history of malignancy is in general a contraindication to living kidney donation, other than carcinoma in situ of the uterine cervix or treated low grade, non- melanotic skin carcinoma.
- Donors with transmissible infections- HIV positive status remains a contraindication for donation. Cytomegalovirus (CMV) and Ebstein-barr virus (EBV) status is measured at some transplant centers and they delay transplant till PCR for CMV becomes negative. Most of the adults are EBV and CMV-positive; most of the children are negative. The risk of post-transplantation lymphoproliferative disorder (PTLD) is the concern in CMV and EBV-negative individuals receiving positive donors. However, the risk is not as high to prohibit renal transplantation (Delmonico et al, 2005). Renal transplantation should be considered using HCV-seropositive grafts for qualified patients with chronic kidney disease (CKD) stage 5 and HCV infection since good information indicates that the transplantation of kidneys from HCV-infected donors results in improved survival compared to wait-listed and dialysis-dependent candidates (Fabrizi et al, 2009). Hepatitis C Virus (HCV) positive donor may be considered for donation to a HCV positive recipient only if the donor PCR is negative, certain genotypes (Genotype 4) are treated and eradicated of the donor and there is no evidence of chronic hepatitis or cirrhosis on liver biopsy. However, there is no data on live kidney transplantation from HCV positive donors. Hepatitis B Virus (HBV) positive status currently is not accepted for donation. However, there are some isolated reports of transplantation by groups in New Zealand (Delmonico et al, 2005). Donors treated for pulmonary TB require a more specific and extensive examination of the urinary tract and the kidneys prior to donation.

5.1.7 Ethical issues

Ethical issues in accepting marginal criteria donors are very complex. The living kidney donation means giving life to a patient on dialysis but at the same time avoiding risks to the donor. An important problem with marginal donors is that these marginal living donors may themselves add up the pool of chronic kidney disease patients in the long run.

At American Transplant Congress 2003, in cases of marginal donor transplantation, a prior sample consent by both donor and recipient was proposed stating expect increase in delayed graft function, expected decrease in graft survival, expected decrease in waiting time, expected increase in survival compared to waiting and benefit of transplant prior to increased morbidity.

It is truly anticipated that the transplantation of ECD and DCD kidneys would result in higher costs. More frequent need for hemodialysis, more hospital readmissions due to poor or late onset graft function and more opportunistic infections in recipients of ECD and DCD kidneys results in higher cost for their initial medical care.

5.2 Marginal cadaveric donor

The Organ Procurement and Transplantation Network instituted a formalized definition of marginal kidneys in 2002 with the advent of the Expanded Criteria Donor (ECD) (Metzger et al, 2003). These deceased donor kidneys were demonstrated to convey a 70% or greater risk for graft loss for transplant recipients relative to an ideal donation and were characterized by a donor age older than 60 yr or older than 50 yr and accompanied by two additional risk factors, including a history of hypertension, elevated terminal donor Creatinine, and cerebrovascular cause of death.

Despite expected higher rate of graft failure compared to SCD kidneys, multiple studies have subsequently shown that kidney transplantation using ECDs is still associated with a substantial reduction in morbidity and improvement in life expectancy when compared with suitable transplant candidates who remained on maintenance dialysis treatment (UNOS Policy 3.5.1, 2002; Institute of Medicine, 1997; Ojo et al, 2001).

6. Donation after cardiac death (DCD)

Another approach to the organ shortage has been the utilization of donors after cardiac death. The recovery of organs from nonheart beating donors is an important, medically effective and ethically acceptable approach to reducing the gap that exists now and will continue to exist in future between the demand for and available supply of organs for transplantation'. A lot of investigators have reported excellent short-term outcomes using these donors, and 10–15% growth in organ donation as a result of the use of DCD donors was demonstrated. Multiple studies have shown that the overall results of DCD (without ECD characteristics) and SCD kidney transplants are comparable (Institute of Medicine, 1997; Ojo et al, 2001; Stratta et al, 2004). A main issue with NHBD is the significantly higher rate of delayed graft function, compared with that associated with heart-beating donor (Keizer et al, 2005).

7. Role of kidney biopsy

Outcomes of ECD kidney transplantation are improved when a pre-implantation biopsy of the donor kidney is evaluated using the scoring system introduced by Karpinski and colleagues (Karpinski et al, 1999). Using this system, donor renal pathology is scored from 0 to 3 (none to severe disease) in 4 areas: glomerulosclerosis, interstitial fibrosis, tubular atrophy, and vascular disease. A donor vessel score of 3/3 is associated with a 100% incidence of delayed graft function and a significantly worse renal function at one year.

8. Patient management: Immunosuppressive protocols

Optimal management is a challenge in ECD kidney transplant recipients. These transplants are feared with increased rates of acute rejections and delayed graft function. Therefore, adequate level of Immunosuppression is desired. Management for an ECD kidney is based on potential nephron-protecting strategies, including cold ischemia time minimization, pulsatile perfusion preservation, immunosuppression focused on nephrotoxicity minimization, and adequate infection prophylaxis. Although calcineurin inhibitors are excellent drugs, the nephrotoxicity they impart is largely responsible for postponing chronic allograft dysfunction and achieve better long-term graft survival. The problem of calcineurin inhibitor-related nephrotoxicity is an even greater concern in older recipients of ECD kidneys. Various strategies of CNI withdrawal, minimization as well as avoidance were utilized by a number of investigators.

- Antibody induction, MMF, steroids.
- MMF monotherapy or MMF plus steroids.
- Antibody induction, sirolimus, MMF, steroids.
- Antibody induction, sirolimus, MMF, steroids.
- Conversion from a calcineurin-inhibitor-based regimen to a sirolimus-based regimen

The potential for CNI-free sirolimus and MMF–based therapy in ECD kidney transplant recipients has not been adequately studied to date. Consequently, extrapolation of the best results obtained with anti–interleukin 2 receptors, MMF, steroids, and moderate exposure to tacrolimus might constitute an advisable strategy (Ekberg et al, 2007).

9. Conclusion

In summary, the use of marginal donors for kidney transplantation increases the numbers of donor kidneys available, results in shorter waiting times, and limits the morbidity and mortality associated with long-term dialysis therapy. These kidneys are known to have worse long-term survival than standard criteria kidneys. Elderly patients with longer waiting times show better survival receiving such kidney than remaining on dialysis therapy. A management protocol for ECD kidney transplantation should be based on potential nephronprotecting strategies like, minimization of cold ischemia time, tailored immunosuppression with early CNI minimization or delayed moderate dose, CNI addition after induction, and adequate infection prophylaxis.

10. References

American Transplant Congress (2003). American Journal of Transplantation 2003:supp3; 49–150.

Bryce Kiberd. Optimizing ECD Utilization Expanded Criteria Donor: Revisited? (2011) http://www.cdha.nshealth.ca/multi-organ-transplant-program/documents, 3 may2011

De Fijter JW, Mallat MJK, Doxiadis IIN et al (2001). Increased immunogenicity and cause of graft loss of old donor kidneys. *J Am Soc Nephrol* 2001; 12: 1538–1546.

De La Vega LS, Torres A, Bohorquez HE, Heimbach JK, Gloor JM, Schwab TR, et al (2004) . Patient and graft outcomes from older living kidney donors are similar to those from younger donors despite lower GFR. *Kidney Int* 2004; 66:1654-61.

Delmonico F, Council of the Transplantation Society (2005). A report of the Amsterdam forum on the care of the live kidney donor: data and medical guidelines. *Transplantation* 2005; 79 (Suppl 6): S53–66.

Duraj F, Tydén G, Blom B (1995) Living-donor nephrectomy: how safe is it? *Transplant Proc1995; 27:803–*804.

Ekberg H, Tedesco-Silva H, Demirbas A, et al.(2007) Symphony comparing standard immunosuppression to low dose cyclosporine, tacrolimus or sirolimus in combination with MMF, daclizumab and corticosteroids in renal transplantation. *N Engl J Med* 357:2562-2575, 2007

Fabrizi F, Messa P, Martin P (2009). Current status of renal transplantation from HCV-positive donors. *Int J Artif Organs*. .2009; 32(5):251-61.

Fehrman-Ekholm I, Duner F, Brink B, Tyden G, Elinder CG (2001). No evidence of accelerated loss of kidney function in living kidney donors; results from a cross-sectional follow-up. *Transplantation2001; 72:444–449*

Foster MH, Sant GR, Donohoe JF, Harrington JT(1991). Prolonged survival with a remnant kidney. *Am J Kidney Dis1991; 17:261–265.*

Gill J, Bunnapradist S, Danovitch G, Gjertson D (2008). Outcomes of Kidney Transplantation from Older Living Donors to Older Recipients. *American Journal of Kidney Diseases* 2008; 52:541-552

Ho KLV, Chow G (2005). Prevalence and early outcome of donor graft lithiasis in living renal transplants at the Mayo Clinic. *J Urol*. 2005; 173(suppl.):439; abstract 1622

Institute of Medicine (1997): Non-Heart-Beating Organ Transplantation: Medical and Ethical Issues in Procurement. Washington, DC: National Academy Press; 1997: 1–35.

Kasiske BL, Bia MJ (1995). The evaluation and selection of living kidney donors. *Am J Kidney Dis* 1995; 26: 387–98.

Kasiske BL, Snyder J (2002). Matching older kidneys with older patients does not improve allograft survival. *J Am Soc Nephrol* 2002; 13: 1067–1072.

Karpinski J, Lajoie G, Cattran D, et al (19990. Outcome of kidney transplantation from high-risk donors is determined by both structure and function. *Transplantation*. 1999; 67:1162-1167.

Kauffman MH, Bennett LE, McBride MA, Ellison MD (1997). The expanded donor. *Transplant Rev* 1997; 11: 165–190.

Keizer KM, de Fijter JW, Haase-Kromwijk BJ, Weimar W (2005). Non-heart-beating donor kidneys in the Netherlands: allocation and outcome of transplantation. *Transplantation* 2005; 79: 1195–9.

Kumar A, Verma BS, Srivastava A, Bhandari M, Gupta A, Sharma RK (2000). Long-term follow-up of elderly donors in a live related renal transplant program. *J Urol* 2000; 163 : 1654-8.

Lee CM, Carter JT, Weinstein RJ et al (1999). Dual kidney transplantation: older donors for older recipients. *J Am College Surgeons* 1999; 189: 82–91.

Metzger RA, Delmonico FL, Feng S, Port FK, and Wynn JJ, Merion RM (2003): Expanded criteria donors for kidney transplantation. *Am J Transplant 3[Suppl 4]: 114–125, 2003*

Merion RM, Ashby VB, Wolfe RA, et al (2005). Deceased-donor characteristics and the survival benefit of kidney transplantation. *JAMA*. 2005; 294:2726-2733.

Michelle A Josephson, Elaine M Worcester (2006). Stone Formers as Living Kidney Donors—Is It Safe? *US Nephrology*, 2006 ;(2):38-41

Moreso F, Seron D, Gil-Vernet S et al (1999). Donor age and delayed graft function as predictors of renal allograft survival in rejection-free patients. *Nephrol Dial Transplant* 1999; 14: 930–935

Najarian JS, Chavers BM, McHugh L, Matas AJ (1992). 20 years or more of follow-up of living kidney donors. *Lancet1992; 340:1354*–1355

Nathan HM, Conrad SL, Held PJ et al (2003). Organ donation in the United States. *Am J Transplant* 2003; 3(Suppl 4): 29–40.

National Kidney Foundation (2011). Chronic kidney disease a major killer in the US. Medscape. http://www.medscape.com/viewarticle/586587

Ojo AO, Hanson JA, Meier- Kriesche, et al. Survival in recipients of marginal cadaveric donor kidneys compared with other recipients and waitlisted transplant candidates. *J Am Soc Nephrol.* 2001; 12:589-97.

Ozdemir FN, Guz G, Sezer S, et al (2000). Ambulatory blood pressure monitoring in potential renal transplant donors. *Nephrol Dial Transplant* 2000; 15: 1038–40

Praga M, Hernandez E, Herrero JC, et al (2000). Influence of obesity on the appearance of proteinuria and renal insufficiency after unilateral nephrectomy. *Kidney Int* 2000; 58: 2111–18.

Prommool S, Jhangri GS, Cockfield SM, Halloran PF (2000). Time dependency of factors affecting renal allograft survival. *J Am Soc Nephrol* 2000; 11: 565-73.

Remuzzi G, Cravedi P, Perna A, et al (2006). Long-term outcome of renal transplantation from older donors. *N Engl J Med.* 2006; 354:343-352.

Schnitzler MA, Whiting JF, Brennan DC, et al (2003). The expanded criteria donor dilemma in cadaveric renal transplantation. *Transplantation.* 2003; 75:1940-1945

Seaquist ER, Goek FC, Rich S, Barbosa J (1989). Familial clustering of diabetic kidney disease: Evidence for genetic susceptibility to diabetic nephropathy. *N Engl J Med* 1989; 320:1161-5.

Smits JM, Persijn GG, van Houwelingen HC, Claas FH, Frei U (2002). Evaluation of the Euro transplant Senior Program. The results of the first year. *Am J Transplant* 2002; 2: 664–670.

Stratta RJ, Rohr MS, Sundberg AK et al (2004). Increased kidney transplantation utilizing expanded criteria deceased organ donors with results comparable to standard criteria donor transplant. *Ann Surg* 2004; 239: 688–697.

Sunga RS, Christensenb LL et al (2008). Determinants of Discard of Expanded Criteria Donor Kidneys: Impact of Biopsy and Machine Perfusion. *American Journal of Transplantation* 2008; 8: 783–792

Toma H, Tanabe K, Tokumoto T, Shimizu T, Shimmura H. (2001) Time-dependent risk factors influencing the long-term outcome in living renal allografts: Donor age is a crucial risk factor for long-term graft survival more than 5 years after transplantation. *Transplantation* 2001; 72: 940-7.

UNOS data base. http://www.unos.org/

UNOS Policy 3.5.1(2002). Expanded Criteria Donor Definition and Point System. Richmond, VA: United Network for Organ Sharing; 2002:1–26.

Voiculescu A, Schlieper G, Hetzel GR et al (2002). Kidney transplantation in the elderly: age-matching as compared to HLA-matching: a single center experience. *Transplantation* 2002; 73: 1356–1359.

Wolfe RA, Ashby VB, Milford EL, Ojo AO, Ettenger RE, Agodoa LYC, Held PJ, Port FK(1999): Comparison of mortality in all patients on dialysis, patients on dialysis awaiting transplantation, and recipients of a first cadaveric transplant. *N Engl J Med* 341: 1725–1730, 1999

3

Donor Nephrectomy

Gholamreza Mokhtari, Ahmad Enshaei,
Hamidreza Baghani Aval and Samaneh Esmaeili
Urology Research Centre, Guilan University of Medical Sciences, Iran

1. Introduction

Donor selection for allografting of a non-paired vital organ, such as the heart, is necessarily limited to cadaveric or possibly xenogeneic sources. In contrast, because of the presence in most normal persons of two kidneys - each with a physiological reserve capable of providing four times the minimal required function - renal transplantation has become an accepted medical procedure using cadaveric and living related or unrelated volunteers as organ sources.

Each of these donor categories presents unique ethical, legal and social implications (Spital, 1991; Woo, 1992).

That must be addressed carefully to protect not only the health and rights of the recipient but also those of the donor.

Of equal importance are the medical aspects of donor evaluation and the technical features of the nephrectomy procedure.

The initial functional capacity of the transplanted kidney is largely independent of immunological factors; however, it is highly dependent on the efficacy of donor preparation and procurement techniques in preventing ischemic injury.

It has been necessary to adapt the surgical procedures to develop combination procurement techniques that provide equal protection for the extra renal organs as well as the kidneys.

2. Living kidney donor

The first successful renal transplant was performed in 1954. With the development of effective immunosuppressive regimens, this observation was extended to less compatible intrafamilial donors and eventually to unrelated donors.

Until the early 1980s, many dialysis patients had doubt to heed cadaver donor transplantation because its morbidity and mortality rates were manifold.

With the introduction of calcineurin inhibitors, monoclonal and polyclonal antibody immunosuppression and other new immunosuppressive agents into clinical regimens, the gap in graft survival between living related and cadaveric renal transplantation narrowed considerably.

Living related donor grafts still have a 10 to 12 % better survival rate at 1 year and a significantly higher probability of function thereafter, however (Cecka and Terasaki, 1998).

Family members as suitable organ donors were recommended. (Delmonico et al., 1990).

The experience of using living unrelated kidneys in transplantation has shown that these organs have a graft survival profile that, in fact approaches that of related donors (Terasaki et al., 1995).

Even with the current widespread application of calcineurin inhibitors and monoclonal and polyclonal antibody immunosuppression, there is a persisting biological advantage of living donor kidneys (living related donor or living unrelated donor) over cadaver donor allograft.

Although short - term graft survival after transplantation from both donor sources is excellent, the 5 year success rate of greater than 80 % that can be attained using living donor kidneys exceeds by 10 to15% of any reported cadaver donor results.

Another justification for using living donors is that the operation can be specifically planned, limiting waiting time on dialysis.

Of greater importance is the ability to perform the transplant when the recipient is in optimal medical condition. This ability is particularly pertinent for diabetic patients, whose condition may deteriorate rapidly on dialysis. Finally, there is the risk that the patient may develop antibody to HLA antigens during prolonged dialysis, especially if intermittent blood transfusions are required.

The final reason for the continued expansion of living donor transplantation is the insufficient supply of cadaver donor organs required to fulfill the needs of renal failure victims awaiting transplantation (Cohen et al., 1998).

For each 1 million of the population, approximately 75 to 80 renal transplants would have to be performed annually to keep pace with the more than 100 new patients diagnosed with end - stage renal disease and previous transplant recipients whose allograft eventually fail.

Even in areas with outstanding cadaver donor retrieval rates or with less strict criteria for donor selection (Kauffman et al., 1997), the number of potential recipients greatly exceeds the supply of donor's kidneys. A steadily growing population of patients is being maintained on dialysis in most areas of the world.

With the extension of minimally invasive techniques to living kidney donation the potential adverse impact of the operation has become less significant.

Although, it was thought that laparoscopic nephrectomy for renal transplantation might have some adverse effects to the donor organ because of prolonged warm ischemic interval, it is known that laparoscopic donor nephrectomy leads to decreases analgesic dose, decreased length of hospitalization, early return to normal daily activity and less surgical morbidity.

Nowadays, new devices are used in laparoscopic nephrectomy, have led to shorten ischemic time. So that its results are now comparable to those achieved after classic open nephrectomy. (Ratner et, al., 1997).

Laparosopic donor nephrectomy (LDN) has become the preferred technique for live donor nephrectomy at most transplant centers in the United States (Ratner et al, 1999; Jacobs et al, 2004).

Survival studies indicate that the 5 year life expectancy of a unilaterally nephrectomized 35 year - old male donors is 99 % compared with 99.3 % normal expectation (Merrill, 1964).

The quality of life after kidney donation has been reported in 979 patients who had donated a kidney for transplantation (Johnson et al., 1997). Most of the responders had an excellent quality of life.

Multivariate analysis of those who did not respond favorably identified the following two factors for negative psychosocial outcome; relatives other than first degree and recipients who died within 1 year of transplantation.

Concern has been raised that healthy human donors might develop hypertension and renal dysfunction years after unilateral nephrectomy. Follow - up studies of hundreds of living donors for 20 years have been unable, however, to identify any convincing evidence of long - term functional abnormalities associated with unilateral nephrectomy (Najarian et. al., 1992).

Regarding to these considerations, living donors continue to be the significant proportion of that donor pool. The proportion varies from less than 5% in some areas to 100% in areas where cadaver donor transplantation is unavailable. At present in U.S. about 27% of transplanted kidneys are obtained from living donors.

3. Medical evaluation and selection of the living donor

Advantages of transplant should be reasonable in comparison with its limited risks and both patient and donor should be justified for accepting it.

All potential donors are first screened for emotional stability and motivation as well as blood group ABO typing.

Incompatibility of ABO blood group between donor and recipient has resulted in irreversible rejection. Because of the extreme shortage of donor kidneys, especially for blood group O recipients, this requirement has been constantly reassessed. Several groups have reported successful results after transplantation of blood group A_2 kidneys into group O recipients (Nelson et.al., 1998). Approximately 20% of blood group A persons are subtyped as A_2. The highly successful transplantation of A_2 kidneys into group O recipients has been explained by the low expression of A determinants in A_2 kidneys compared with A_1 kidneys.

Potential donors remaining after initial screening process are evaluated to confirm excellent general health and bilateral renal function (kasiske et. al., 1996).The basic criteria for a renal donor are an absence of renal disease, an absence of transmissible malignancy, and an absence of active infection.

Many of the studies are directed toward detection of exterarenal pathology. This medical evaluation may reveal significant but treatable problems of which the donor was unaware. (Table 1) (Ko, et al. 2001)

Family conference with transplant-dialysis team ABO blood group, tissue typing, leukocyte cross match, ± mixed lymphocyte culture
History, physical examinations, serial blood pressure determinations
Cell blood count, coagulation profile, BUN, serum creatinine, FBS, cytomegalovirus antibody, human immunodeficiency virus antibody, hepatitis B and C testing, cholesterol, triglycerides, calcium, phosphorus, urine analysis, urine culture, 24-hour urine protein
Chest radiograph, intravenous pyelogram or ultrasound electrocardiogram
Aortogram or digital subtraction angiography and/or three-dimensional computed tomography

Table 1. Evaluation of living donors.

The remaining studies are concerned with the quality of renal function and the clarification of any anatomical abnormalities in either kidney. It must be determined that the non-donated kidney is normal.

Final selection of the donor, if several medically suitable relatives are available is made on the basis of histocompatibility testing. Selection also may be determined on the basis of age (avoiding elderly volunteers) or on less objective factors, such as the special social obligations of particular family member.

It is now clear that living unrelated donor kidneys provide significant physiological and long term survival advantages and are being accepted with increasing frequency. In most centers donation for monetary compensation is not allowed (Childress, 1996; Quinibi 1997).

The imaging of kidneys prior to nephrectomy performs by several methods, including: ultrasound (US); conventional angiography (CA); digital subtraction angiography (DSA); computed tomography (CT) and magnetic resonance imaging (MRI), each of which has innate problems. A single modality to assess vasculature, renal parenchyma and urinary drainage is preferred. The pre-nephrectomy anatomy which most anticipates complications during the transplant procedure is the presence or absence of variant arteries (Stephen Munn, 2010).

For the living donor who has been identified by these criteria, the classic gold standard aortogram has been the final diagnostic study scheduled. The ability to visualize data obtained with CT or MRI in a three-dimensional method carefully reconstructing the images, isolating arteries, veins or parenchymal structures has assisted surgical planning. Surgical goals are to minimize warm ischemia time, to preserve renal vessels, and to preserve ureteral blood supply.

Magnetic resonance imaging and angiography provide suboptimal information on renal vascular anatomy (Kok NF, et al., 2008).

Arvine-Berod and et al compared the sensitivity of computed tomography angiography (CTA) and magnetic resonance angiography (MRA) in preoperative renal vascularisation in living kidney donors. They determined that MRA is less sensitive than CTA in living kidney donors especially in the detection of multiple renal arteries. (Arvine-Berod A, et al., 2011)

4. Post operative care and complications

We administer a first generation cephalosporin for 24 hours, beginning 1 hour before surgery.

Most of patients are ready for discharge from the hospital in 3 to 4 days and for return to employment by 4 weeks.

Urine culture, renal function tests and a complete blood count are reassessed before discharge. The patient then has follow - up evaluations at increasing intervals.

The perioperative mortality rate for kidney donors is estimated to be 0.30 % (kasiske et al., 1996). Approximately 20 deaths have been reported after living donor allograft donation over 35 years (Jones et al., 1993). Other complications of the kidney donor procedure are generally minimal and easily remediable (Johnson et al., 1997).

The current overall complication rate is approximately 2 % (Bia et al., 1995).

Most complications occur in the perioperative period, with atelectasis, urinary infection, wound problems and prolonged bowel dysfunction accounting for the majority.

One of the most dangerous complications is thrombophlebitis with possible life-threatening pulmonary embolus.

Fatal cases of hepatitis, myocardial infarction and depression, leading to alcoholism have been reported.

Longer term morbidity should be minimal. Endogenous creatinine clearance rates rapidly approach 70 to 80 % of the preoperative level, and reports of late renal failure have been extremely rare. An important factor is the exclusion during the selection process of pathology or potential pathology in the donors.

The short and long - term morbidity of donor nephrectomy are generally considered to be low enough, and probability of successful graft outcome high enough, to make the risks acceptable for fully informed donors.

The decrease of worsening donor and noticeable successful results of transplantation from unrelated living donors caused some centres became interested to donation from strangers (Spital, 1994). According to our experience, male donors have better prognosis and survival compared with females.

5. Cadaver kidney donor

If a suitable living donor is not available, most patients with end-stage renal failure should be considered for cadaveric renal transplantation, not only because transplantation is more cost-effective but also because true rehabilitation seldom is achieved on long-term dialysis (Evans et al., 1985). Although the long-term success rates remain inferior to those achieved with interfamilial transplantation, projections indicate that cadaver donor allograft currently have a 1-year graft survival rate of greater than 85% and graft half-life (time to loss of 50% of currently surviving grafts) has improved to at least 10 years (Cecka and Terasaki, 1998).

Present methods of preservation may permit 72 hours maintenance of the cadaver donor kidney in a condition sufficiently viable to allow return of function after revascularization. Opportunities are present for evaluation of the physiological and bacteriological condition of the donor kidney and for pursuing histocompatility selection after the organ is removed from the cadaver. Because of these factors and increasingly widespread establishment of the definition of brain death guidelines that allow removal of organs that are more likely to be physiologically healthy, cadaver donor renal allograft continue to account for approximately

75% of reported transplants. The total number is limited only by the unsolved worldwide problem of persisting barriers to organ donation (Cohen et al., 1998).

6. Evaluation of the potential cadaver kidney donor

The ideal donor is a young, previously healthy individual who has sustained a fatal head injury or cerebrovascular accident.

Transplantation of kidneys from small pediatric donors is possible, although the technical aspects are more exacting. When kidneys are obtained from a pediatric donor less than 3 years of age, most groups recommend en bloc transplantation of both organs into a single adult recipient. We have reported a successful En Bloc bilateral kidney, Aorta, and Vena Cava Transplantation from a 3 years old deceased boy to an adult recipient in our center in Guilan University of Medical Sciences, Iran. (Fig. 1) (Mokhtari et al., 2010)

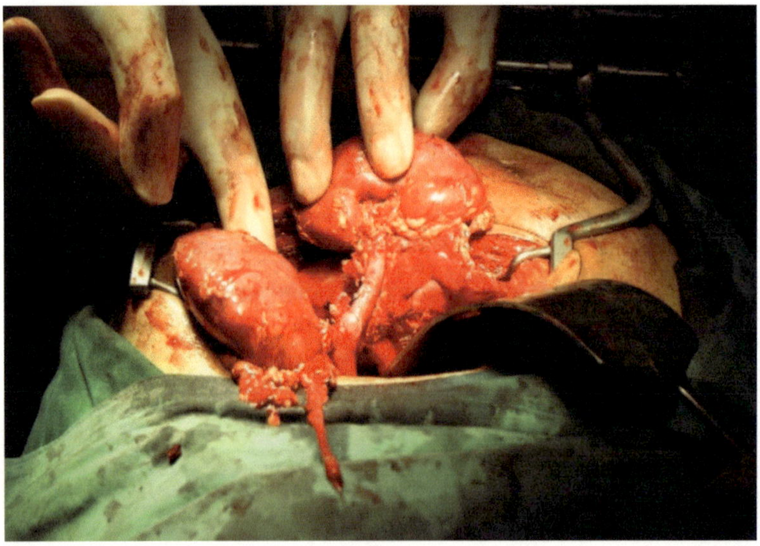

Fig. 1. En-bloc kidneys after transplantation (recipient). After irreversibility of brain damage is established, maintenance of renal blood flow and function without any complication and adequate hydration is important. Minor terminal elevations of blood urea nitrogen and creatinine levels are not unusual and do not necessarily exclude the donor.

A major concern for the donor team is the risk of transmitting infection with the allograft into an immunosuppressed recipient.

Diagnosis of irreversible coma, or brain death, which has been recognized by neurologists and neurosurgeons, has presented a set of circumstances that of great potential benefit to patients needing organ allografts. The concept and definition of brain death do not depend in any way on transplantation.

The discontinuation of respiratory support and other extraordinary therapy for patients who have been declared dead after careful assessment of brain function should be considered a humane and necessary act without regard to the possibility of such a person serving as an organ donor.

After extensive assessment of such patients, neurologists and neurosurgeons universally have agreed that once functional death of the brain stem occurs, there is no chance for partial recovery, and artificial support should be withdrawn.

7. Nonhuman kidney donor

The need for kidneys is growing steadily, whereas organ donation has leveled off or decreased in some regions. This situation has resulted in a rapidly escalating demand for medical and economic resources to support long-term peritoneal dialysis or hemodialysis programs. Because the supply of such resources is limited, constant efforts must be made to improve the efficacy and increase the number of transplants performed. The latter is determined primarily by the number of donor organs available.

Nonhuman (xenogenetic) donors represent a possible alternative source of transplantable organs. Beginning in the earlry1900$_s$, several isolated attempts were made on to transplant kidneys from various animal donors into patients with renal failure. If a successful approach to the use of such organs could be established, an unlimited pool of donors free of most of the legal and moral issues associated with the use of human organs could be made available.

The major obstacle to such an approach has been the increased intensity of the rejection response elicited by the more diverse genetic relationship between donor and recipient (Ko, et al. 2001).

For several reasons, there is renewed interest in the possibility that xenotransplantation could provide the solution for the shortage of human donor organs. The first reason for this enthusiasm is the increasingly successful use of genetic engineering to produce transgenic animals expressing recombinant molecules designed to moderate the immune response (Bhatti et al., 1999; Schmoeckel et al., 1998; Waterworth et al., 1998; Zaidi et al., 1998). Another reason for the renewed optimism regarding xenotransplantation has been the demonstration in preclinical primate models that tolerance of allograft can be produced without the need for long-term immunosuppression (Kirk et al., 1999).

8. References

Arvine-Berod A, Bricault I, et al. (2011) Preoperative assessment of renal vascular anatomy for donor nephrectomy: Is CT superior to MRI?. Prog Urol.; 21(1): 34-9.

Bhatti FN, Schmoeckel M, et al. (1999). Three-month survival of HDAFF transgenic pig hearts transplanted into primates. Transplant Proc.; 31(1-2):958.

Bia, M.J., Ramos, E.L., et al. (1995). Evaluation of living renal donors: the current practice of US transplanted centers. Transplantation. 60, 322.

Cecka, J.M. and Terasaki, P.I. (1998). The UNOS Scientific Renal Transplant Registry-1998. Clin Transplant. 1.

Childress, J. (1996). The gift of life: ethnical issues in organ transplantation. Bull. Am.Coll.Surg.81,8.

Cohen, B., McGrath, S.M., et al. (1998). Trends in organ donation. Clin. Transplant. 12, 525.

Delmonico, F.L., Fuller, T.C. and Cosimi, A.B. (1990). 1000 renal transplants at the Massachusetts General Hospital: improved allograft survival for high-risk patients without regard to HLA matching. Clin Transplant. 247, 53.

Evans, R.W., Manninen, D.L., et al. (1985). Living related kidney donors: a 14-year experience. Ann. Surg. 203, 637.

Johnson, E.M., Remucal, M.J., et al. (1997). Complications and risks of living donor nephrectomy. Transplantation 64, 1124.

Jacobs S, Cho E, Foster C, et al. (2004). Laparoscopic live donor nephrectomy: The University of Maryland 6-year experience. *J Urol* ; 171:47.

Jones, J., Payne, W.D., et al. (1993). The living donor-risks, benefits, and related concerns. Transplant. Rev. 7, 115.

Kasiske, B.L., Ravenscraft, M., et al. (1996). The evaluation of living renal transplant donors: clinical practice guidelines. Ad Hoc Clinical Practice Guidelines Subcommittee of Patient Care and Education Committee of the American Society of Transplant Physicians. J. Am.Soc.Nephrol. 7, 2288.

Kauffman, H. M., Bennett, L.E., et al. (1997). The expanded donor. Transplant. Rev. 11, 165.

Kirk AD, Burkly LC., et al. (1999). Treatment with humanized monoclonal antibody against CD154 prevents acute renal allograft rejection in nonhuman primates. Nat Med. 5:686-93.

Ko, S.C. D., and Cosimi, A.B. (2001). The donor and donor nephrectomy. In: Morris P.J. Kidney Transplantation (2001). Chapter 7, 89-105.

Kok NF, Dols LF, et al. (2008) complex vascular anatomy in live kidney donation: imaging and consequences for clinical outcome. Transplantation; 85(12): 1760-5.

Mereill, J.P. (1964). Moral problems of artificial and transplanted organs. Ann. Intern.Med. 61, 335.

Mokhtari G., Pourreza F., et al. (2010). En Bloc Bilateral Kidney, Aorta, and Vena Cava

Transplantation From a Deceased Pediatric Donor to an Adult Recipient: A Case Report. UroToday International Journal. 3(5), doi:10.3834/uij.1944-5784.2010.10.04.

Najarian, J.S., Chavers, B.M., et al. (1992). 20 years or more of follow-up of living kidney donors. Lancet 340, 807.

Nelson, P.W., Landreneau, M.D., et al. (1998). Ten-year experience in transplantation of A2 kidneys into B and O recipients. Transplantation 65, 256.

Quinibi, W. (1997). Commericially motivated renal transplantation: results in 540 patients transplanted in India. The living Non-Related Renal Transplant Study Group. Clin. Transplant. 11, 536.

Ratner, L.E., Kavoussi, L.R., et al. (1997). Laparoscopic assisted live donor nephrectomy--a comparison with the open approach. Transplantation. Jan 27;63(2):229-33.

Ratner LE, Montgomery RA, (1999). Kavoussi LR: Laparoscopic live donor nephrectomy: The four-year Johns Hopkins University experience. *Nephrol Dial Transplant*; 14: 2090.

Schmoeckel, M., Bhatti, F.N., et al. (1998). Orthotopic heart transplantation in a transgenic pig-to-primate model [published erratum appears in transplantation 1998 Oct 15; 66(7), 943]. Transplantation 65, 1570.

Spital A. (1994)Unrelated living kidney donors. An update of attitudes and use among U.S. transplant centers. Transplantation. 27;57:1722-6.

Stephen Munn. (2010). Assessment of donor kidney anatomy. NEPHROLOGY; 15, S96–S98.

Terasaki PI, Cecka JM, et al. (1995). High survival rates of kidney transplants from spousal and living unrelated donors. N Engl J Med. ;333:333-6.

Waterworth, P.T., Dunning, J., et al. (1998). Life-supporting pig-to-baboon heart xenotransplantation. J.Heart Lung Transplant. 17, 1201.

Woo, KT. (1992). Social and cultural aspects of organ donation in Asia. Ann Acad Med Singapore.; 21:421-7.

Zaidi A, Schmoeckel M., et al. (1998). Life-supporting pig-to-primate renal xenotransplantation using genetically modified donors. Transplantation. 27; 65:1584-90.

4

Renal Transplantation and Urinary Proteomics

Ying Wang, Li Ma, Gaoxing Luo, Yong Huang and Jun Wu
[1]*State Key Laboratory for Trauma, Burn and Combined Injury, Institute of Burn Research, Southwest Hospital, Third Military Medical University, Chongqing*
[2]*Chongqing Key Laboratory for Disease Proteomics, Chongqing*
China

1. Introduction

Urine is the terminal metabolites of bloodstream which is produced by filtration of glomerulus, and re-absorption, secretion and excretion of the renal tubule and collecting tubule (Figure 1), so that proteins found in serum may also be identified in urinary proteins. Urinary composition and properties can reflect the status of the entire urinary system, especially the changes in the type and quantity of proteins in the urine that carry information of the occurrence and development as well as prognosis of a variety of diseases of the urinary system, urine can also reflect relevant situation of other organs of the body. The source of urine is simple, convenient and non-invasive, easily accepted by patients, with no discomfort and contraindications. Therefore, uroscopy is one of the most common and important methods used to diagnose kidney and urinary tract diseases. In this sense, urinary proteome analysis can be used for the diagnosis and / or prognosis indicators of diseases.

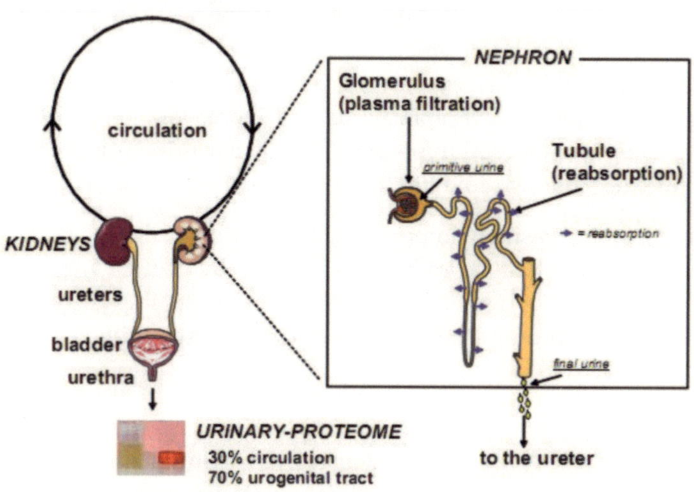

Fig. 1. 70% of the urinary proteins and peptides originate from the kidney and the urinary tract, whereas the remaining 30% originates from the circulation (Davis et al, 2001).

2. Methods of uroscopy

For diseases of urinary system, uroscopy is an important basis for diagnosis and is also of very important reference value for the diagnosis of certain systemic diseases and diseases of other organs of the body which affect the changes of urine, such as diabetes, blood diseases, liver and gallbladder diseases, epidemic hemorrhagic fever, etc. Meanwhile, the laboratory tests of urine can also reflect the treatment efficacy and prognosis of some diseases.

2.1 Urine routine examination

Uroscopy includes items of routine uroscopy, mid-stream urine culture (MSU), urinary three cups test, Addis count, quantitative test of urine protein and so on. The usually popular saying of "uroscopy" most often refers to routine uroscopy, and it is one of the most popular tests of routine examination. The test items included in routine uroscopy are visual inspection and biochemical tests, etc., wherein visual inspection refers to directly observation of the color and appearance of urine with naked eyes; biochemical tests refers to the urinary biochemical tests, which are often carried out with urine analyzer in hospital. The test items by urine analyzer are: urine protein, urine sugar, urine three bile pigments (urine bilirubin, urobilinogen and urobilin), urine volume, urine ketone, urobilinogen, urine specific gravity, and urine sediment. Compared with serum and other body fluid samples, the protein composition of urine is relatively simple, stable and easy to be analyzed, and can be used for the detection of many human diseases, especially diseases of urinary system. Therefore, regular urine examination is of great significance to detect urinary tract diseases.

2.2 Special urine examination

With the rapid development of molecular biology, the examination methods of urine changed from simplification to diversification. For example: 1. ELISA kits for detection of HIV antibodies in urine specimens, WB diagnostic kits for detection of HIV-1 antibodies in urine; 2. fluorescently labeled DNA probes for detection of the four kinds of chromosomal abnormalities associated with bladder cancer; 3. pregnancy test strip for detection of Human Chorionic Gonadotropin (hCG); 4. Streptococcus pneumonia antigen detection technique for screening of invasive pneumococcal infections; 5 K powder urine test board for detection of occult blood; 6 urine test kits for rapid detection of heroin.

Uroscopy is playing an increasingly important role in the clinical application, and more and more attention is being paid to it in product test and product R & D. Therefore, the study on urine has become a popular research direction, in which study on urine proteins is particularly prominent, including studies on specific proteins and whole proteomics.

3. Urinary proteomics

At the same time of proteomics study extensively extending into various fields of the medical community, urinary proteomics has also made great progress, and has achieved important research results in finding early diagnostic markers of various diseases of urinary tract and other systems and exploring the mechanisms of disease development.

3.1 Study status of normal urinary proteomics

In 1996, Marshall et al proposed the concept of urinary proteomics, which is to use the high-throughput of proteomics technologies and systematically to analyze and identify all proteins in urine and study their biological functions. They applied proteomics technologies to analyze the composition of normal urinary proteins for the first time. First, normal urine was condensed through dye precipitation, and then analysed by 2-dimensional electrophoresis (2-DE), but no protein was identified.

In 1997, Heine et al employed reversed phase chromatography (RP) and ion exchange chromatography to purify and separate peptides. Combining with high performance liquid chromatography-electrospray ionization-mass spectrometry (HPLC-ESI-MS), they analyzed the spectra of peptides and proteins of normal urine, and 34 high-abundance proteins were identified, including albumin, apolipoprotein, immunoglobulin, collagen, procollagen.

In 2001, Spahr et al identified 751 peptide sequence and 124 proteins using liquid chromatography–tandem mass spectrometry (LC-MS/MS). Compared with 2-DE, LC-MS/MS is much quicker in analysis and identification, but it could not be used to quantitatively analyze the difference in protein content between different samples.

In 2002, Thongboonkerd et al analyzed normal adult urinary proteins isolated by acetone extraction and ultracentrifugation using 2-DE, discovered 67 spots by gel imaging, and identified 47 proteins by matrix assisted laser desorption ionization/time of flight mass spectrometry (MALDI-TOF-MS), including transport proteins, adhesion molecules, complement components, molecular chaperones, receptors, enzymes, matrix proteins, and signal-related proteins using MALDI-TOF-MS. The proteins and membrane proteins isolated by ultracentrifugation in this experiment can not be obtained by conventional acetone extraction, indicating that complete urinary protein mapping could not be obtained by using a single separation method.

In 2004, Pieper et al, by combining MALDI-TOF-MS with 2-D LC/ESI-MS/MS, separated nearly 140 protein spots and identified 150 unique urinary proteins, a third of which were classified as original plasma proteins in circulation. In 2004, Schaub et al analyzed normal urine using surface-enhanced laser-desorption/ionization time-of-flight mass spectrometry (SELDI-TOF-MS) and found that there were differences in protein composition for female midstream urine and first voided urine samples, while there were no such differences in male urine samples.

In 2004, Weissinger et al analyzed the urinary proteomes of 57 healthy volunteers, 16 patients with minimal change disease (MCD), 18 patients with membranous glomerulonephritis (MGN), and 10 patients with focal segmental glomerulosclerosis (FSGS) by capillary electrophoresis mass spectrometry (CE-MS). They identified 173 peptides with more than 90% probability, and 690 peptides with more than 50% probability from healthy individuals. Based on these data, they established a "normal" polypeptide pattern in healthy individuals. Peptides found in the urine of patients differed significantly from the normal controls. These differences allowed the distinction of specific protein spectra in patients with different primary renal diseases.

In 2004, Oh et al carried out proteomics analysis on the urine of 40 healthy adults (equal number of male and female) after precipitation trichloroacetic acid. In addition to some potential-dependent protein spots, the urinary protein spots on 2-DE gel of male and female were almost identical (Figure 2), which can be used as standard 2-DE urinary protein profiles, providing a foundation for analyzing and looking for novel specific biomarkers for diseases in the future.

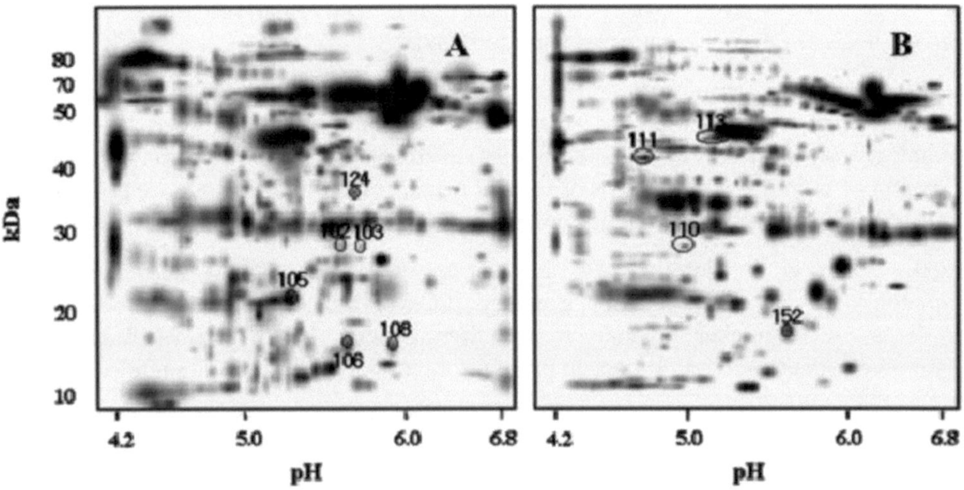

Fig. 2. Comparison of (A) female and (B) male urinary proteins separated on 2-D gels. Male and female specific proteins are indicated with circles (Oh et al,2004).

In 2005, Sun et al identified 226 special urinary proteins in combination 1-DE with 1-D LC/MS/MS, 1-D LC/MS/MS, or 2-D LC/MS/MS, and discussed the proteins identified by different methods. In 2005, Castagna et al confirmed 383 special gene products from urinary proteins enriched on coating beads with hexamer peptide ligand library in combination with linear ion trap-Fourier transform mass spectrometry (LTQ FTMS).

In 2006, Adachi et al employed 1-D sodium dodecyl sulfate polyacrylamide gel electrophoresis (SDS-PAGE) and RP-HPLC for protein separation, and then used LTQ FTMS and LTQ Orbitrap-MS to analyze trypsin digested pepdides. Finally, 1543 proteins and their fragments were identified in the urine of healthy individuals. Further research showed that most of the proteins in the urine were membrane proteins, which may derive from external secretion. In 2010, Li et al identified 1310 non-redundant high-confidence proteins using integrated multidimensional liquid chromatography (IMDL) and multidimensional liquid chromatography (MDLC).

In summary, good results have been achieved in normal urinary proteomics, the proteome profiles of healthy population have been gradually improved and supplemented. At the same time, the methods and techniques for urinary proteomics have also been further developed and optimized. However, the identification consistency of normal urine proteins by researchers is low, and the reliability of the results remains to be verified. The establishment of profiles of normal urinary proteomes plays an important role in screening different markers of urine differentiation for a variety of disease states.

3.2 Urinary proteomics technologies

The commonly used technologies for protein isolation and identification in urinary proteomics include SDS-PAGE, 2-DE, LC-MS, SELDI-TOF-MS, CE-MS (Figure 3,Figure 4). Currently, proteomics technologies have been extensively used in clinical diagnosis and various fields of biological study.

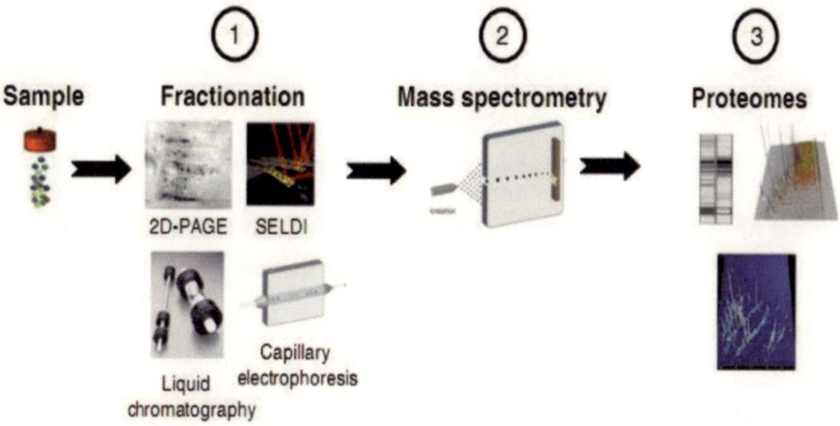

Fig. 3. Proteome analysis of urine requires fractionation to reduce complexity of the sample. 1 Fractionation can be obtained by different chromatographic techniques or by the specific absorption of a set of proteins on a surface. 2 These fractions are subsequently analyzed by MS where the relative abundance of the different proteins and peptides is determined. 3 Informatics treatment of the protein data in combination with the fractionation (example: migration time on a capillary or LC column) parameters yields protein profiles representing the (partial) proteincontent of samples. SELDI-TOF-MS, 2-D-PAGE (Caubet et al, 2010).

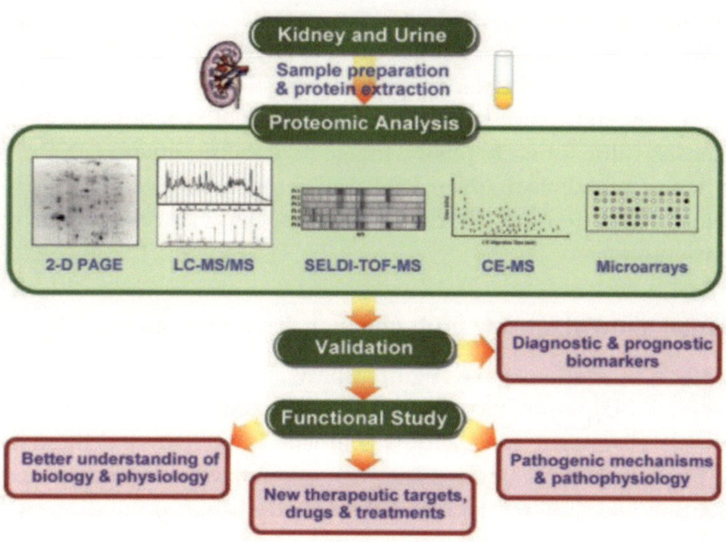

Fig. 4. Schematic summary of methodologies and applications of renal and urinary proteomics. 2-D PAGE; LC-MS/MS, SELDI-TOF-MS; CE-MS. (Thongboonkerd , 2010)

3.3 Significance and problems of urinary proteomics

Urinary proteomics related to the huge protein networks has exhibited widely application in many areas. The therapeutic intervention target molecules have demonstrated a valuable impact for the diagnosis and treatment technology, and have become a powerful weapon for clarifying the mechanisms, diagnosis, prevention and control of major human diseases. Although rapid developments have already been achieved in urinary proteomics technologies, some urgent problems still need to be solved, such as (1) the low amount of proteins in normal urine, imperfect enrichment techniques, and different urinary protein sample preparation methods, which can affect the isolation and identification of urinary proteins; (2) the determination of the best collection time of urine samples: the available studies have shown that urinary proteins in urine samples collected at different times show significant difference; (3) the elimination of various ions and high-abundance proteins without losing low-abundance proteins; (4) the analysis of extremely acidic, alkaline, small, large, low-abundance, and highly hydrophobic proteins using proteomics technologies; (5) the lack of adequate standard urine profiles for different diseases, and the further improvement of urinary protein data and bioinformatics; (6) the establishment of standard urine protein preparation and analytical methodology.

The broad prospects of urinary proteomics are beyond doubt, and urinary proteomics involves a large network of proteins, with the continuous development of science and technology of today, the above problems will gradually be resolved.

4. Urinary proteomics and diseases

With the development of front research in life sciences and the emergence of cutting-edge new technologies, proteomics has entered into a brand new era of studying functional proteomics in large scale and high-throughput, and could play an important role in the study of major diseases. Back in the late 1990s, people have begun to identify urinary proteins. The available studies have shown that survivin and cox2-2 proteins in urine are valuable for the diagnosis of early bladder cancer; transforming growth factors TGF-β1 and laminin (LN) have some relevance to breast cancer; the detection of podocalyxin has a very important diagnostic value for early renal damage in diabetic patients; AQP-2 protein plays a key role in water metabolism disorder in patients with liver cirrhosis; AQP-2 has diagnostic value in hypertension. Studies on disease biomarkers are the most popular hotspot in urinary proteomics.

4.1 Developmental trend of urinary proteomics in renal diseases

As early as the 1990s, researchers have begun urinary proteomics in renal diseases, and have found some special diagnostic biomarkers and characteristic spectra. Compared with traditional methods, diagnostic specificity was greatly improved, and these methods were easily accepted by patients. In renal diseases, such as renal cancer, glomerular disease, acute renal transplantation rejection, researchers have already begun urine diagnostic biomarker related study. But no significant achievement and dramatic breakthrough were reported. Therefore, researchers need make more efforts to actively promote the progress of research in this area.

The identification of urinary proteomes shows great potential in diagnosis and monitoring of renal diseases, and is the important direction of developing non-invasive diagnosis and monitoring for renal diseases. Another important goal for proteomic research is to apply newly discovered biomakers into clinical laboratory testing. This method is convenient, rapid, repeatable, and non-invasive. The entire process only takes 3 to 4 hours, greatly reducing the time for histopathologic examination, which makes great contribution to improve the post-operative care level after renal transplantation. Renal transplantation was the earliest developed and also the most mature organ transplantation currently, which provides a second life chance for patients with advanced renal failure. However, transplantation rejection is still an insurmountable obstacle in the field of transplantation.

4.2 Renal transplantation and acute rejection

Acute rejection (AR) is the most common form rejection in clinical. It can occur at any time after renal allograft transplantation, but mostly occurs in the 3 months after transplantation, while within the first month is the most common. AR is not only a vital factor to influence the long-term survival of the kidney transplanted, but also the major reason to cause the early graft damage, long-term graft dysfunction, and chronic graft nephropathy. Until now, to carry out transplantation renal biopsy and pathological histology is the only way to confirm definite diagnosis. However, these methods cause not only pain in patients but also a certain degree of renal damage. Furthermore, rejection is a continuous biological process occurred under the use of immunosuppressant, and the diagnosis by renal biopsy is only based on the tissue samples at a certain time. For some patients, immunological changes could not be observed in rejection even if a pathological examination has been carried out and it is difficult to differentiate from the damages caused by the use of immunosuppressant, and the diagnosis takes two to three days. Thus, it is urgently need a frequently used and non-invasive detection method for early detection of markers of allograft damages.

4.3 Acute renal allograft rejection status of proteomics

Clarke et al analyzed the urinary proteins from renal transplantation patients with AR (17 recipients) and without rejection (15 recipients) using SELDI-TOF-MS. Significant differences were observed at 6.5KD, 6.7 KD, 6.6 KD, 7.1 KD and 13.4 KD between the two groups, while 10.0 KD and 3.4 KD were found to have a sensitivity of 83% and a specificity of 100% in diagnosing AR. It was also found that several groups of proteins specifically appeared in the urine of AR patients, which are likely to serve as diagnostic markers of AR.

O'Riordan et al studied the urine of renal transplantation patients using SELDI-TOF-MS. 3 proteins with peak value at 4.7kDa, 25.6kDa and 19.0kDa, sensitivity between 90.5 % ~ 91.3% and specificity between 77.2 % ~ 83.3 %, were screened out, which could serve as important biomarkers for distinguishing of AR patients from stable renal function patients. For the follow-up study, two peptides, ß-defensin -1 (4.7KD) and Alpha 1-antichymotrypsin (4.4KD), were indentified. Compared with patients with stable renal function after transplantation, ß-defensin -1 decreased in the urine of AR patients while Alpha 1-antichymotrypsin increased ($P < 0.05$). The study showed that the ratio of ß-defensin -1 and Alpha 1-antichymotrypsin in urine might be a potential new biomarker for diagnosing AR after renal transplantation.

To use SELDI-TOF-MS, Schaub et al found three peak clusters in 17 AR patients among 18 renal transplant patients, four out of 22 stable transplant patients, zero out of 28 control patients. The follow-up study showed that theses peak clusters derived from non-trypsin attached from of urine ß2-micglobulin (ß2-m). Thus, ß2-m may be use as acute tubular injury biomarker, becoming one of the standards of non-invasive early AR diagnosis.

Reichelt et al analyzed the urine of 13 renal biopsy confirmed AR patients and 10 renal transplant patients without pathological symptom of rejection by using SELDI-TOF-MS, and two biomarkers, 25.71kDa and 28.13kDa, were found, the diagnostic sensitivity was 90% and 93% respectively, and the specificity was 80% and 85% respectively. SELDI-TOF-MS appears to be a promising new diagnostic tool for distinguishing renal transplant patients with AR from those without rejection or healthy volunteers.

Jia et al chose urine as the object to find biomarkers for AR using 2-DE-MS and Westernblot assay. They obtained 30 protein spots with significant decline trend by MS, and identified 16 protein spots. Among them, three proteins, alpha-1-antichymotrypsin, tumor rejection antigen gp96, and Zn-Alpha-2-Glycoprotein associated with immune rejection, which may be candidate biomarkers for early clinical diagnosis of AR after renal transplantation.

Freue et al studied the plasma proteome collected from 32 patients with and without renal biopsy confirmed AR after renal transplantation using iTRAQ-MALDI-TOF/TOF. They found that 18 plasma proteins to be related to inflammation could be potential plasma biomarkers. Plasma biomarkers may be used to monitor post-transplant and permit effectively therapeutic intervention to minimize graft damage.

A large number of studies showed that some special biomarkers found in the urine of patients with AR after renal transplantation had a certain degree of reproducibility. However, above mentioned studies still need to design reasonably to improve the sensitivity and specificity of the results so that these potential biomarkers could be used for clinical screening.

4.4 Proteomics in AR in renal transplantation and current problems

Renal transplantation is the main way to treat end-stage renal diseases. With the application of immunosuppressant, the survival rate for renal transplantation has been increased step by step. However, there is still rejection after renal transplantation. Currently, renal biopsy is still the main basis for diagnosis, but mostly biopsy is only carried out when symptoms occur to the patients, diagnosis can not be made in advance, and there are some risks for renal biopsy itself. The ideal way is to find some specific indicators in urine or blood to make diagnosis. The advantage of this kind of diagnosis is that it is non-invasive, and the change of some biological indicators in body fluid appeared earlier than clinical symptoms, so diagnosis can be made in advance by taking advantage of these indicators. Even if urinary proteomics can not completely replace renal biopsy to become a "golden standard", it may still be used as an early screening tool so that renal biopsy will be minimized and unnecessary renal biopsy will be avoided. Taking into consideration of the high cost of protein analysis, the proteins identified in different laboratories still need to be further confirmed. Thus, the use of urinary proteins to monitor patients of renal transplantation is difficult to be carried out clinically within a short period of time.

5. Developmental direction of proteomics

With the rapid development of proteomics and its extensive application in many areas, proteomics technologies have been applied to a variety of life sciences. Proteomic research subjects include prokaryotic microorganisms, eukaryotic microorganisms, plant, animals, and human being, involving many important biological phenomena, such as signal transformation, cell differentiation, and protein folding. Therefore, the new research direction is the inexorable development trend of proteomics.

5.1 Quantitative proteomics

At present, life sciences have entered the post-genomic era. The research focuses have shifted from the discovery of genetic information to functional analysis, attempting to qualitatively and quantitatively study the full set of proteins of a certain biological sample expressed under specific conditions. It is a research hotspot in post-genomic era. With the continuous deepening of research and development of experimental techniques, quantitative proteomics has become hot research topics. The focus of quantitative proteomics is the accurate quantitation of the complex proteins from biological samples. For special proteomes, their physical and chemical properties are highly complicated because the dynamic range of protein expression is large. Thus high-throughput and high sensitivity experimental platform, represented by biological mass spectrometry, is the effective means and key technology for proteomics research.

The performance indicators of biological mass spectrometry, such as resolution, sensitivity, speed, accuracy, reproducibility, and dynamic range, have continuously improved as the development of proteomics. However, technological advances could not solve all the problems. Furthermore, complex steps are used from sample preparation to data analysis, which will introduce not ignorable system errors, and as well as seriously affect the accuracy of quantitative analysis. Currently, the analysis strategies of quantitative proteomics based on biological mass spectrometry are as follows: fluorescent two-dimensional difference gel electrophoresis (2-D DIGE), isotope coded affinity tagging (ICAT), isobaric tags for relative and absolute quantitation (iTRAQ), stable isotope labeling with amino acids in cell culture (SILAC), chemical labeling with amino acids, and comparison of the difference of peptide mass spectra. Quantitative methods include relative and absolute quantitation. Relative quantitative proteomics, also known as comparative proteomics, refers to the comparative analysis of relative changes of protein expression in cells, tissues or body fluids under different physiological and pathological conditions. Absolute quantitative proteomics is to determine the quantity or concentration of each protein in cells, tissues or body fluids. Absolute quantitation of proteins is a method to compare particular peptide elements of a sample against a spiked in isotopic labeled synthetic analogue.

Proteomics quantitative information can be used to understand the functions of proteins in interaction network. The analysis of the absolute amount of clinical biomarkers could help us determine the occurrence and development of diseases, and this provides practical guidance for the clinical diagnosis and treatment of diseases.

5.2 Phosphoproteomics

Recently, protein post-translational modification has gradually become one of research hotspots in proteomics. Protein phosphorylation is a reversible post-translational modification which plays an important role in cell proliferation, cell differentiation, cell signal transduction, regulation, transcription and translation, protein complex formation, and protein degradation. Therefore, the identification of phosphorylated proteins is an important part of research on post-translational modification. However, it is difficult to use mass spectrometry to directly detect phosphorylated proteins because of their low abundance. To solve this problem and enhance the signal response of phosphorylated peptides/proteins in mass spectra, we need to enrich phosphorylated peptides/proteins. The widely used and newly established isolation and enrichment methods of phosphoproteomics mainly include: antibody enrichment, kinase-specific enrichment, affinity enrichment, chemical modification, multi-chromatography separation and enrichment.

Li et al identified 31 phosphorylated proteins and 51 specific peptides from normal urine using proteomics methods. The rapid development of quantitative phosphoproteomics methods and technologies has laid a solid foundation for the study of spatial and temporal dynamics of protein phosphorylation and better understanding of biological functional of regulatory networks. As an important part of proteomics research, quantitative phosphoproteomics will meet great challenges in technologies and methods because of the unique characteristics of phosphorylated proteins. Phosphoproteomics will become an important study direction in the future.

5.3 Glycoproteomics

Glycosylation is one of the most common and important post-translational modification of proteins. It is currently known that at least one half of mammal proteins are glycoprotein, which widely distributed in various cells and tissues, especially abundant in the cell surface and body fluids. Protein glycosylation has important biological functions, such as participation in cell adhesion and signal transformation, influence on the secretion and stability of proteins, elimination of the aging proteins in plasma, immune and inflammatory response, and recognition of egg and sperm. Protein glycosylation is of great significance in diseases, especially in the occurrence, development and metastasis of tumors. In a particular state, the amount of glycoprotein and /or the change of sugar chain structure of glycoprotein reflect the change of physiological or pathological states, such as the autoimmune diseases caused by sugar chain abnormity of immunoglobulin (Ig), rheumatoid arthritis, IgA nephropathy, thyroiditis, systemic lupus erythematosus, and AIDS.

In 2006, Wang et al identified 225 glycoprotein enriched by ConA lectin from the urine of normal young volunteers using LTQ. Currently the discovered biomarkers of a variety of known diseases are glycoprotein, such as prostate specific antigen which could serve as suggestive biomarker for prostate cancer, tumor antigen CA125 etc.

Hence, researches on glycoprotein have great biological significance and application prospect. Glycoproteomics has begun to attract more and more attention. In recent years, with the rapid development of proteomics technologies, glycoproteomics has also gained considerable progress. At current stage, researches on glycoproteome are mainly focused on the development and utilization of methodology. The existing enrichment methods, such as lectin affinity chromatography, solid phase capture based on chemical reaction, are relatively mature, and are currently the most widely applied methods for glycoprotein enrichment. Although the research methods of glycosylation sites have been improved gradually, to solve the main problems existed still depends on the further development of mass spectrometry. We believe that, as the development of technologies, glycoproteome will play a greater role in further improvement of proteome expression, the discovery of biological markers in disease proteomics, and the research of drug targets.

6. Conclusion

For many patients with end-stage renal failure, renal transplantation is their first choice, the prognosis is good, but long-term survival rate has not yet achieved great improvement. Each patient should insist on taking immunosuppressant after renal transplantation, which is essential for the long-term prognosis of renal transplantation. Therefore, it is urgently needed for a non-invasive testing method to be used repeatedly for the early detection of biomarkers of allograft injury. Although current diagnostic methods have made some progress, none of them is absolutely reliable for clinical application. The combined application of many methods may lead to the increase of the diagnostic sensitivity and specificity. Its exact clinical application value needs to be further confirmed. In short, new diagnostic methods will continue to emerge as the development of technologies. Timely and accurate detection of AR through non-invasive or low-invasive methods is the future research direction. Although some progress has already made in this area, there is still no reliable, less invasive, and costless method that can be applied to clinical practice. Urinary proteomics technologies have the potential to reveal the complex pathophysiology, and are expected to become a powerful tool to solve this problem. Researches based on large scale samples are expected to provide proof for clinical application.

7. References

Theodorescu, D; Wittke, S. & Ross, MM. (2006). Discovery and validation of new protein biomarkers for urothelial cancer: a prospective analysis, *Lancet Oncology*, Vol.7, No.3, (March 2006), PP. 230–240, ISSN: 1470-2045

Fliser, D; Novak, J. & Thongboonkerd,V. (2007). Advances in urinary proteome analysis and biomarker discovery. *Journal of the American Society of Nephrology*, Vol.18, No.4, (February2007), pp.1057–1071, ISSN: 1046-6673

Muller, GA; Muller, CA. & Dihazi, H. (2007). Clinical proteomics-on the long way from bench to bedside? *Nephrol Dial Transplant*, Vol. 22, No.5, (February2007), pp.1297–1300, ISSN: 0931-0509

Roelofsen, H; Alvarez-Llamas, G. & Schepers, M. (2007). Proteomics profiling of urine with surface enhanced laser desorption/ionization time of flight mass spectrometry. *Proteome Science*, Vol.5, No.2, (October 2006), pp.1-9, ISSN:1477-5956

Yates, JR; Ruse, CI. & Nakorchevsky, A. (2009). Proteomics by Mass Spectrometry: Approaches, Advances, and Applications. *Annual Review of Biomedical Engineering*, No.11, (April 2009), pp. 49–79, ISSN: 1523-9829

Yarmush, ML& Jayaraman, A. (2002). Advances in proteomic technologies. *Annual Review of Biomedical Engineerin*, No.4, (March 2002), pp.349–73, ISSN: 1523-9829

VidalJr, BC ; Bonventre, JV & Honghsu, SI. (2005). Towards the application of proteomics in renal disease diagnosis. *Clinical Science*, Vol.109, No.5, (November 2005), pp.421–430, ISSN: 1470-8736

Davis, MT; Spahr, CS & McGinley, MD. (2001). Towards defining the urinary proteome using liquid chromatography-tandem mass spectrometry II. Limitations of complex mixture analyses. *Proteomics,* Vol.1, No.1, (January 2001), pp.108–117, ISSN: 1615-9861

Cutillas, PR; Norden, AGW & Cramer, R. (2003). Detection and analysis of urinary peptides by on-line liquid chromatography and mass spectrometry: application to patients with renal Fanconi syndrome. *Clinical Science,* Vol.104, No.5, (November 2002), pp.483–490, ISSN: 1470-8736

Tiensiwakul, P. (1998). Urinary HIV-1 antibody patterns by Western blot assay. *clinical laboratory science,* Vol.11, No.6, (November 1998), pp.336-338, ISSN: 0091-7370

Oelemann, WMR; Lowndes, CM & Veríssimo da Costa, GC. (2002). Diagnostic Detection of Human Immunodeficiency Virus Type 1 Antibodies in Urine: a Brazilian Study.*Journal of Clinical Microbiology,* Vol.40, No.3, (December 2001), pp. 881–885, ISSN: 0095-1137

Neuman, MI & Harper, MB. (2003). Evaluation of a Rapid Urine Antigen Assay for the Detection of Invasive Pneumococcal Disease in Children. *PEDIATRICS,* Vol.112, No.6, (Febuary 2003), pp.1279-1282, ISSN: 0031-4005

Neithardt,AB; Dooley, SL & Borensztajn, J. (2002). Prediction of 24-hour protein excretion in pregnancy with a single voided urine protein-to–create-nine ratio. A*merican journal of obstetrics and gynecology,* Vol.186, No.5, (May2002), pp.883 -886, ISSN: 0002-9378

Duggan, B & Williamson, K. (2004). Molecular markers for predicting recur-rence progression and outcomes of bladder cancer. *Current Opinion in Urology,* Vol.14, No.5, (September 2004), pp. 277 -286, ISSN: 1473-6586

Ohsawa, I; Taiji, N & Yukihiro, K (2004). Detection of urine survivin in 40 patients with bladder cancer. *Journal of Nippon Medical School,* Vol.71, No.6, (December 2004), pp. 379-383, ISSN: 1345-4676

Shariat, SF; Casella, R & Khoddami, SM · (2004). Urine detection of survivin is a sensitive marker for the noninvasive diagnosis of bladder cancer. *Journal of Urology ,* Vol.171,No.2, (Febuary 2004), pp.626-630, ISSN: 1677-5538

Elliot, S; Goldsmith, P & Knepper, MA. (1996). Urinary excretion of aquaporin-2 in humans: A potential marker of collecting duct responsiveness to vasopressin. *Journal of American Society Nephrology,* Vol.7, No.3, (1996), pp.403-409, ISSN: 1046-6673

Ivarsen, P; Frokiaer, J & Aagaard, NK. (2003). Increased urinary excretion of aquaporin 2 in patients with liver cirrhosis. *Gut,* Vol.52, No.8, (March 2003), pp.1194-1199, ISSN: 1468-3288

Bonventre, JV & Massachusetts, B. (2002). The kidney proteome: A hint of things to come. *Kidney International,* Vol.62, (2002), pp.1470 –1471, ISSN: 0058-2238

Marshall, T & Williams, K. (1996). Two-dimensional electrophoresis of human urinary proteins following concentration by dyeprecipitation. *Electrophoresis,* Vol.17, No.7, (April 1996), pp.1265-72, ISSN: 1265-1272

Heine, G; Raida, M & Forssmann, WG. (1997). Mapping of peptides and protein fragments in human urine using liquid chromatography-mass spectrometry. *Journal of Chromatography. A,* Vol.776, No.1, (July 1997), pp.117-24, ISSN: 0021-9673

Spahr, CS; Davis MT & Mcginley, MD. (2001). Towards defining the urinary proteome using liquid chromatography-tandem mass spectrometry I. Profilingan unfractionated tryptic digest. *Proteomics,* Vol.1, No.1, (January 2001), pp.93-107, ISSN: 1615-9861

Thongboonkerd, V; McLeish, KR & Arthur, JM. (2002). Proteomic analysis of normal human urinary proteins isolated by acetone precipitation or ultracentrifugation. *Kidney International,* Vol.62, No.4, (May 2002), pp.1461–1469, ISSN: 0085-2538

Pieper, R; Gatlin, CL & McGrath, AM. (2004). Characterization of the human urinary proteome: a method for high-resolution display of urinary proteins on two-dimensional electrophoresis gels with a yield of nearly 1400 distinct protein spots. *Proteomics*, Vol.4, No.4, (February 2004), pp.1159-1174, ISSN: 1615-9861

Schaub, S; Wilkins, J & Weiler, T. (2004). Urine protein profiling with surface-enhanced laser-desorption/ionization time-of-flight mass spectrometry. *Kidney International*, Vol.65, No.1, (August 2003), pp.323-332, ISSN: 0085-2538

Weissinger, EM; Wttke, S & Kaiser, T. (2004). Proteomic patterns established with capillary electrophoresis and mass spectrometry for diagnostic purposes. *Kidney International*, Vol.65, No.6, (January 2004), pp.2426–2234, ISSN: 0085-2538

Oh, JS; Pyo, JH & Jo, EH. (2004). Establishment of a near-standard two-dimensional human urine proteomic map. *Proteomics*, Vol.4, No.11, (September 2004), pp.3485–3497, ISSN: 1615-9861

Sun, W; Li, F. Wu S & Wang, X. (2005). Human urine proteome analysis by three separation approaches. *Proteomics*, Vol.5, No.18, (May 2005), pp.4994-5001, ISSN: 1615-9861

Castagna, A; Cecconi, D & Sennels, L. (2005). Exploring the hidden human urinary proteome via ligand library beads. *Journal of Proteome Research*, Vol.4, No.6, (October 2005), pp.1917-1930, ISSN: 1535-3893

Adachi, J; Kumar, C & Zhang, YL.(2006). The human urinary proteome contains more than 1500 proteins, including a large proportion of membrane proteins. *Genome Biology*, Vol.7, No.9, (May 2006), pp.R80, ISSN:1465-6906

Khan, A & Packer, NH. (2006). Simple urinary sample preparation for proteo-mic analysis. *Journal of Proteome Research*, Vol.5, No.10, (September 2006), pp.2824–2838, ISSN: 1535-3893

Thongboonkerd, V; Chutipongtanate, S & Kanlaya, R. (2006). Systematic evaluation of sample preparation methods for gel-based human urinary proteomics: Quantity, quality, and variability. *Journal of Proteome Research*, Vol.5, (2006), pp.183–191, ISSN: 1535-3893

Jürgens, M; Appel, A & Heine G. (2005). Towards characterization of the human urinary peptidome. *Combinatorial chemistry & high throughput screening*, Vol. 8, No.8 , (December 2005), pp.757–765, ISSN:1386-2073

Metzger, J; Schanstra, JP & Mischak, H. (2009). Capillary electrophoresis–mass spectrometry in urinary proteome analysis: current applications and future developments. *Analytical and Bioanalytical Chemistry*, Vol.393, No.5, (March 2008), pp. 1431–1442, ISSN: 1618-2642

Hampel, DJ; Sansome, C & Sha, M. (2001). Toward proteomics in uroscopy: urinary protein profiles after radiocontrast medium administration. *Journal of the American Society of Nephrolog*, Vol.12, No.5, (June 2000), pp.1026-35, ISSN: 1046-6673

Clarke, W; Silverman, BC & Zhang, Z. (2003). Characterization of Renal Allograft Rejection by Urinary Proteomic Analysis. *Annals of Surgery*, Vol.237, No.5, (2003), pp. 660-664, ISSN: 0003-4932

O'Riordan, E;Orlova, TN & Mei, JF. (2004). Bioinformatic Analysis of the Urine Proteome of Acute Allograft Rejection. *Journal of the American Society of Nephrolog*, Vol.15, No.12, (March 2004), pp.3240-3248, ISSN: 1046-6673

Schaub, S; Rush, D & Wilkins, J. (2004). Proteomic-based detection of urine proteins associated with acute renal allograft rejection. *Journal of the American Society of Nephrolog*, Vol.15, No.1, (January 2004), pp.219-227, ISSN: 1046-6673

Schaub, S; Wilkins, JA & Antonovici, M. (2005). Proteomic-based identification of cleaved urinary ß2-m microglobulin as a potential marker for acute tubular injury in renal allografts. *American Journal of Transplantation*, Vol.5, No.4, (June 2005), pp: 729-738, ISSN: 1600-6143

Reichelt, O; Müller, J & Von Eggeling, F. (2006) .Prediction of renal allograft rejection by urinary protein analysis using ProteinChip Arrays (surface-enhanced laser desorption/ionization time-of-flight mass spectrometry). *Urology*, Vol.67, No.3, (2006), pp.472-485, ISSN: 0090-4295

O'Riordan, E; Orlova, TN & Podust, VN. (2007). Characterization of urinary peptide biomarkers of AR in renal allografts. *American Journal of Transplantation*, Vol.7, No.4, (December 2002), pp.930-40, ISSN: 1600-6143

Jia, X; Gan, C & Xiao, K. (2009). Detection of urinary biomarkers for early diagnosis of acute renal allograft rejection by proteomic analysis. *Proteomics Clinical Applications*, Vol.3, No.6, (December 2008), pp.694-704, ISSN: 1862-8354

Freue, GV; Sasaki, M & Meredith, A. (2010).Proteomic signatures in plasma during early acute renal allograft rejection. *Molcular & Cellular Proteomics*, Vol.9, No.9, (May 2010), pp. 1954-67, ISSN: 1535-9476

Caubet, C; Lacroix, C & Decramer, S. (2010).Advances in urinary proteome analysis and biomarker discovery in pediatric renal disease. *Pediatric Nephrology*, Vol.25, (2009), pp.27-35, ISSN: 0931-041X

Shao, C; Wang, Y & Gao, YH. (2011). Applications of urinary proteomics in biomarker discovery. *Science China Life Sciences*, Vol.54, No.5, (May 2010), pp.409–417, ISSN: 1674-7305

Thongboonkerd, V. (2010). Current status of renal and urinary proteomics: ready for routine clinical application? *Nephrology Dialysis Transplantation*, Vol.25, No.1, (September 2009), pp.11-16, ISSN: 0931-0509

Traum, AZ & Schachter, AD. (2007). Proteomic Analysis in Pediatric Renal Disease. *Seminars Nephrology*, Vol.27, No.6, (December 2007), pp.652-7, ISSN:0270-9295

Thongboonkerd, V. (2008). Renal and Urinary Proteomics: Methods and Protocols. *Proteomics Clinical Applications*, ISBN: 978-3-527-31974-9, USA

Cutillas, PR ; Norden, AGW & Cramer, R. (2004). Urinary proteomics of renal Fanconi syndrome. *Contributions to Nephrology*, Vol.141, (2004), pp. 155–169, ISSN: 0302-5144

Ong, SE & Mann, M. (2005). Mass spectrometry-based proteomics turns quantitative. *Nature Chemical Biology*, Vol.1, No.5, (September 2005), pp.252-262, ISSN:1552-4450

Gygi, SP; Rist, B & Gerber, SA. (1999). Quantitative analysis of complex protein mixtures using isotope-coded affinity tags. *Nature Biotechnology*, Vol.17, No.10, (July 1999), pp.994-999, ISSN: 1087-0156

Neilson, KA; Ali, NA & Muralidharan, S. (2011). Less label, more free: approaches in label-free quantitative mass spectrometry. *Proteomics*, Vol.11, No.4, (January 2011), pp. 535-553, ISSN: 1615-9861

Mayya, V & Han, DK. (2009). Phosphoproteomics by mass spectrometry: insights, implications, applications and limitations. *Expert Review of Molcular Diagnosis*, Vol.9, No.7, (2009), pp.695-707, ISSN: 1473-7159

Li, QR; Fan, KX & Li, RX. (2010). A comprehensive and non-prefractionation on the protein level approach for the human urinary proteome:touching phosphorylation in urine. *Rapid Communications in Mass Spectrometry*, Vol.24, (September 2009), pp. 823–832, ISSN: 1097-0231

Zhou, F; Galan, J& Geahlen, JL. (2007). A Novel Quantitative Proteomics Strategy To Study Phosphorylation-Dependent Peptide Protein Interactions. Journal of Proteome Research. Vol.6, No.1, (November 2006), pp.133-140, ISSN: 1535-3893

Wang, L; Li, F & Sun, W. (2006), Concanavalin A-captured glycoproteins in healthy human urine. *Molecular & Cellular Proteomics.* Vol.5, No.3, (November 2005), pp.560–562, ISSN: 1535-9476

5

Renal Explantation Techniques

Marco Antonio Ayala- García[1,2], Éctor Jaime Ramírez-Barba[3,4,5],
Joel Máximo Soel Encalada[1], Beatriz González Yebra[1,5]
[1]*Hospital Regional de Alta Especialidad del Bajío*
[2]*HGSZ No. 10 del Instituto Mexicano del Seguro Social, Delegación Guanajuato*
[3]*Instituto de Salud Pública del Estado de Guanajuato*
[4]*Secretaria de Salud del Estado de Guanajuato*
[5]*Universidad de Guanajuato*
México

1. Introduction

The demand for kidneys for transplantation has increased significantly in recent years. This increase is, at least in part, due to improvements in therapies that minimize tissue rejection, as well as to more inclusive selection criteria for kidney recipients. The high demand for organs also places challenges on surgeons, requiring them to be familiar with more diverse sources of organ donors. Currently, there are three main sources of kidneys for explantation: cadaveric donors with brain death, non-heart-beating donors, and live donors.

Kidney explantation from a cadaveric donor with brain death can be performed following one of two main approaches: 1) multi-organ explantation using the classic technique or with total abdominal evisceration, or 2) by explanting the kidneys only.

In renal explantation from non-heart-beating donors two techniques can be applied: *in situ* perfusion or cooling of the body with cardiopulmonary bypass.

To obtain a kidney from a live donor, either traditional open surgery or laparoscopy is performed. The latter can be carried out in a transperitoneal or retroperitoneal fashion, with endless variations that take advantage of recent technological improvements.

Surgical transplantation teams within medical institutions should be capable of performing renal explantation from both cadaveric and live donors, and should have in place organizational strategies that are most appropriate for each particular case, complying with the following:

1. Simplicity; the procedures should be easy to perform.
2. Effectiveness; the procedures should best preserve the integrity of the organs.
3. Efficiency; the procedures are carried out using only those resources that are strictly necessary.

This chapter describes each one of the renal explantation techniques, as well as the back-table procedures, i.e. preparation of the renal graft after explantation for further implantation of the organ in the recipient.

2. Renal explantation from cadaveric donor with brain death

Renal explantation from a cadaveric donor with brain death may be performed during multi-organ extraction using the traditional technique or with total abdominal evisceration. Modifications to these techniques, such as quick removal or combined liver-pancreas explantation do exist, but their detailed description is beyond the scope of this chapter.

Exclusive renal explantation from a cadaveric donor with brain death can also be performed, if necessary, when limitations exist due to special circumstances, including:

1. The quality of the facilities available
2. The specific guidelines of different organ transplant programs.
3. The viability of other organs in the cadaveric donor.
4. The need for further approval procedures for the removal of certain organs.

All surgical organ explantation procedures on cadaver must meet the following basic principles:

1. Adequate exploration and dissection to detect anomalies.
2. Cannulation and perfusion with preservation fluids *in situ.*
3. Extraction without damage to organs and with unscathed vascular pedicles.

2.1 Classic multi-organ explantation

This technique was described in 1984 by Starzl, and is based on the dissection of all of the organ vascular pedicles, prior to their perfusion, such that explantation takes place shortly after perfusion. In general, this technique is carried out by independent surgical teams, with one team per organ. It is essential that all surgeons adhere to the pre-approved procedures, with the following order of participation:

Cardiac Surgery Team
Lung Surgery Team
Liver Surgery Team
Pancreatic Surgery Team
Renal Surgery Team
Corneal Team
Musculoskeletal Team

2.1.1 Description of the classical multi-organ extraction technique

The donor is placed in the supine position with arms in forced abduction. A nasogastric tube and a Foley catheter in urethra are placed. Body hair shaving and antisepsis are performed from chin to mid-thigh. Sterile drapes are placed, and two suction devices are installed, one for the thoracic phase and a second one for the abdominal phase. Six thousand (6000) cc of preservation fluid should be available, at a temperature of 0 to 4 $^{\circ}$ C, as well as sterile crushed ice. The cardiac or hepatic team starts the surgery by performing a sternotomy and an incision from the xiphoid process to the pubis, with or without bilateral subcostal extension (Fig. 1), allowing access to all thoracic and abdominal organs. After opening the peritoneum, the round ligament is transected and ligated, and the falciform ligament is sectioned with electrocautery until the origin of the right and left triangular ligaments is reached.

In the thoracic phase, a perfect hemostasis of the sternal branches should be accomplished when performing the sternotomy. A Finochietto sternal retractor is put in place before sectioning both pleurae vertically. A short right and left frenectomy improves thoracic and abdominal removal. This is done with electric scalpel, while the lung, pericardium and liver are protected by the hands of the assistant. The opening of the pleura is useful for correction of a possible hypoventilation.

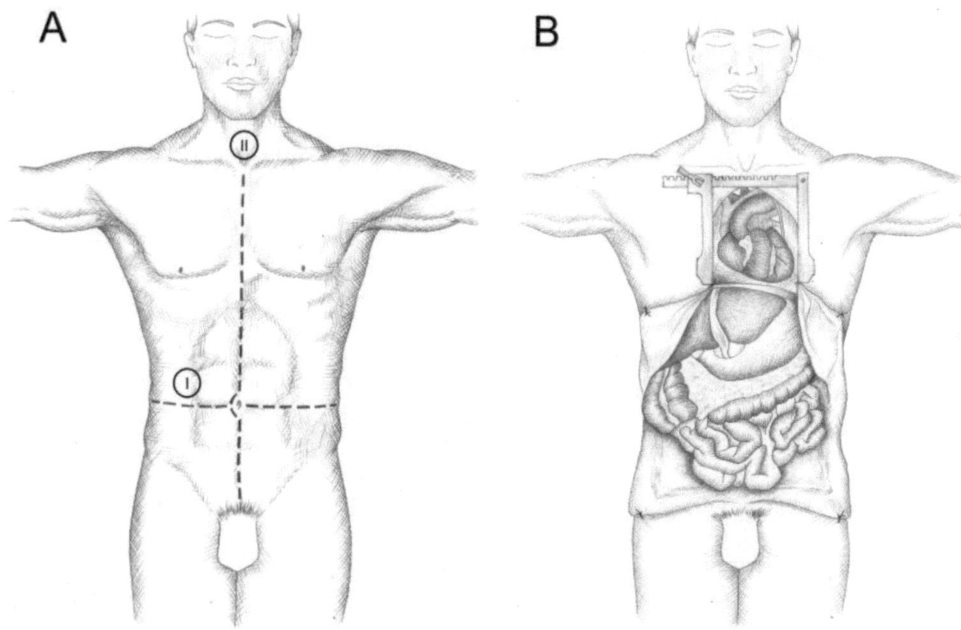

Fig. 1. (A) Sternotomy and midline laparotomy with (I) or without (II) bilateral subcostal extension. (B) Exposure of the thoracoabdominal organs.

The cardiac team opens the pericardium and inspects the heart for vascular or contractility abnormalities. If the organ is deemed adequate for transplantation the team informs the transplant coordinator, such that logistic arrangements related to transplantation procedures can be followed.

The hepatic team inspects the liver, assessing its consistency, color, presence of trauma or other pathology, and the presence of possible vascular abnormalities, especially arterial abnormalities. When applying digital pressure on the parenchyma, a healthy liver rapidly regains its color; when this does not happen, a biopsy will be needed to evaluate steatosis. Injury in more than 60% of the hepatocytes indicates a greatly increased risk of primary dysfunction of the organ, and thus it is rejected for explantation. If after performing this inspection the liver is considered viable for transplantation, the procedure continues and the transplant coordinator is informed. The ascending colon is greatly mobilized by sectioning the right parietocolic and a Kocher maneuver is performed to access the abdominal aorta and inferior vena cava, both of which are dissected and controlled with a thick ligation on their caudal origins (Fig. 2). The inferior mesenteric artery is tied and sectioned.

The pancreatic team sections the gastrocolic ligament and obtains hemostasis by successive ligations, from the right to the left colic flexures, along the greater curvature of the stomach. To the left this maneuver is continued with section of the gastrosplenic ligament and of the short vessels. This allows uncovering of the omentum and exposure of the tail of the pancreas, which can be explored. A normal pancreas has a yellow-orange coloration, is flexible and presents little or no edema. A significant peripancreatic edema that dissects the glandular lobes points to an initial acute pancreatitis, which rules out the explantation of the pancreas. After hanging down the right and left colonic flexures, the vascular pedicles of the mesocolon are dissected and sectioned at their origin, between two ligatures. This maneuver allows the lowering of the colonic frame and exposure of the entire pancreas (Fig. 3).

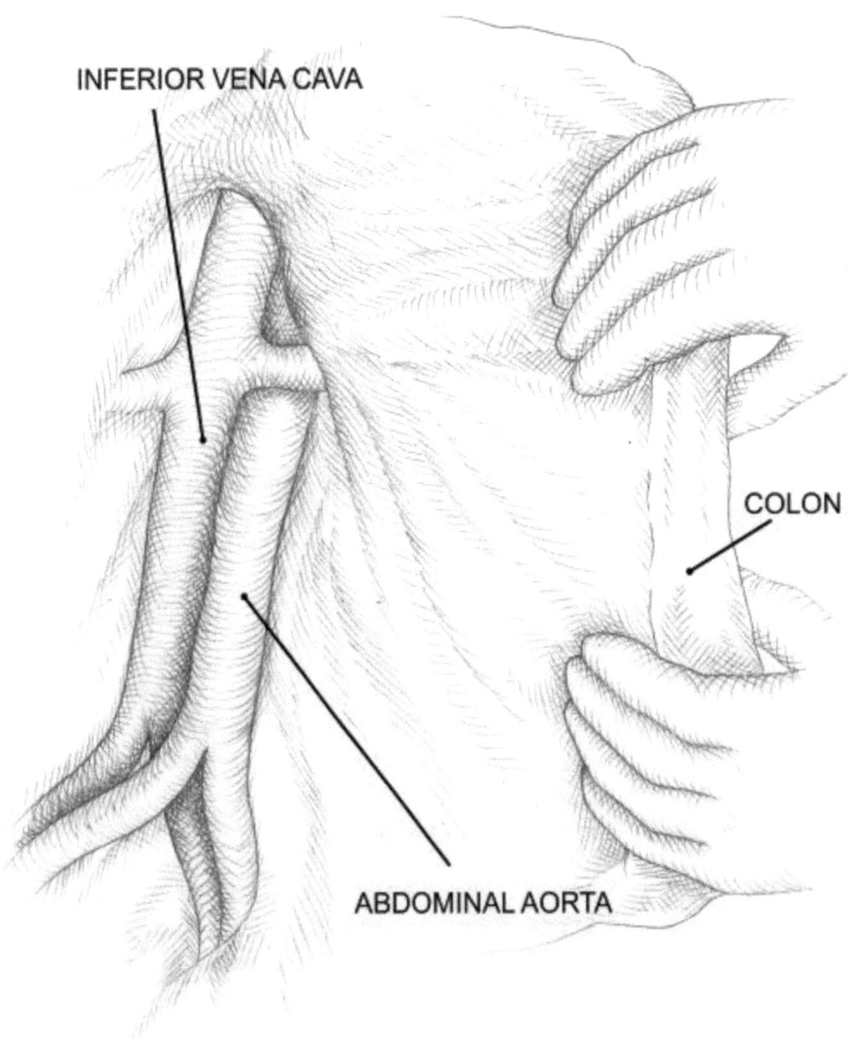

Fig. 2. Kocher maneuver, access to the abdominal aorta and inferior vena cava.

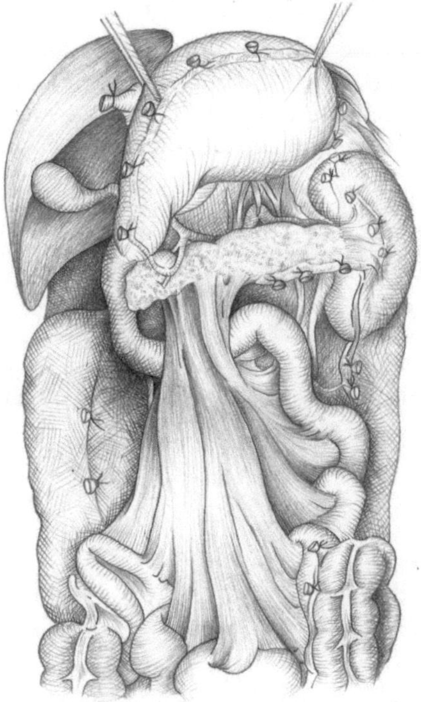

Fig. 3. Downward displacement of the colon, exposing all of the subdiaphragmatic organs.

The hepatic team intervenes further; it identifies and dissects the superior mesenteric artery from its aortic origin to about 3-4 cm distally, to check for the possible presence of an anomalous right hepatic artery. The elements of the hepatic hilum are dissected and the left gastric artery is dissected in search of a left hepatic artery. The left triangular ligament is transected with electrocautery and the left lobe of the liver is moved to the right. A dissection of the supraceliac abdominal aorta is performed, sectioning the right crus of the diaphragm. Once it has been surrounded, the aorta is controlled with a tourniquet, for its subsequent clamping. The gallbladder is opened and rinsed with saline solution.

After the dissection of all of the vascular elements described above, heparinization of the cadaver takes place, by the administration of 300 U/kg of intravenous heparin. Cannulation of the inferior mesenteric vein is performed just below the inferior edge of the pancreas, at about 2 cm, using a probe of 18 to 20 Frens. The end of this probe is placed at the origin of the portal vein, firmly fixing it to the vein above and below its point of entry. Cannulation of the abdominal aorta is performed just above the iliac bifurcation, with a 24 Frens probe in adults and a 16 Frens probe in children. Similarly, cannulation of the vena cava is performed, to allow for venous drainage, thus preventing edema of various organs and facilitating their cooling.

The cardiac team simultaneously cannulates the ascending aorta and the pulmonary artery, through cardioplegia and pulmoplegia needles, respectively. The cardiac team then clamps the thoracic aorta, while the supraceliac aorta is clamped by the hepatic team. The perfusion of the abdominal organs is initiated by means of the cannulas located in the aorta and inferior mesenteric vein, while the cardioplegic perfusion starts through the ascending aorta, and the pulmoplegic perfusion through the pulmonary artery (Fig. 4). Six thousand (6000) cc of preserving solution is commonly used: 1000 cc in the ascending aorta, 1000 cc in the pulmonary artery, 2000 cc in the abdominal aorta, and 2000 cc in the inferior mesenteric vein.

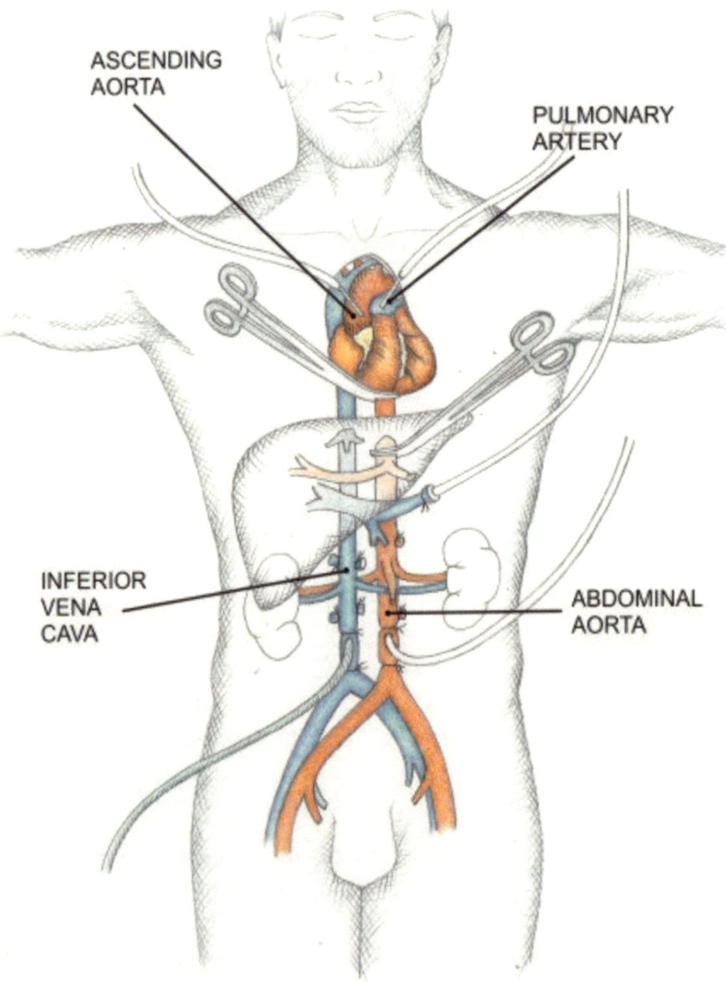

Fig. 4. In situ hypothermic perfusion.

At this point the mechanical ventilator is disconnected from the endotracheal tube. Once the thoracic aorta is occluded, the decompression of the heart chambers is performed via the inferior vena cava, by partially severing the left atrial appendage. The lack of a "universal" preservation solution makes it necessary to separate the cooling territories of heart, lungs and abdominal organs. The thoracic and abdominal cavities are simultaneously irrigated with crushed ice to further accelerate the cooling.

The cardiac team removes the heart, severing the pulmonary veins, the superior and inferior vena cava, the aorta, and the pulmonary arteries. Special care should be taken with the section of the pulmonary artery, as there should be enough tissue left in both the lung and heart grafts.

The pulmonary team sections the pericardium up to the pulmonary hilum, leaving wide margins. The trachea is clamped as proximally as possible, and a staple line is placed above the 5th tracheal ring (6-8 cm). The trachea is then sectioned between the clamp and the staple line. The triangular ligaments are severed on both hemithorax, as well as the posterior mediastinal soft tissue, allowing the explantation of the lungs as a block.

After removing the heart and lungs, the hepatic team waits until the liver is adequately perfused. This is apparent by the discoloration of the organ, and should take approximately 10 to 15 minutes. The removal of the liver depends intimately on that of the pancreas, because the arteries of these organs originate from a common celiac trunk. Additionally, when a right hepatic artery originates from the superior mesenteric artery, the latter is also a common origin for both hepatic and pancreatic vessels. The issue that arises is whether the celiac trunk should accompany the liver or the pancreas. It all depends on the distribution of the arteries of the liver. If one right and one left hepatic arteries do exist, taking the celiac trunk with the liver may allow taking of the gastrohepatic trunk to the potential implantation site for the right hepatic artery (gastroduodenal stump or splenic ostium).

The gastroduodenal artery and the common bile duct are transected at the level of the duodenum, so that the portal vein is exposed. The perfusion of the inferior mesenteric vein is stopped, the cannula is withdrawn and the vein is tied along the bottom edge of the pancreas. The portal vein is transected. If the celiac trunk accompanies the liver, the aorta is transected between the origin of the celiac trunk and the superior mesenteric artery; the axis of the section should be very oblique, upwards and backwards, to avoid the risk of injury to a renal artery. The infrahepatic vena cava is transected just above the confluency of the renal veins. The right diaphragm and retrocaval tissue are sectioned, which exposes the whole liver and allows its extraction.

The pancreatic team rejoins the surgical field and transects the duodenum between two rows of surgical staples (TA55) immediately below the pylorus and then at the angle of Treitz. The superior mesenteric pedicle is tied and severed at the bottom edge of the third duodenal portion. The origin of the superior mesenteric artery is freed from its lymphatic surroundings and is meticulously tied because it can be the source of considerable lymphatic leakage on the revascularized graft. The superior mesenteric artery is sectioned at the level of the aorta, becoming free of the pancreas.

Once the heart, lungs, liver and pancreas are explanted from the cadaver, the renal team gets involved. The perfusion of preservation solution to the kidneys can be maintained throughout the previous phase, to avoid heating and thereby injury. Both ureters are dissected and sectioned at their distal end, close to the bladder. The aorta and inferior vena cava are sectioned distally to the insertion of the perfusion cannulas. All lumbar vessels and retroaortic tissue are sectioned in a cranial direction. Finally, the adhesions of the kidneys to the retroperitoneum are sectioned. This fully releases the kidneys, which can then be extracted for subsequent packaging in preservation solution and back-table preparation.

After all useful organs have been explanted, the following tissues are also recovered: iliac vessels that may be needed for vascular reconstruction of both the liver and kidneys, and spleen material for Human Leukocyte Antigen (HLA) system studies. At this time the corneal team intervenes, and finally the musculoskeletal team. At some facilities skin is also removed, and this is the last explantation procedure to be performed.

The reconstruction of the cadaver must be very careful. This step is as important as any of the above, as it is essential to preserve the dignity and integrity of the cadaver (Fig. 5). This procedure should allow delivering of the body of the donor in the following fashion: 1) all incisions performed for the removal of organs and tissues should be sutured, 2) no tubes or catheters should remain, 3) the body should be clean, with particular care in removing all blood stains, 4) the eyes should be closed, 5) limbs from where skeletal or muscle tissue was explanted should be properly covered, 6) a sign should be placed indicating whether skeletal or muscle tissue was obtained, and that prostheses were placed accordingly, 7) the body should be covered with a sheet or placed inside a bag.

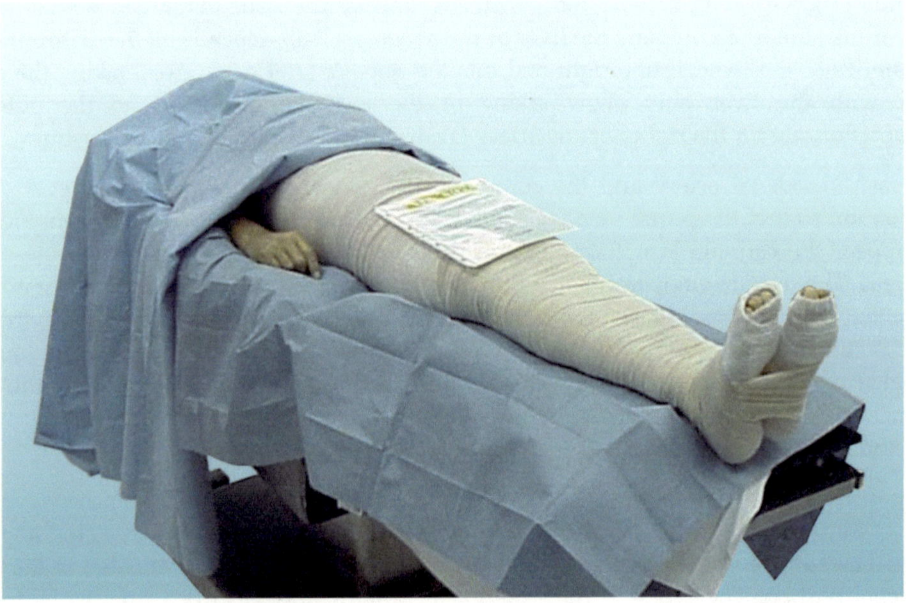

Fig. 5. Dignity of the cadaver.

2.2 Total abdominal evisceration

Developed by Nakazato in 1992, this technique is based on the minimal possible manipulation of the donor body, which is limited to the insertion of cannulas for infusion of preservation fluids. The organs are then dissected out and most of the surgical procedures on the organs are performed at the bench "*ex vivo*". Two surgical teams are involved in this method, a thoracic team and an abdominal team, and they each operate in two distinct phases: the dissection of the corpse and the dissection of organs *ex vivo*.

2.2.1 Dissection on the cadaver

The donor is placed in the supine position as in the classical technique, catheters are placed and antisepsis and shaving are performed. With preservation fluid and sterile crushed ice available, a sternotomy and midline laparotomy are performed with bilateral subcostal extension (Fig. 1). Both the thoracic and abdominal organs are approached and inspected, and their potential viability or any contraindications are communicated.

Once the decision to proceed has been made both the thoracic and abdominal teams work simultaneously. The thoracic team performs the opening of the pericardium, dissection of large vessels, and identification of ascending aorta and pulmonary artery, if lung explantation is going to be performed. The abdominal team identifies the superior mesenteric vein at the root of the mesocolon, identifies the infrarenal aorta just above the origin of the iliac arteries and dissects the descending thoracic aorta before widely opening the left diaphragm. At this level the aorta is covered by only the pleura and has no branches. Once these maneuvers have been performed, which should take approximately 15 to 30 minutes, heparin is administered intravenously at a dose of 300 U/kg. The perfusion cannulas are then put in place.

In the thorax, the cardioplegic cannula is inserted into the aortic root. When the lungs are to be removed, the insertion of the cannula is performed at the level of the pulmonary artery. In the abdomen, the insertion of the cannula (18 to 20 Frens in adults, 14 to 16 Frens in children) is performed at the level of the inferior mesenteric vein. There is also insertion of a cannula into the distal aorta (20 to 24 Frens for adults and 14 to 16 Frens for children). Also, the inferior vena cava is cannulated for venous drainage.

After performing the maneuvers described above both teams are ready to start the infusion and coordinated extraction of the respective organs, in the following order: First, simultaneous clamping of thoracic and abdominal aorta, and establishment of large venous drainage through the cannula placed in the vena cava, with sectioning of the infracardiac vena cava. Perfusion of the preservation fluids is started, at the following ratios: 1000 cc for the heart, 1000 cc for the lung, and 4000 cc for the abdomen. After the organs have been perfused, the removal of the heart and lungs is performed, just as in the classical technique. In the abdomen all of the mesocolon is sectioned, and the colon is mobilized. The jejunum is transected at the level of the ligament of Treitz with a stapling device (GIA™ or PLC™) and the small intestine mesentery is sectioned, after which the small bowel and colon are externalized from the abdomen. Both ureters are identified and distally sectioned. The left diaphragm insertion and left parietocolic are transected. The stomach, spleen, pancreas and left kidney are moved toward the midline. The right diaphragm insertion and right parietocolic are then transected, following mobilization toward the midline of the liver, pancreas and right kidney. The distal thoracic esophagus is identified and sectioned with a stapling device and the thoracic aorta is transected just above the clamp placed at that level, which remains in the closed position to allow the continuous perfusion of the abdominal organs. The posterior diaphragm and all retroperitoneal tissue posterior to the aorta are then sectioned. The infrarenal aorta and vena cava are sectioned distally to the insertion site of the perfusion cannula.

The organ complex consisting of the liver, stomach, duodenum-pancreas-spleen, and kidneys is introduced into a pan with saline solution and crushed ice. The explantation is now completed, and as in the classical technique, additional tissues are recovered and the final preparation of the corpse is secured. This explantation technique takes about 15 to 30 minutes, such that the overall duration of surgical procedures in the donor will be no longer than 45 to 60 minutes. This relatively short time significantly simplifies logistics and makes total abdominal evisceration particularly advisable in cases where the maintenance of the donor body is complicated.

2.2.2 Dissection *ex vivo*

2.2.2.1 Separation of renal block

The abdominal specimen is dissected from its posterior face. The aorta is sectioned throughout its entire length, thereby identifying the origins of all visceral arteries and their possible anomalies. The anterior side of the aorta is sectioned between the orifices of the renal arteries and superior mesenteric artery. The hepatorenal ligament is sectioned, followed by identification of the infrahepatic vena cava, which is sectioned just above the outlet of the renal vessels. The pancreatorenal ligament is transected. The kidneys are then ready for back-table surgery.

2.2.2.2 Separation of the liver from the pancreas-duodenum-spleen complex

The superior mesenteric artery is identified and dissected to check for the presence of a right hepatic artery which, if present, is preserved as part of the hepatic specimen. The celiac trunk is identified and dissected, after which the splenic and left gastric arteries are identified and sectioned, provided that there are no anomalies in the left hepatic artery. The specimen is turned over, in order to dissect it by its anterior or ventral face. When the pancreas is to be explanted, the common bile duct, gastroduodenal artery and portal vein are distally sectioned from right to left, just above the outlet of the coronary vein. Otherwise, the sectioning is performed at the junction with the superior mesenteric vein. The stomach is separated by cutting the gastrohepatic ligament, and the duodenum is sectioned with a stapling device when the pancreas is to be explanted. Otherwise, the liver can be separated from the rest of the specimen at this point.

2.3 Exclusive renal explantation from cadaveric donor

This technique follows the principles of the classical multi-organ explantation described by Starzl, and kidney transplant surgeons are invariably well versed in this approach. It is used when limitations are imposed on the surgical team by outside factors, such as the hospital, the specific organ transplantation programs that may be active in the facility, the quality of the other organs in the donor, or the unavailability of the authorizations necessary to explant organs other than the kidneys.

2.3.1 Description of the exclusively renal explantation technique

The cadaveric donor is placed on the operating table in the supine position, with the arms in forced abduction, and a Foley catheter is placed in the urethra. Shaving and antisepsis of the abdominal wall is performed, sterile fields are placed and the abdominal cavity is accessed by means of a medial xifopubic laparotomy with bilateral subcostal extension. The right colon is greatly mobilized by cutting the right parietocolic, and a Kocher maneuver is performed, the small bowel is mobilized superiorly until it is only held together by the mesenteric vessels. Following these maneuvers the abdominal aorta and inferior vena cava can be accessed, dissected, and controlled with a thick ligature in its caudal origins (Fig. 2). The inferior mesenteric artery is ligated and sectioned. The right kidney is identified and is freed from the fascia of Gerota. The same dissection is done with the left kidney, ending with the creation of a window on the left sided colonic mesentery. At this point there is no attempt to identify and dissect the renal arteries or veins. The hilum is left untouched.

During this dissection, the surgeons look for several anomalies that might be present, such as:

1. Congenital malformations and anatomical variations of the kidneys, such as horseshoe kidney.
2. Iliac arterial branches to the lower kidney poles.
3. Precava branches of the lower pole of right kidney.
4. Postaortic left renal vein.

The superior mesenteric artery is sectioned. The lymph nodes near the stump of the superior mesenteric artery are sectioned in order to place the vascular clamp 1 cm above the origin of said artery. The hepatic hilum is dissected and the portal vein is ligated. The donor is heparinized intravenously at a dose of 300 U/kg. The aorta and the cava are ligated distally and are proximally cannulated, and the perfusion of preservation fluids through the aorta is started. The aorta is clamped above the superior mesenteric artery, while the drainage of blood is allowed from the cannula in the abdominal vena cava. It is often necessary to open the diaphragm and cut the infracardiac vena cava, allowing abundant venous drainage. As a consequence of this maneuver blood contaminates the abdominal cavity, and thus constant suction will be required within the cavity. Should it be desirable to keep blood away from the abdominal cavity, a sternotomy could be performed as part of the initial approach (Fig. 1), thus preserving the integrity of the diaphragm and restricting blood to the thoracic cavity, where constant suction with two sets of aspiration equipment should be ensured. The abdominal cavity is irrigated with crushed ice prepared with normal saline to further accelerate cooling, while 4 liters of preservation solution is infused through the aorta (Fig. 6). Subsequently the ureters are clipped in their more distal portion using Kelly forceps, near the bladder, are cut at this level, and dissected in the distal to proximal direction. The abdominal aorta and inferior vena cava are sectioned, above the site of their initial ligation, and are sectioned below the diaphragm. The complete specimen including aorta and vena cava is extracted, together with the kidneys and ureters. The iliac vessels are removed, as they may be required for vascular reconstructions, and splenic tissue is obtained for studies of the HLA system. Everything is placed in cold solution with crushed ice. The specimen consisting of both kidneys will subsequently be subjected to back-table surgery. The abdominal cavity is then sutured, and the cadaver is left clean, removing any catheters and tubes. The corpse is treated as described previously.

3. Renal explantation from non-heart-beating donor

In recent years, the possibility of obtaining organs for transplantation from donors in asystole has been reconsidered. Following the work of García-Rinaldi in 1975, *in situ* perfusion of cadaveric kidneys by cold infusion made directly through a catheter via the femoral artery into the aorta has successfully been applied. This approach has allowed a significant reduction in the time of warm ischemia, thus overcoming the main limitation of non-heart-beating donors, i.e. the poor preservation of the organs, which are often subjected to long periods of warm ischemia. "Warm ischemic time" is defined as the time elapsed from the moment of circulatory arrest until the cooling of the organ, and includes the time elapsed both with and without effective cardiopulmonary resuscitation maneuvers. In contrast, "cold ischemic time" involves the time elapsed from the moment of cold perfusion until revascularization is achieved, once the organ is implanted in the recipient.

Following García-Rinaldi, many authors have implemented these methods with good results, and the inclusion of this group of donors in organ procurement programs is increasingly being recommended. Other variations to this protocol have also emerged, such as that of Koyama, who has used body hypothermia by cardiopulmonary bypass with good results in non-heart-beating donors.

The sources of non-heart-beating donors are diverse, and after the Maastricht workshop in 1995 four categories have been defined:

Category 1: Donors that reach the hospital as cadavers (after traffic accidents or other causes, patients have cardiac arrest during transport to the hospital, without application of cardiopulmonary resuscitation maneuvers. These donors are considered cadavers upon arrival to the hospital).

Category 2: Recipients of ineffective cardiopulmonary resuscitation (CPR, includes most non-heart-beating donors, and can originate from within the hospital or from outside sources).

Category 3: Donors where cardiac arrest is expected (patients with irreversible brain damage, but that do not meet the criteria for brain death donors. The donors are taken to the operating room, where the life support measures are interrupted, and cardiac arrest is expected). This group raises many ethical considerations and is not accepted in many countries.

Category 4: Donors with brain death that are part of organ donation programs, and who suffer cardiac arrest in the course of the diagnostic procedures or while awaiting for explantation equipment to become available.

3.1 Selection criteria for donors

Selection criteria for potential non-heart-beating organ donors include:

1. Age between 7 and 55.
2. Cause of death should be known or suspected, ruling out those donors who have died as a consequence of personal violent acts (due to potential interference with judicial investigations)
3. Thoracic or abdominal injuries with massive bleeding should be absent
4. Ischemic time without effective CPR of less than 30 minutes.
5. Ischemic time with effective CPR of up to 2 hours.
6. A total warm ischemic time, including the time with and without cardiopulmonary resuscitation maneuvers, of up to 2 and a half hours.
7. The criteria applicable to donors with brain death

3.2 Initial procedures

The procedure for removal of organs from non-heart-beating donors begins after the diagnosis of death by the medical team that has treated the patient, at which point the cadaver is considered as a potential donor. At this point it is necessary to accurately assess the length of warm ischemia suffered by the organs, from the time of cardiac arrest until the beginning of cardiopulmonary resuscitation, and from the beginning of these maneuvers until the onset of cold recirculation. Initially, mechanical ventilation and cardiac massage on the body is continued, in order to maintain the best possible perfusion of the organs, and the heparinization of the donor begins (300 U/kg body weight). Simultaneously, blood samples are obtained to perform laboratory measurements, with emphasis on the plasma serology information that will be necessary for the selection of the recipient. Some authors (Booster MH et al, 1993) recommend the use of phentolamine (0.125 mg/kg) to induce vasodilatation of the renal vessels prior to the infusion, and thus facilitate the rapid decrease in temperature. The femoral artery and vein are catheterized by surgical dissection and cold perfusion of organs is started. Some groups (González MM et al, 1994; Szostek M et al, 1995) have reported good results using mechanical ventilation and cardiac massage for the maintenance of the donor until the moment of explantation.

3.3 Techniques for perfusion *in situ*

Renal perfusion was traditionally achieved by gravity, with perfusion of cold preservation solution through the femoral artery (*in situ* perfusion), and exsanguination via the femoral vein. García Rinaldi et al. used a catheter with a double balloon and triple lumen, placed in the aorta via the femoral artery, thus achieving isolation of renal circulation. Surface cooling of the kidneys has been added to this methodology, by continuous hypothermic peritoneal infusion, which reduces the temperature in the kidney and protects renal microvasculature in case of ineffective cold perfusion. This is especially important in cases when perfusion lasts a relatively long time. Improvements have also been made by adding pressure to the preservation fluid. Anaise has shown that when 70 mmHg of pressure is used, the drop in temperature is faster and more effective (up to 15 degrees Celsius in 5 minutes). Lower pressure would increase the release of renin-angiotensin, which could cause an increase in renal vascular resistance, thus promoting a decrease in renal blood flow and poor hypothermia.

3.4 Body cooling with cardiopulmonary bypass

In this procedure, cannulation of the femoral artery and vein is performed, allowing connection to an extracorporeal circulation system with a membrane oxygenator and heat exchanger (Fig. 6). A Fogarty balloon is placed through the contralateral femoral artery to interrupt blood flow above the level of the superior mesenteric artery. This prevents the flow of blood from the donor and of preservation solution above this level, ensuring a temperature differential between both chambers. Priming and premedication of the extracorporeal circulation system is achieved with 2 g fosfomycin, 8 mg pancuronium, 300 mg hydrocortisone, 2000 cc of Ringer-Lactate, 500 cc hydroxyethyl starch, 200 cc of molar bicarbonate serum, and 30,000 U of heparin.

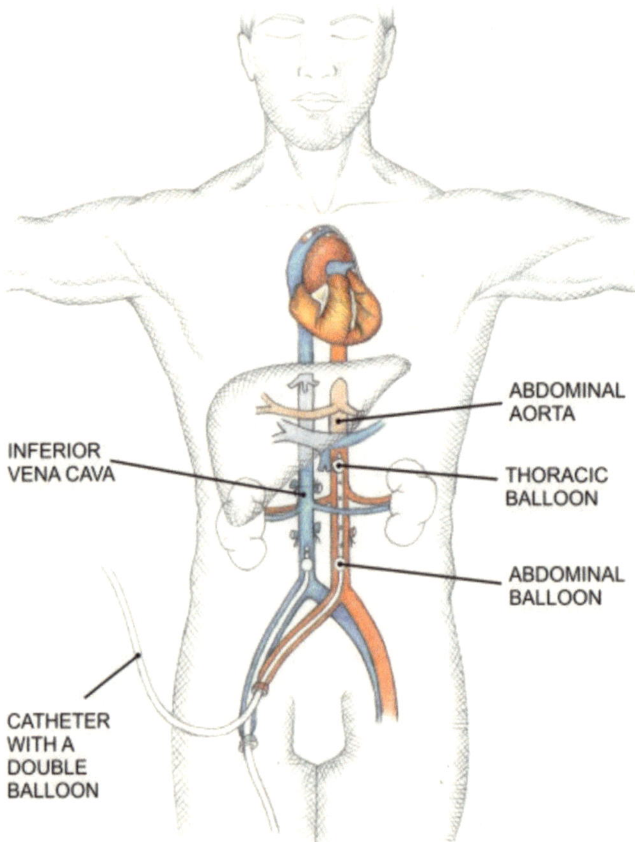

Fig. 6. Cannulation of the femoral artery and vein in the non-heart-beating donor.

The main difference between the *in situ* perfusion technique and body cooling with cardiopulmonary bypass is that in the latter the blood volume of the donor is maintained, without exsanguination. This ensures the reversibility of the process, and therefore its universal applicability, including in cases where it is necessary to wait for further authorization before confirming the deceased as an organ donor. In the two techniques used (*in situ* perfusion and body cooling with cardiopulmonary bypass), the donor is transferred to the operating room after obtaining court approval, and the kidney explantation is performed and, where appropriate, that of the liver and other tissues. The techniques used are the same previously described in this chapter for brain-dead cadaver donors.

3.5 Final procedures

More so than for other types of donor, in the non-heart-beating donor, the assessment of organ viability is crucial. This is achieved through macroscopic examination, and through biopsies. Biochemical determinations after death will provide very little guidance regarding kidney function, due to post-mortem cytolysis. Research in this area is currently focused on the metabolism of adenine nucleotides. Through these studies, the correlation between cellular energy status (adenine nucleotides) and post-transplant functionality has been established, both in renal and hepatic transplants obtained from non-heart-beating donors.

4. Explantation of kidneys from living donors

Because of the large numbers of patients awaiting kidneys worldwide, public health systems have invested more effort in promoting donation from living individuals. One of the factors that traditionally have discouraged potential living donors is the need to undergo an open nephrectomy, which can cause significant pain and scarring. Open nephrectomy was the first to be applied to living donors, starting in the mid twentieth century.

The advent of laparoscopic procedures in almost all branches of surgery, including urology, opened new possibilities for increasing the number of living kidney donors. Patients are able to return to work sooner, suffer less pain, and find the minimal scarring more aesthetically acceptable. In 1991 Clayman et al. introduced the use of laparoscopic urological procedures for curative nephrectomy. Later, in 1995, Ratner et al. described laparoscopic nephrectomy, initially transperitoneal, for the purposes of transplantation. Also in 1995 Yang et al. published the retroperitoneal procedure, and thereafter a host of variations to these techniques have emerged, increasingly taking advantage of the significant technological advances in surgery. The currently used surgical techniques for kidney explantation from living donors are described below.

4.1 Open nephrectomy with classic lumbar sectioning

This technique is safe for the donor and for the kidney graft, and is used as the "gold standard" for the evaluation of new techniques. The live donor is placed in the lateral position, and the operating table is flexed at the level of the umbilicus to achieve complete flank exposure (Fig. 7). A 15 to 20 cm incision is made on the flank below the 12th rib, and a retroperitoneal dissection is performed. After ligation of the renal vessels the kidney can be removed and placed in cold preservation solution, so that back-table surgery can be performed. This procedure allows for a very short time of warm ischemia. The main disadvantages of this approach are related to the significant surgical wounding of the abdominal wall, which causes pain, prolonged hospital stays, poor aesthetics of the wound, and a slow convalescence.

4.2 Minimally invasive open donor nephrectomy

After the introduction of the laparoscopic donor nephrectomy, there was increasing interest in developing a minimally invasive modification of the classical open donor nephrectomy, and subsequently the muscle-sparing mini-incision donor nephrectomy was developed. This operation can be performed via an anterior, flank or posterior approach with an incision of approximately 7 cm. With the donor placed in a lateral decubitus position and the operation table maximally flexed, a horizontal skin incision is made anterior to the 11th rib toward the umbilicus. The fascia and muscles of the abdominal wall are carefully split between the muscle fibres avoiding harm to the intercostal nerves between the internal oblique and transverse abdominal muscles. The peritoneum is displaced medially and Gerota's fascia is opened on the lateral side of the kidney. The working space is limited, therefore long instruments are used. The kidney is meticulously dissected and arterial and venous structures are identified. After dissection, the ureter is divided and sutured distally. The renal artery and vein are clamped and ligated. This approach provides the safety of the conventional open technique. This minimally invasive open donor nephrectomy results in reduced blood loss, hospital stay and incision-related complications compared with the classical open donor nephrectomy. There is only a marginal increase in operation time without compromising graft and recipient survival.

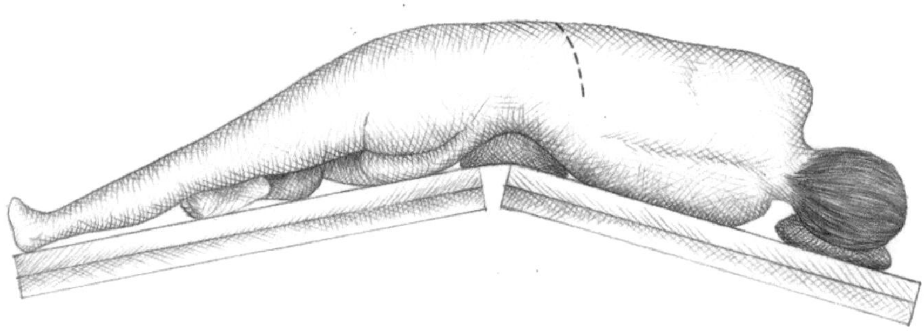

Fig. 7. Living donor position in the open nephrectomy.

4.3 Laparoscopic nephrectomy

With the donor in the lateral position and the operating table maximally flexed, 4 trocars are inserted in the following fashion (Fig. 8): 1) a 12 mm port at the umbilical level in the midclavicular line, 2) a 10 or 12 mm port at the umbilical level, 3) a 5 mm port between the umbilicus and the xiphoid process, and 4) a 12 mm port, 2 cm away from the symphysis pubis (the wound for this port will be incorporated into the Pfannenstiel incision, through which the kidney will be removed from the abdominal cavity). The abdomen is insufflated to 12 mmHg. The colon is mobilised and displaced medially. Gerota' s fascia is opened and the renal vein and ureter, with sufficient periureteral tissue, are identified and dissected. The renal artery is identified. Branches of the adrenal, gonadal and lumbar veins are clipped and divided. The ureter is clipped distally and divided. Then, a low transverse suprapubic (Pfannenstiel) incision or midline incision is made creating a gate for extraction of the kidney. The renal artery and vein are divided using an endoscopic stapler or clips. The kidney is extracted through the extraction incision, and flushed with preservation fluid and stored on ice. Extraction of the kidney can be performed directly through the incision or by using a special endoscopic specimen retrieval bag.

Disadvantages of this technique include the steep and long learning curve, the risk of bowel injury from trocar insertion or during instrumentation, internal hernias or hernia through trocar sites and intestinal adhesions. Injuries to the lumbar vein, renal artery and aorta, pneumomediastinum, splenic injury, and adrenal/retroperitoneal haematomas have been reported.

Conversion rate from laparoscopic to open surgery is 1.8% (range 0 to 13.3%). Approximately half of the conversions to open surgery are due to bleeding or vascular

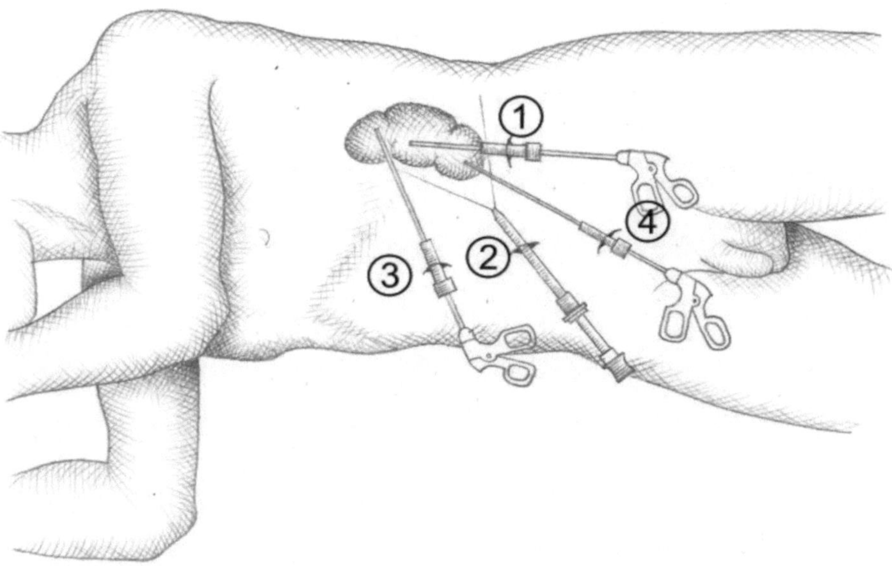

Fig. 8. Living donor position and placement of trocars for laparoscopic nephrectomy.

injury. The laparoscopic technique results in a shorter vascular pedicle when compared with the open donor nephrectomy. The warm ischaemia time and operating time for laparoscopic donor nephrectomy are substantially longer than those achieved in open donor nephrectomy.

4.4 Hand-assisted laparoscopic nephrectomy

This technique incorporates one port for the hand. Hand-assisted laparoscopic donor nephrectomy was first utilized in order to minimize the learning curve of the total laparoscopic donor nephrectomy (Fig. 9). In addition, the hand port provides increased safety to laparoscopic donor nephrectomy, because rapid control of eventual massive blood loss from major blood vessels is possible.

Different incisions for hand introduction have been described, such as a Pfannenstiel incision, a midline supraumbilical, periumbilical, or infraumbilical incision. The hand port can be used partly or totally during the operation.

The hand-assisted laparoscopic donor nephrectomy is done transperitoneally. After open dissection of the distal ureter and gonadal vein through a 7 to 8 cm Pfannenstiel incision the nondominant operator's hand is introduced through a hand port and two trocars are placed. The insufflation pressure is maximally 12 mmHg. The right or left colon is then mobilized. The renal vein and artery are identified and the kidney is mobilized from the surrounding tissue. After transecting the ureter distally, the renal artery is transected with metal clips or an endoscopic stapler which is used to transect the renal vein. The kidney is extracted through the Pfannenstiel incision and flushed and preserved with cold preservation fluid. Potential disadvantages are higher costs because of the hand port, a worse ergonomic

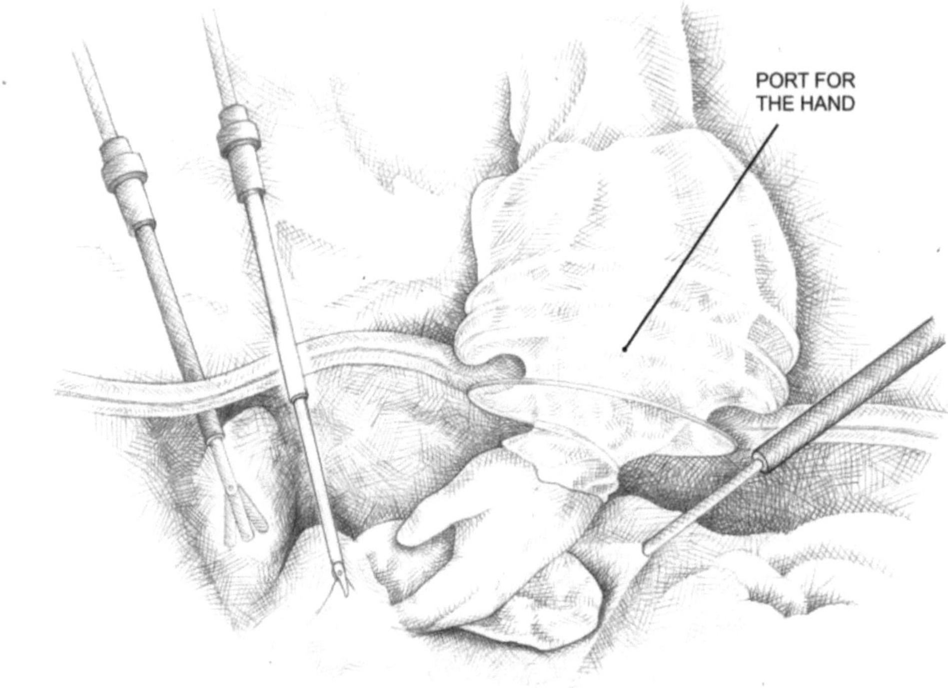

Fig. 9. Hand-assisted laparoscopic donor nephrectomy.

position for the surgeon during operation, a higher rate of wound infections and increased traumatic injury to the transplant as a consequence of manipulation. Conversion to open surgery is 2.97% in the hand-assisted group. The most common causes for conversion to open surgery include intraoperative haemorrhage or vascular injury, difficult kidney exposure or an obese donor, vascular staple malfunction, adhesions and loss of pneumoperitoneum. Potential advantages of hand-assisted laparoscopic donor nephrectomy over conventional laparoscopy include the ability to use tactile feedback, less kidney traction, rapid control of bleeding, fast kidney removal and shorter warm ischaemic periods.

4.5 Laparo-endoscopic single-site (LESS) donor nephrectomy

In this technique a single port is used (Fig. 10). There are two variants, the transperitoneal, which involves a 7 cm periumbilical incision, and the retroperitoneal, which utilizes a 6 cm incision in the groin, below the "bikini line". The instruments and lens for dissection and sectioning of renal hilar vessels and the ureter are introduced through the single port. The same port is later used to remove the kidney.

4.6 Robotic-assisted donor nephrectomy

Robotic-assisted donor nephrectomy can be performed with or without hand assistance. The Da Vinci robotic system has three components: a console, a control tower and the surgical

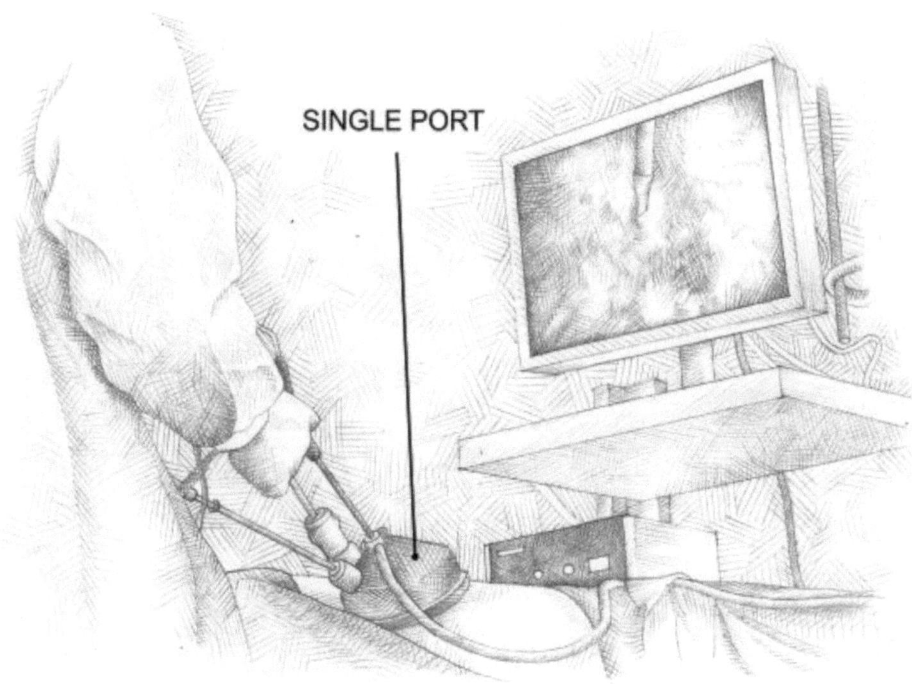

Fig. 10. Laparoendoscopic single-site (LESS) donor nephrectomy.

arm cart (Fig. 11). The donor nephrectomy is performed with the patient placed in a decubitus position. The operating table is flexed to maximize the exposure of the kidney during the procedure. Four trocars are placed in the left or right side of the abdomen to allow placement of three articulated robotic arms, the robotic camera, and the standard laparoscopic instrument used for retraction and dissection during the procedure. The left or right colon is mobilized medially to expose the kidney. Dissection of Gerota' s fascia, perirenal tissue and vascular structures are performed as described above.

The advantage of this technique is that the movement of the articulated arm of the robot reproduces the action of the human wrist, which provides more mobility. A potential disadvantage is the costs.

4.7 Use of natural orifices

An innovative approach to spare the donors of some of the surgical consequences of the donation, and thus increase the pool of living donors, relies on avoiding sectioning of the abdominal wall altogether, by removing the kidney through the vagina. This technique has been used before for the purpose of treating a diseased kidney, and has subsequently been proposed as an option for explantation from living donors. This method represents, at this point, just a preliminary proposal, and several objections have been raised, but it is worth mentioning it as one more possible alternative.

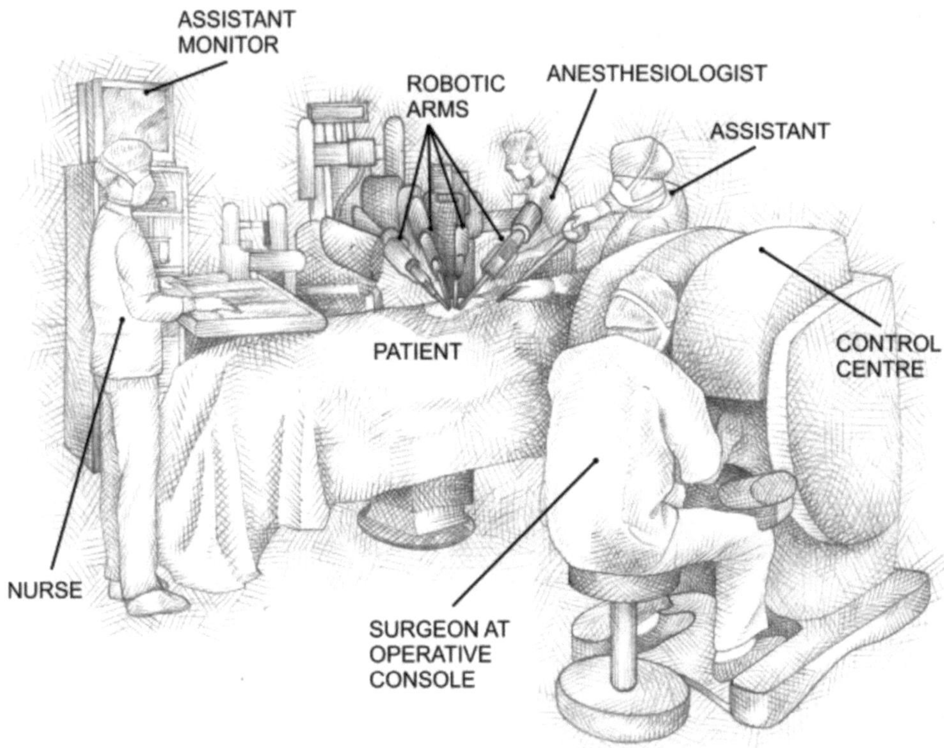

Fig. 11. Da Vinci robotic system.

5. Back-table preparation

The purpose of back-table on the explanted kidney is to examine the organ and prepare, under hypothermic conditions (4 ° C), the vascular ends for the subsequent vascular anastomosis. Perinephric fat is removed, without damaging the renal vessels or ureter. It is best not to dissect close to the hilum. The vessels that do not lead to or from the kidney are ligated. Arterial branches are completely dissected and, before being ligated, lack of flow to the kidney and ureter must be ensured. If the specimen was obtained from a cadaveric donor, it is placed such that its posterior face is visible. The aorta and the vena cava are opened (Fig. 12), the emergence of both renal vessels is identified, and through them, proper perfusion of the kidney with preservation solution is ensured. The emergence of both renal vessels is dissected and separated from the aorta, leaving behind an ample Carrel patch. There is a difference in the length of the vein and the artery in the right kidney (the vein being shorter). Many surgeons use the vena cava to extend the right renal vein, thus compensating for this difference in length, in order to prevent bending of the renal artery after transplantation. An alternative approach used by some surgeons is to cut the artery and perform an end-to-side anastomosis in the transplant, without a Carrel patch. The kidneys are subsequently packaged in sterile plastic bags (doubly bagged), with preservation solution, and then placed on ice for transport or preservation until the time of transplantation.

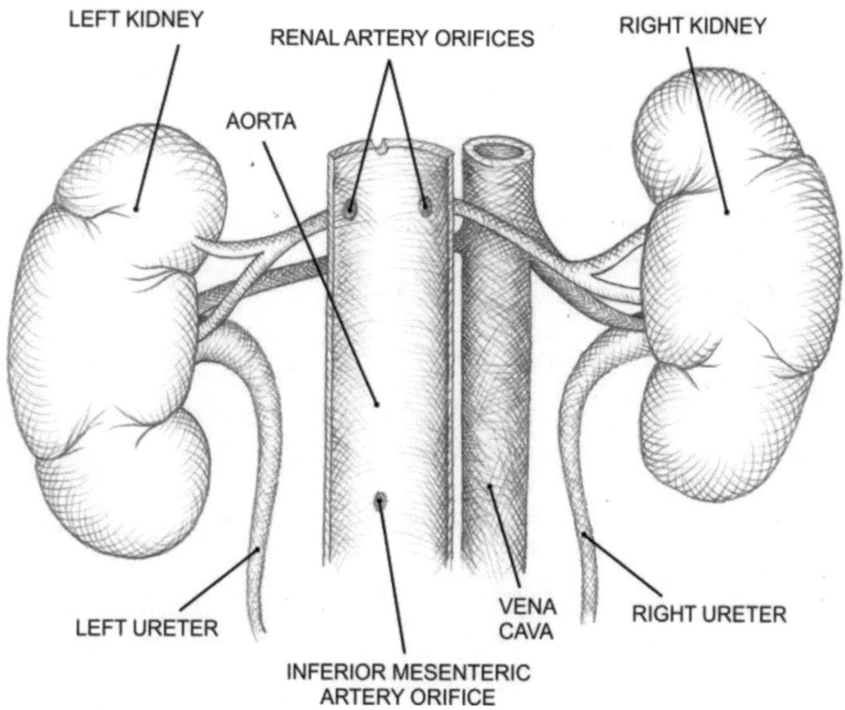

Fig. 12. Posterior view of the kidneys. The aorta is divided in the posterior midline.

6. Conclusions

There are multiple techniques and approaches to renal explantation, whose application will depend on, among other factors:

1. Type of donor.
2. Preferences and experience of the surgical team that will perform the explantation.

Some general guidelines to be considered in choosing the most appropriate renal explantation procedure are shown in Table 2.

Studies that have compared the evolution of transplanted organs and documented the outcomes of both the classical explantation approach and the total abdominal evisceration have found no differences between these two methods.

The kidney-only explantation procedure from cadaveric donor, and the back-table preparation are the two basic techniques that must be mastered by all renal transplant surgeons, because they are the basis on which all other renal explantation techniques for cadaveric donors are based.

Successful kidney explantation from non-heart-beating donors requires perfect organization and coordination between different disciplines, both within and outside the hospital unit, to ensure the quality of the process and therefore the usefulness of the organs procured for transplantation.

TYPE OF DONOR	EXPLANTATION TECHNIQUE	VARIANTS	COMMENTS
Cadaver with brain-death	Classic multi-organ extraction		Requires coordination with different surgical teams.
	Total abdominal evisceration		Indicated when time for extraction is limited (unstable donor)
	Kidney-only extraction		Used when explantation of other organs is not granted
Non-heart-beating donor	Perfusion *in situ*	With or without continuous hypothermic peritoneal perfusion	Requires a perfect organization and coordination between different disciplines inside and outside the hospital
	Body cooling with cardiopulmonary bypass		
Live donor	Open nephrectomy	Classic lumbar opening	The gold standard for evaluation of other kidney explantation techniques from live donors
		Muscle-sparing mini-incision donor nephrectomy	Reduced blood loss, hospital stay and incision-related complications
	Laparoscopy	Laparoscopic nephrectomy	Shortens hospitalization time, requires less analgesia, improves the aesthetics of the wound and ensures quick return to normal activities
		Hand-assisted laparoscopic nephrectomy	There is less kidney traction, better bleeding control, the kidney is removed faster, reduces the warm ischemia and surgical time
		Transperitoneal or retroperitoneal laparo-endoscopic single-site (LESS) donor nephrectomy	Technically complex procedures
		Robotic-assisted donor nephrectomy	High costs
		Use of natural orifices	It would only be applicable to female patients (vaginal route). Risk of infections

Table 2. Techniques for explantation of kidneys for transplantation.

In selecting techniques for kidney explantation from living donors, the following factors are to be considered: operating time, postoperative complications, postoperative pain, warm ischemic time, surgical aesthetics and prognosis of renal function in the recipient.

Any newly proposed approach or technique for renal explantation must:

1. Be technically feasible.
2. Prove to be as safe as the technique that it seeks to replace.
3. Be demonstrably innocuous to the graft and to the recipient.

7. Acknowledgment

We would like to thank Luis Felipe Alemón Soto and Juan José Lozano García for their help in the preparation of this chapter.

8. References

Anaise, D.; Yland, MJ.; Waltzer, WC.; Frischer, Z.; Hurley, S.; Eychmuller, S. & Rapaport, FT. (1969). Flush Pressure requirements for optimal cadaveric donor Kidney preservation. *Transplantation Proceedings*, Vol.20, No.5, (October 1988), pp.891-894, ISSN 0041-1337.

Anaya, R.; Rodríguez, F. & Toledo, L. (1999). Preservación de órganos, In : Introducción al trasplante de órganos y tejidos, Cuervas-Mons V & del Castillo-Olivares JL (Ed.), pp. 107-134, Arán Ediciones S.A., ISBN 84-86725-49-6, Madrid, España

Anaya, F. (1980). Innovaciones tecnológicas en la donación en asistolia. *Nefrologia*, Vol.16, No.2, (February 1996), pp. 96-106, ISSN 0211-6995

Abecassis, M. & Corry, R. (1965). An update on páncreas transplantation. *Advances in surgery*, Vol. 26, No. 1 (September 1993), pp. 163-188, ISSN 0065-3411

Allaf, M.; Singer, A.; Shen, W.; Green, I.; Womer, K.; Segev, D. & Montgomery, R. (2000). Laparoscopic live donor nephrectomy with vaginal extraction. *American Journal of Transplantation*, Vol.10, No.6, (June 2010), pp. 1473-1477, ISSN 1600-6143

Booster, M.; Wijnen, R.; Ming, Y.; Vroemen, J. & Kootstra, G. (1969). In situ perfusion of kidneys from non-heart beating donors: The Maastricht protocol. *Transplantation Proceedings*, Vol.25, (February 1993) pp.1503-1504, ISSN 0041-1337

Clayman, R.; Kavoussi, L.; Soper, N.; Dierks, S.; Merety, K.; Darcy, M.; Long, S.; Roemer, F.; Pingleton E. & Thomson, P. (1985). Laparoscopic nephrectomy. *New English Journal of Medicine*, Vol.324, No.19, (May 1991), pp. 1370-1371, ISSN 0022-5347

Chin, E.; Hazzan, D.; Edye, M.; Wisnivesky, J.; Herron, D.; Ames, S.; Palese, M.; Pomp, A.; Gagner, M. & Bromberg, J. (1991). The first decade of a laparoscopic donor nephrectomy program: Effect of surgeon and institution experience with 512 cases from 1996 to 2006. *Journal of American College of Surgeons*, Vol.209, No.1, (July 2009), pp. 106-113, ISSN 1072-7515

Dols, L.; Kok, N.; Terkivatan, T.; Tran, T.; d'Ancona, F.; Langenhuijsen, J.; Zur, I.; Alwayn, I.; Hendriks, M.; Dooper, I.; Weimar, W. & Ijzermans, J. (2000). Hand-assisted retroperitoneoscopic versus standar laparoscopic donor nephrectomy: Harp-trial. *BMC Surgery*, Vol.10, No. 1, (March 2010), pp. 11, ISSN 1471-2482

Dols, L.; IJzermans, J.; Wentink, N.; Tran, T.; Zuidema, W.; Dooper, I.; Weimar, W. & Kok, N. (2000). Long-Term Follow-up of a Randomized Trial Comparing Laparoscopic and Mini-Incision Open Live Donor Nephrectomy. *American Journal of Transplantation*, Vol.10, No.11, (November 2010), pp. 2481-2487, ISSN 1600-6143

Garcia-Rinaldi, R.; Lefrak, E.; Defore, W.; Feldman, L.; Noon G.; Jachimczyk, J. & DeBakey, M. (1985) In situ preservation of cadaver Kidneys for transplantation: Laboratory observations and clinical application. *Annals of Surgery*, Vol.182, No.5, (November 1975), pp.576-584, ISSN 1528-1140

Gjertsen, H.; Sandberg, A.; Wadstrom, J.; Tyden, G. & Ericzon, B. (1969). Introduction of hand assisted retroperitoneoscopic living donor nephrectomy at Karolinska

University Hospital Huddinge. *Transplantation Proceedings*, Vol.38, No.8, (October 2006), pp. 2644-2645, ISSN 0041-1345

González, M.; García, J.; García C. et al. Trasplante de riñón procedente de donantes en asistolia. *Actas Urológicas Espanolas*, Vol.18, (1994), pp. 433-436, ISSN 1699-7980

Halgrimson, W.; Campsen, J.; Mandell, M.; Kelly, M.; Kam, I. & Zimmerman, M. (1995). Donor complications following laparoscopic compared to hand-assisted living donor nephrectomy: An analisis of the literature. *Urology*, Vol.70, No.6, (January 2007), pp. 1060-1063, ISSN 0090-4295

Horgan, S.; Vanuno, D.; Sileri, P.; Cicalese, L. & Benedetti, E. (1969). Robotic-assisted laparoscopic donor nephrectomy for kidney transplantation. *Transplantation*, Vol.73, No.9, (May 2002), pp. 1474-1479, ISSN 0041-1337

Ho, Y.; Won, H.; Koon, R.; Sang, H.; Young, Ch.; Woong, Han. & Won, Chang. (1960). Laparoendoscopic Single-Site Nephrectomy Using a Modified Umbilical Incision and a Home-Made Transumbilical Port. *Yonsei Medicine Journal*, Vol.52, No.2, (March 2011), pp.307-313, ISSN 0513-5796

Koyama, I.; Hoshino, T.; Nagashima, N.; Adachi, H.; Ueda, K. & Omoto, R. (1969). A new approach to kidney procurement from non heart beating donors: core cooling on cardiopulmonary bypass. *Transplantation Proceedings*, Vol.21, No.1, (February 1989), pp.1203-1205, ISSN 0041-1337

Leventhal, J.; Kocak, B.; Slavalaggio, P.; Koffron, A.; Baker, T.; Kaufman, D.; Fryer, J.; Abecassis, M. & Stuart, F. (1945). Laparoscopic donor nephrectomy 1997 to 2003: lessons learned with 500 cases at a single institution. *Surgery*, Vol. 136, No. 4, (October 2004), pp. 881-890, ISSN 0039-6060

Matas, A.; Bartlett, S.; Leichtman, A. & Delmonico, F. (2000). Morbidity and mortality after living kidney donation, 1999–2001: Survey of United Stated transplant centers. *American Journal of Transplantation*, Vol.3, No.7, (July 2003), pp. 830-834, ISSN 1600-6143

Mahdavi, P.; Bowman, R.; Tenggardjaja, C.; Jellison, F.; Ebrahimi, K. & Baldwin, D. (1969). A Novel Bridging Hand-Assisted LESS Donor Nephrectomy Technique. *Transplantation*, Vol.90, No.7, (October 2010), pp. 802-804, ISSN 0041-1337

Minnee, R.; Bemelman, W.; Donselaar, K.; Booij, J.; ter Meulen, S.; ten Berge, I.; Legemate, D.; Bemelman, F. & Idu, M. (1969). Risk Factors for Delayed Graft Function After Hand-Assisted Laparoscopic Donor Nephrectomy. *Transplantation Proceedings*, Vol.42, No.7, (July 2010), pp. 2422-2426, ISSN 0041-1345.

Nicholson, M.; Kaushik, M.; Lewis, G.; Brook, N.; Bagul, A.; Kay, M.; Harper, S.; Elwell, R. ; Veitch, P. & Hosgood, SA. (1969). Health-Related Quality of Life After Living Donor Nephrectomy: A Randomized Controlled Trial of Laparoscopic Versus Open Nephrectomy. *Transplantation*, Vol.91, No.4, (February 2011) pp. 457-461, ISSN 0041-1337

Nanidis, T.; Antcliffe, D.; Kokkinos, C.; Borysiewicz, C.; Darzi, A.; Tekkis, P. & Papalois, V. (1985). Laparoscopic versus open live donor nephrectomy in renal transplantation: a meta-analysis. *Annals of Surgery*, Vol.247, No.1, (January 2008), pp. 58-70, ISSN 1528-1140

Nakazato, P.; Concepcion, W.; Bry, Limm, W.; Tokunaga, Y.; Itasaka, H.; Feduska, N.; Esquivel, C. & Collins, G. (1945). Total abdominal evisceration: An en bloc technique for abdominal organ harvesting. *Surgery*, Vol.111, No.1, (January 1992), pp. 37-47, ISSN 0039-6060

Nicholson, M.; Elwell, R.; Kaushik, M.; Bagul, A. & Hosgood, S. (1969). Health-related quality of life after living donor nephrectomy: a randomized controlled trial of laparoscopic versus open nephrectomy. *Transplantation*, Vol.91, No.4, (February 2011) pp. 457-461, ISSN 0041-1337

Rane, A.; Ahmed, S.; Kommu, S.; Anderson, C. & Rimington, P. (1945). Singleport "scarless" laparoscopic nephrectomies: The United Kingdom experience. *British Association of Urological Surgeons*, Vol.104, No.2, (July 2009), pp. 230, ISSN 1464-410X

Ratner, L.; Ciseck, L.; Moore, R.; Cigarroa, F.; Kaufman, H. & Kavoussi, L. (1969). Laparoscopic live donor nephrectomy. *Transplantation*, Vol.60, No.9, (November 1995), pp. 1047-1049, ISSN 0041-1337

Ratner, L. & Pescovitz, M. (2000). Giving birth to an operation: laparoscopic live donor nephrectomy with vaginal extraction. Is this misconceived?. *American Journal of Transplantation*, Vol.10, No.6, (June 2010), pp. 1347-1348, ISSN 1600-6143

Renoult, E.; Hubert, J.; Ladrière, M.; Billaut, N.; Mourey, E.; Feuillu, B. & Kessler, M. (1909). Robot-assisted laparoscopic and open live-donor nephrectomy: a comparison of donor morbidity and early renal allograft outcomes. *Nephrol Dial Transplant*, Vol.21, No.2, (February 2006), pp. 472-477, ISSN 1460-2385

Starzl, T.; Hakala, T.; Shaw, B.; Hardesty, R.; Roshental, T.; Griffith, B.; Iwatsuki, S. & Bahnson, H. (1909). A flexible procedure for multiple cadaveric organ procurement. *Surgery, Gynecology & Obstetrics*, Vol.158, No.3, (March 1984), pp. 223-230, ISSN 0039-6087

Starzl, T.; Miller, C.; Broznick, B. & Makowka, L. (1909). An improved technique for multiple organ harvesting. *Surgery, Gynecology & Obstetrics*, Vol.165, No.4, (October 1987), pp. 343-348, ISSN 0039-6087

Starzl, T.; Todo, S.; Tzakis, A.; Alessiani, M.; Casavilla, A.; Abu, K. & Fung, J. (1909). The many faces of multivisceral transplantation. *Surgery, Gynecology & Obstetrics*, Vol.172, No.5, (May 1991), pp. 335-344, ISSN 0039-6087

Szostek, M.; Danielewicz, R.; Lagiewska, B. Pacholczyk, M.; Rybicki, Z.; Michalak, G.; Adadynski, L.; Walaszewski, J. & Rowinski, W. (1969). Successful transplantation of kidneys harvested from cadaver donors at 71 to 259 minutes following cardiac arrest. *Transplantation Proceedings*, Vol.27, No.5, (October 1995), pp.2901-2902, ISSN 0041-1345

Sundqvist, P.; Feuk, U.; Haggman, M.; Persson, A.; Stridsberg, M. & Wadstrom, J. (1969). Hand-assisted retroperitoneoscopic live donor nephrectomy in comparison to open and laparoscopic procedures: a prospective study on donor morbidity and kidney function. *Transplantation*, Vol.78, No.1, (July 2004), pp. 147-153, ISSN 0041-1337

Troppmann, C.; Daily, M.; McVicar, J.; Troppmann, K. & Perez, R. (1969). The transition from laparoscopic to retroperitoneoscopic live donor nephrectomy: A matched pair pilot study. *Transplantation*, Vol.89, No.7, (April 2010), pp. 858-863, ISSN 0041-1337

Van der Merwe, A.; Bachmann, A. & Heyn, C. (2005). Retroperitoneal LESS Donor Nephrectomy. *International Brazilian Journal of Urology*, Vol.36, No.5, (October 2010), pp. 602-606, ISSN 1677-6119

Yang, S.; Park, D.; Lee, D.; Lee, J. & Park, K. (1917) Retroperitoneal endoscopic live donor nephrectomy: report of 3 cases. *Journal of Urology,* Vol.153, No.6, (June 1995) pp.1884-1886, ISSN 0022-5347

Wadstrom, J.; Lindstrom, P. & Engstrom, B.(1969). Hand-assisted retroperitoneoscopic living donor nephrectomy superior to laparoscopic nephrectomy. *Transplant Proceedings*, Vol.35, No.2, (March 2003), pp. 782-783, ISSN 0041-1345

6

Renal Transplantation in Patient with Fabry's Disease Maintained by Enzyme Replacement Therapy

Taigo Kato
Department of Urology,
Osaka University Hospital
Japan

1. Introduction

Fabry's disease (FD) is a rare inborn error of glycosphingolipid catabolism can lead to renal failure. The life expectancy is reduced for both genders, and the major causes of death include cardiac death, stroke, or the consequences of end stage of renal disease. This article summarizes the current knowledge about FD and the treatment of kidney transplantation and enzyme replacement therapy in FD.

2. About Fabry's disease

FD is a rare sphingolipidosis related and X-linked disorder of glycosphingolipid catabolism caused by deficient lysosomal α-galactosidase A activity(Fig.1). Deficiency of the enzyme leads to progressive accumulation of the glycosphingolipid globotriaosylceramide (Gb3) in vascular endothelia, heart tissue, connective tissue, peripheral nerves, and the kidneys (Table.1, Fig.2). Male patients typically develop painful acroparesthesia followed by proteinuria, renal failure, cardiac hypertrophy and cerebral white matter lesions. Females are carriers and may present a wider range of symptoms(Fig.3,4). The incidence has been estimated to be 1:117,000 live births and 1:50,000 males. Registries of dialysis patients from the United States and Europe indicate that FD is the cause of end-stage renal disease (ESRD) for approximately 0.2% of patients on dialysis(Fig.5). Renal disease of some form occurs in most patients, with ESRD a common manifestation in hemizygous males that may develop by the fourth to fifth decade of life. The clinical course in heterozygous female patients involves a delayed onset of symptoms and milder progression, although some female patients present with symptoms similar to those seen in classically affected male patients. The analysis of 197 kidney transplant recipients with FD indicates that they have superior graft survival and similar patient survival compared with patients with other causes of ESRD. However, Fabry patients had a higher risk of death compared with a matched cohort of patients with other causes of ESRD. The median lifespan is 50 years for affected male patients and 70 years for female patients. Current therapy for ESRD in patients with FD involves renal transplantation and enzyme replacement therapy (ERT).

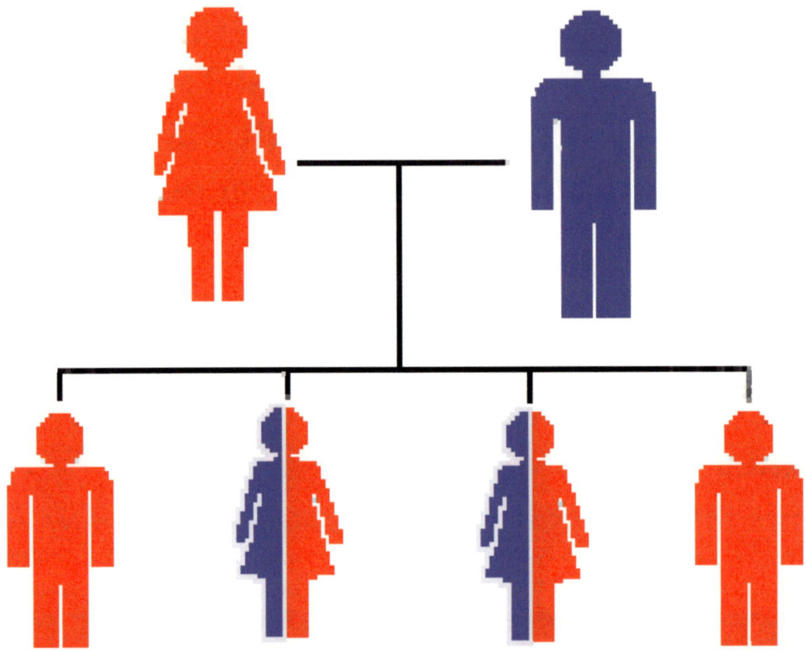

Fig. 1. If a male with Fabry disease and an unaffected (non-carrier) female have children, all of their daughters will be Fabry carriers and none of their sons will be affected with Fabry disease.

Disease		Accumulated material	Deficient enzyme
GM 1 gangliosidosis		GM 1 ganglioside	β-galactosidase
GM 2 gangliosidosis	Tay-Sachs Disease	GM 2 ganglioside	β-hexosaminidase
	Sandhoff Disease	GM 2 ganglioside	β-hexosaminidase
Metachromatic Leukodystrophy		Sulfatide	arylsulfatase A
Ferber Disease		Ceramide	Ceramidase
Gaucher Disease		Glycocerebroside	β-glucocerebrosidase
Niemann-Pick Disease		Phosphorylcholine Ceramide	Sphingomyelinase
Krabbe Disease		galactocerebroside	β-galactosidase A
Fabry Disease		**globotriaosylceramide**	**α-galactosidase A**

Table 1. The classification of sphingolipidosis.

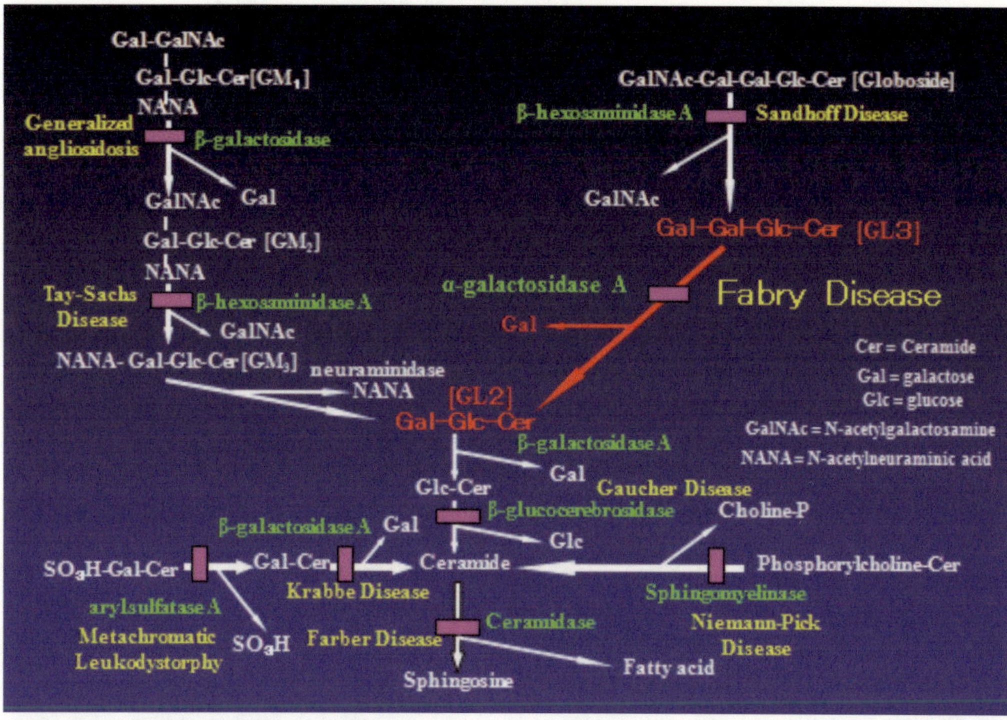

Fig. 2. The classification of sphingolipidosis.

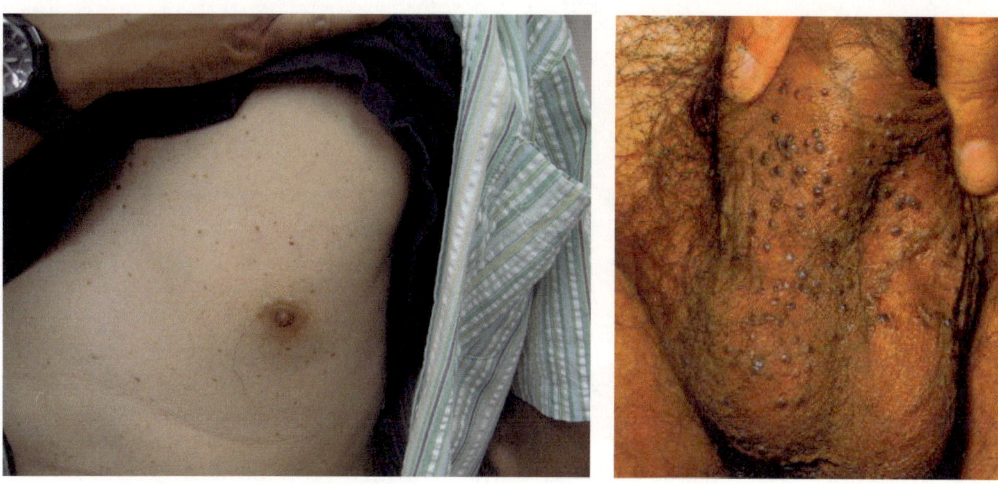

Fig. 3. Clinical features of Fabry's disease; angiokeratomas.

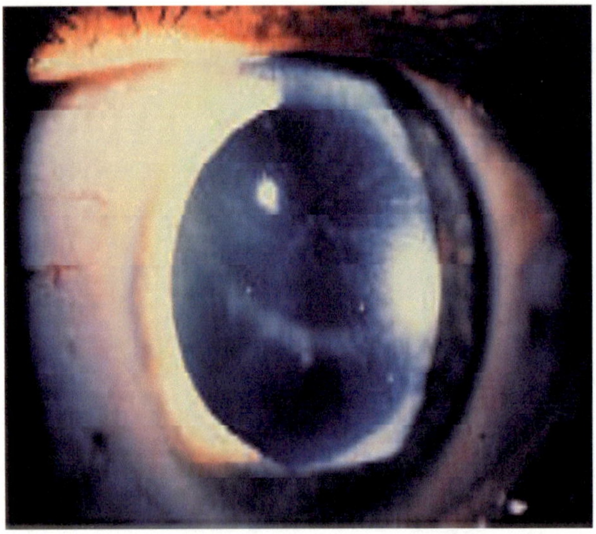

Fig. 4. Clinical features of Fabry's disease; corneal and lenticular opacities.

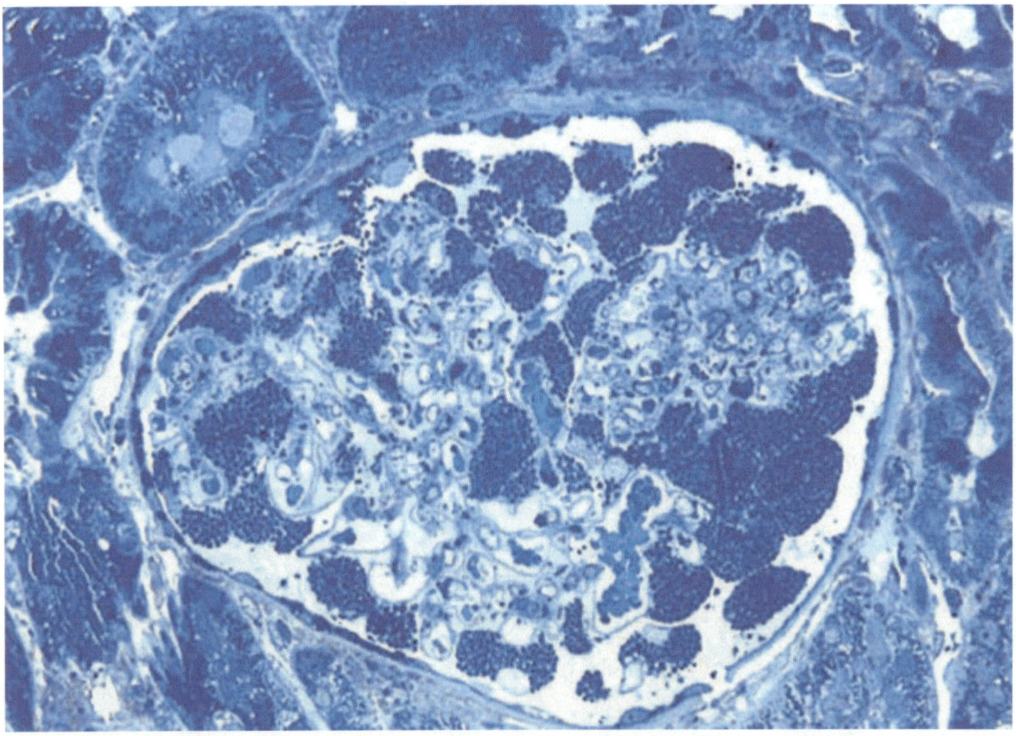

Fig. 5. Ultra structural changes in glomerulus with FD with myelin-like inclusions and subendothelial deposits.

3. Renal transplantation in patient with Fabry's disease

Renal transplantation was known to be effective for FD, as previous reports demonstrated that the procedure provided equivalent 5-year patient and graft survivals, as well as improvement of overall prognosis in patients with ESRD due to FD. In contrast, another study found that a renal allograft could not repair the deficient enzyme activity of α-galactosidase A and noted that the accumulation of Gb3 impaired renal function, which might signify the possibility of recurrence of FD in the renal allograft. According to a previous study from the European Dialysis and Transplant Association/European Renal Association Registry, graft survival at 3 years in 33 patients with FD was not considered as inferior to that of patients with other nephropathies (72% vs. 69%), and patient survival after transplantation was comparable to that of patients aged under 55 years with non-Fabry nephropathies. Excellent graft and patient survival were also reported from the US Renal Data System Registry. FD is therefore not considered a contraindication for renal transplantation. Although a case study has shown that the disease may recur in the transplanted organ, another case study has shown no evidence of disease recurrence in a renal biopsy 8 years after transplantation. A further case study showed extensive Fabry-related renal changes in a renal biopsy from a patient who had received a graft from his sister who was heterozygous for the disease.

4. The efficacy of enzyme replacement therapy (ERT)

Enzyme replacement therapy (ERT) for the treatment of Fabry's disease was first performed in the 1970s, however, open-label phase 2 trials were not performed until the 2000s. ERT using recombinant human alpha-galactocidase A (generic names agalsidase alpha and agalsidase beta) was approved for use in Europe in 2001 and in the United States in 2003. Initial randomised controlled trials (RCT) showed that 69% of the treatment group was free of renal microvascular endothelial deposits of globotriaosylceramide (primary endpoint) versus no change in the placebo group after 20 weeks ($p < 0.001$). Although there did not appear to be a difference in quality of life as assessed by the SF-36, another RCT showed a statistically significant decrease in pain severity and improvement in quality of life (primary outcome). This study also showed improvement in renal architectural distortion (mesangial diameter) ($p = 0.01$) and increase in creatinine clearance ($p = 0.02$). In a more recent, larger RCT, 42% of placebo patients versus 27% of treated patients had clinical events (defined as renal, cardiac or cerebrovascular event or death); the time to first clinical event adjusted for baseline proteinuria favoured agalsidase beta but included the null (hazard ratio 0.47, CI: 0.21–1.03; $p< 0.06$). Although overall the results were less than overwhelming, treatment effect was greater in patients with preserved renal function. There are no data currently regarding ERT and affect on mortality.

Moreover, a purified recombinant α-galactosidase A enzyme (Fabrazyme®) was synthesized and administration in non-transplanted FD patients was reported to markedly reduce serum ceramide levels. A detailed report revealed few serious adverse events in a total of 401 patients receiving long-term treatment; as in this study, most adverse events consisted of mild infusion reactions. Patients given recombinant α-GalA at 1 mg/kg once every two weeks showed decreased microvascular endothelial deposits of Gb3 in skin over a period of 20 weeks and plasma Gb3 also decreased. In addition, in patients who received ERT for 30-36 months, serum creatinine and estimated glomerular filtration rate values remained stable, while the level of plasma Gb3 remained in a normal range after ERT. More recently, Cybulla et al. explored the effects of agalsidase alfa in transplant patients with FD. Allograft function of 20 patients from the Fabry Outcome Survey registry was analyzed after approximately 3.5 years (median) of agalsidase alfa therapy at the standard dose of 0.2 mg/kg every other week. After 2 years of ERT, there was a slight but nonsignificant increase in serum creatinine (1.4 mg/dl at baseline versus 1.6 mg/dl) and a decrease in eGFR (59.2 ml/min/1.73 m2 at baseline versus 51.1 ml/min/1.73 m2 at 2 years). Similar to the previously mentioned study, proteinuria remained stable during this time period. In contrast, ERT may be less effective to improve renal or cardiac function in cases with progressive damage to tissue, as it would likely be difficult to recover the function. Therefore, renal transplantation in conjunction with ERT might achieve better improvement of the graft and overall survival of FD patients.

Mignani et al. reported that plasma Gb3 was decreased by 23-50% after ERT in renal transplant patients with FD. In addition, Inderbitzin et al. treated a patient with persistent FD-related acroparesthesia and found that ERT for 100 months after renal transplantation resulted in an excellent clinical course. In another study, Mignani et al. also reported 3 patients who underwent ERT after renal transplantation, who had maintained renal function and improved cardiac function. In each of those cases, ERT was performed after renal transplantation, whereas we previously reported a rare case of successful cadaveric renal transplantation in patient with FD maintained by ERT with an excellent clinical course. We treated a 48-year-old male patient with a typical clinical history of FD from childhood (intermittent fever, cutaneous angiokeratoma, pain attacks in arms and legs). At the age of 25, renal function disorder with proteinuria was pointed out and hemodialysis started at 26 years old. He was diagnosed with FD based on deficient lysosomal α- galactosidase A activity at the age of 46 and began ERT by injection of recombinant α-galactosidase e.g. Agalsidase beta at 1mg per kg bodyweight once every two weeks in August 2004. After the induction of ERT, he still had diffuse angiokeratoma of the body and intermittent abdominal pain. Echocardiographic evaluation suggested hypertrophic obstructive cardiomyopathy with left ventricular hypertrophy.

On December 17, 2005, cadaveric renal transplantation was performed (Fig.6) for the patient. The initial immunosuppressive agents were cyclosporine, mycophenolate mofetil, steroids, and basiliximab, with the cyclosporine trough levels kept at 100-150 ng/ml. No rejection or other complications appeared during the immediate follow-up period, and he withdrew from hemodialysis 23 days after transplantation. At discharge, serum creatinine was reduced to about 1.9 mg/ml and was at a steady-state level. At the same time, the disappearance of the skin lesions and abdominal pain was noticed. At 12 and 24 months after transplantation, graft biopsies were performed, as the serum creatinine level increased to 2.2～2.3 mg/dl. Histological results demonstrated acute cellular rejection, however, there were no abnormal deposits of accumulated glycosphingolipids in the glomerular podocytes or tubular epithelial cells. Electron microscopy revealed normal glomerular cells with a slight increase in the mesangial matrix (Fig.7).

There were no dense deposits. The acute rejection responded to intravenous deoxyspergualin and serum creatinine decreased to 2.0 mg/dl. Since transplantation, ERT has been continued once every two weeks and no complications as a result of that therapy have been recognized.

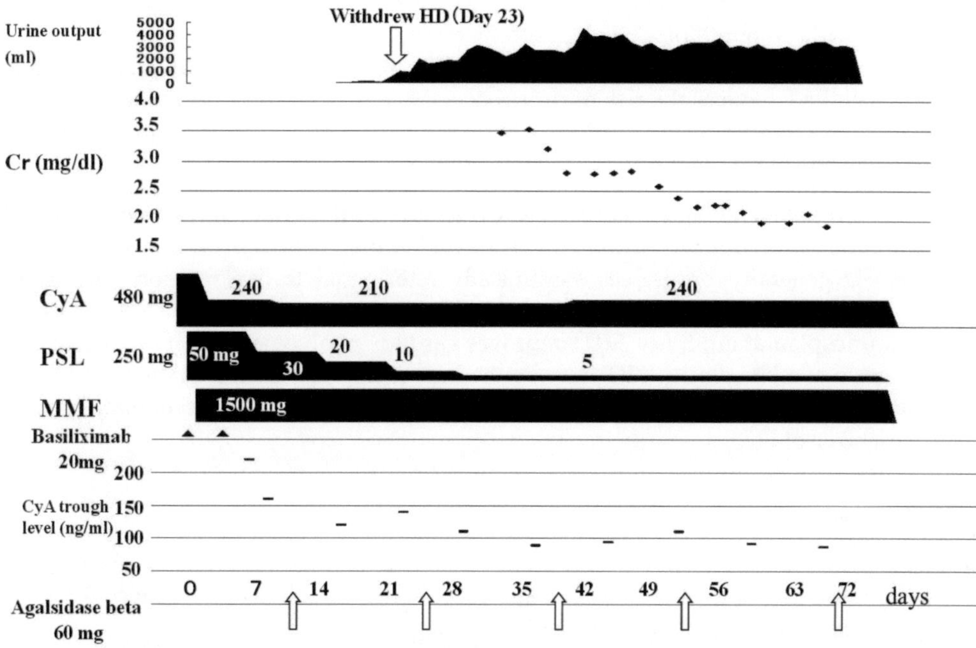

Fig. 6. Clinical course of the patient. Cr creatinine; CsA, cyclosporine; HD, hemodialysis; MMF, mycofenolate mophetil; PSL, predonisolone.

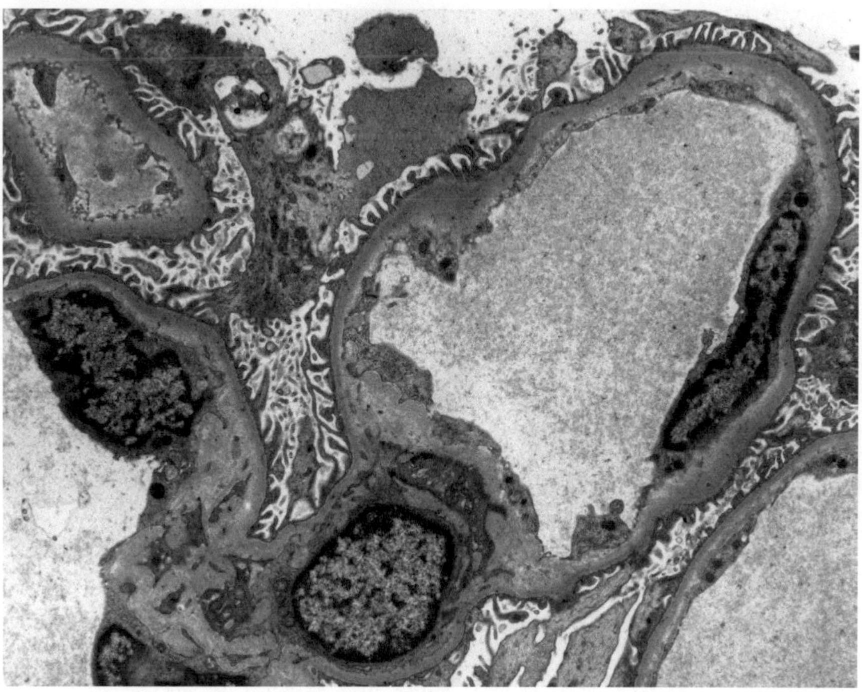

Fig. 7. Electron microscopy of normal glomerulus from kidney graft. Occasional foci of podocyte fusion are present.

The recurrence of FD in patients with a transplanted kidney has rarely been reported. Findings of small amounts of Gb3 deposits in renal grafts have been limited to vascular endothelial cells and tubular epithelial cells. We consider that renal transplantation combined with ERT reduces the risk of recurrence of FD in a transplanted kidney. However, further data are required to confirm whether such treatment will confer long-term renoprotective effects on renal transplantation.

An important problem facing FD patients is that a successful kidney graft survives for 10-15 years, however, cardiovascular complications related to metabolic disease may occur during that time. FD generally progresses systemically after renal transplantation and cardiac ceramide deposition ultimately determines the fate of these patients in the second decade after renal transplantation. Since ERT improves cardiac involvement in FD patients, renal transplantation combined with ERT may be the best therapy for ESRD at the present time. Additional clinical studies are needed to determine the effects of this combination on the overall prognosis of FD.

5. Conclusion

Renal transplantation is effective for FD and improves patient and graft survivals as well as overall prognosis in patients with ESRD due to FD. And ERT is well tolerated in patients with FD who have undergone renal transplantation.

In summary, some studies indicate that kidney transplantation and ERT are viable option for patients with ESRD due to FD. Although ERT appears to stabilize renal function, further data are required to confirm whether such treatment will confer long-term renoprotective effects on kidney transplant patients.

6. References

Andrade J, Waters PJ, Singh RS(2008): Screening for Fabry disease in patients with chronic kidney disease: limitations of plasma alpha-galactosidase assay as a screening test. *Clin J Am Soc Nephrol* 3:139–145

Banikazemi M, Bultas J, Waldek S. (2007) Agalsidase-beta therapy for advanced Fabry disease: a randomized trial. *Ann Intern Med* ; 146:77–86.

Chimenti C, Morgante E, Tanzilli G.(2008) Angina in Fabry disease reflects coronary small vessel disease. *Circ Heart Fail* ; 1: 161–169.

Cybulla M, Walter KN, Schwarting A, Divito R, Feriozzi S, Sunder-Plassmann G; European FOS Investigators Group.(2009). Kidney transplantation in patients with Fabry disease. *Transpl Int.* ;22(4):475-81.

Desnick RJ, Ioannou YA, Eng CM α-galactosidase A deficiency: Fabry disease. In: Scriver CR, Beaudet AL, Sly WS, Valle D, eds. The metabolic and molecular bases of inherited disease. 8th ed. Vol. 3. New York: McGraw-Hill, 2001:3733-74.

Elliott PM, Kindler H, Shah JS(2006) Coronary microvascular dysfunction in male patients with Anderson-Fabry disease and the effect of treatment with alpha galactosidase A. *Heart* ; 92: 357–360.

Eng CM, Guffon N, Wilcox WR. (2001) Safety and efficacy of recombinant human α-galactosidase A replacement therapy in Fabry's disease. *N Engl J Med* 345;9-16

Inderbitzin D, Avital I. (2005) Kidney transplantation improves survival and is indicated in Fabry's disease. *Transplantation Proceedings* 37;4211-4214

Karras A, De Lentdecker P, Delahousse M(2008) Combined heart and kidney transplantation in a patient with Fabry disease in the enzyme replacement therapy era. *Am J Transplant*; 8: 1345–1348.

Kato T, Nishimura K, Ichikawa Y. (2009) Deceased renal transplantation in patient with Fabry's disease maintained by enzyme replacement therapy. *Int J Urol* 16:650

Kleinert J, Kotanko P, Spada M(2009) Anderson-Fabry disease: a case-finding study among male kidney transplant recipients in Austria. *Transpl Int* 22: 287–292

Koskenvuo JW, Hartiala JJ, Nuutila P.(2008) Twenty-four-month alphagalactosidase A replacement therapy in Fabry disease has only minimal effects on symptoms and cardiovascular parameters. *J Inherit Metab Dis*; 31: 432–441.

Kotanko P, Kramar R, Devrnja D(2004) Results of a nationwide screening for Anderson-Fabry disease among dialysis patients. *J Am Soc Nephrol* 15: 1323–1329

MacDermot KD, Holmes A, Miners AH(2001) Anderson-Fabry disease: Clinical manifestations and impact of disease in a cohort of 98 hemizygous males. *J Med Genet* 38: 750–760

MacDermot KD, Holmes A, Miners AH(2001) Anderson-Fabry disease: Clinical manifestations and impact of disease in a cohort of 60 obligate carrier females. *J Med Genet* 38: 769–775

Maslauskiene R, Bumblyte IA, Sileikiene E.(2007) The prevalence of Fabry's disease among male patients on hemodialysis in Lithuania (a screening study). *Medicina (Kaunas)* 43 Suppl 1: 77–80.

Mehta A, Ricci R, Widmer U.(2004) Fabry disease defined: baseline clinical manifestations of 366 patients in the Fabry Outcome Survey. *Eur J Clin Invest*; 34: 236–242.

Merta M, Reiterova J, Ledvinova J(2007) A nationwide blood spot screening study for Fabry disease in the Czech Republic haemodialysis patient population. *Nephrol Dial Transplant* 22: 179–186

Mignani R, Feriozzi S, Pisani A. (2008) Agalsidase therapy in patients with Fabry disease on renal replacement therapy: a nationwide study in Italy. *Nephrol Dial Transplant* May ;23(5):1628-1635

Mignani R, Gerra D, Maldini. (2001) Long term survival of patients with renal transplantation in Fabry's disease. *Contrib Nephrol.* Vol 136;pp229-233

Mignani R,Panichi V,Giudicissi A.(2004) Enzyme replacement therapy with agalsidase beta in kidney transplant patients with Fabry disease. *Kidney Int* 66:1279-1282

Ojo A, Meier-Kriesche HU, Friedman G.(2000) Excellent outcome or renal transplantation in patients with Fabry's disease. Transplantaion 69;2337

Porsch DB, Nunes AC, Milani V(2008): Fabry disease in hemodialysis patients in southern Brazil: prevalence study and clinical report. *Ren Fail* 30:825–830

Rasaiah VI, Underwood JP, Oreopoulos DG(2008) Implementation of high-throughput screening for Fabry disease in Toronto dialysis patients. *Nephrol Dial Transplant* Plus 1: 129–130

Schiffmann R, Ries M, Timmons M, Flaherty JT, Brady RO.(2006)Long-term therapy with agalsidase alfa for Fabry disease: safety and effects on renal function in a home infusion setting. *Nephrol Dial Transplant*. 21(2):345-54

Sessa A, Meroni M, Battini G. (2002) Renal transplantation in patients with Fabry disease. *Nephron;*91:348-351

Shah T, Gill J, Malhotra N, Takemoto SK, Bunnapradist S. (2009) Kidney transplant outcomes in patients with Fabry disease. *Transplantation.* 27;87(2):280-5.

Spinelli L, Pisani A, Sabbatini M, Petretta M, Andreucci MV, Procaccini D. (2004) Enzyme replacement therapy with agalsidase beta improves cardiac involvement in Fabry's disease. *Clin Genet* 66;158-165.

Terryn W, Poppe B, Wuyts B (2008): Two-tier approach for the detection of alpha-galactosidase A deficiency in a predominantly female haemodialysis population. *Nephrol Dial Transplant* 23:294–300.

Tsakiris D, Simpson HK, Jones EH(1996) Report on management of renale failure in Europe, XXVI,: Rare diseases in renal replacement therapy in the ERA-EDTA Registry. *Nephrol Dial Transplant* 11[Suppl 7]: S4–20

Waldek S. (2003) PR interval and the response to enzyme-replacement therapy for Fabry's disease. *N Engl J Med* ; 348: 1186–1187.

Weidemann F, Niemann M, Breunig F.(2009) Long-term effects of enzyme replacement therapy on Fabry cardiomyopathy: evidence for a better outcome with early treatment. *Circulation* ; 119: 524–529.

Whybra C, Kampmann C, Willers I(2001) Anderson-Fabry disease: Clinical manifestations of disease in female heterozygotes. *J Inherit Metab Dis* 24: 715–724

Wilcox WR, Banikazemi M, Guffon N. (2004) Long-term safety and efficacy of enzyme replacement therapy for Fabry Disease. *Am.J.Hum.Genet.*75;65-74

7

Polymorphism of RAS in Patients with AT1-AA Mediated Steroid Refractory Acute Rejection

Geng Zhang and Jianlin Yuan
Department of Urology, Xijing Hospital
Fourth Military Medical University, Xi'an
China

1. Introduction

Acute rejection is one major reason of the graft loss in renal transplantation. Most of the allograft rejections are due to the existence of the antibodies. The importance of the series tests of HLA and HLA antibodies associated with transplantation has been widely recognized. Although considerable rejection episodes can be explained by the appearance of the donor specific anti-HLA antibodies (DSA), it is reported that even in the case of 'ideal' HLA identical donor grafts transplanted into 'ideal' recipients, 23% are rejected within 10 years [1]. So effect of HLA antibodies accounts for only some of the immunological failures of allograft and there must be large fraction of undetected antibodies against non-HLA mismatches.

Despite various ways were used in the prevention of acute rejection, pulse steroid treatment remains the first-line therapy of all immumosuppresion projects and has a 60 to 70% success rate [2]. There are still recipients suffered from steroid refractory acute rejection (SRAR) and get worse. These rejections typically have an aggressive clinical course and are associated with graft loss [3]. Some of the patients would have to return to blood dialysis immediately and part of them die from complications. We detected antibodies in these patients and found that some of them do not have HLA antibodies and one of their marked characteristics is malignant hypertension. We presumed this is a special type of rejection. Thus, both immunologic and non-immunologic mechanisms for this specific type of rapid renal allograft dysfunction have to be considered.

In case of the SRAR is appeared in a small part of the renal transplantation recipients, we presume that the genetic factors are involved it. It is reported that single nucleotide polymorphism (SNP) of some immune response related genes is involved in the development the acute rejection. The SNP of some genes can affect their functions by the changing either cytokine production or amino acid sequence. And the structure and function of some critical components would be altered concomitantly. The characteristic change of related proteins would finally induce the immune response and then trigger the rejection process.

Hypertension has been found to be an independent contributor in the progression of renal allograft failure in some studies [4, 5]. The presence of genetic abnormalities in blood pressure regulation could promote post-transplant hypertension and by that contribute to a more rapid loss of renal allograft function. The recipients' blood pressure levels may depend on several factors, such as graft function, type, and dosage of immunosuppressive agents applied, previous rejection episodes, recurrence of the underlying nephropathy, and a previous history of hypertension [6]. The renin– angiotensin–aldosterone system (RAS) is a proteolytic cascade with an important role in blood pressure regulation and maintenance of fluid and electrolyte balance [7]. It was also reported that over activation of the RAS is linked to poor long-term renal transplant function and decreased graft survival times [8]. RAS polymorphisms associated with hypertension in certain groups have been identified [9]. We hypothesis that the occurrence of SRAR may be due to the over activating of RAS in a special group of recipients. And therefore, genes of the RAS deserve consideration. Among these the angiotensinogen (AGT), angiotensin-converting enzyme (ACE), angiotensin type 1 receptor (AT1R), and aldosterone synthase (CYP11B2) genes are of particular interest. Yet the prevalence and distribution, alone or combined, of the M235T-AGT, I/D-ACE, A1166C-AT1R, or -344C/T-CYP11B2 polymorphisms and their relation with SRAR has not been well studied.

In the studies of immunologic mechanism of acute vascular rejection, some data suggested that agonistic angiotensin type 1 (AT1) receptor autoantibodies (AT1-AA) may contribute to the pathogenesis of the rejection [10]. Some experiments implicated the role of renin-angiotensin system in the regulation of specific immune responses and immune-mediated renal injuries [11]. And AT1 receptor blockade appeared to effectively attenuate the agonistic activity of the antibodies.

So the SRAR may be a kind of specific rejection, whose origin, mechanism and results and treatment are all different from other types of rejections. Therefore, this study tried to determine whether or not gene polymorphisms of RAS are associated with steroid refractory acute rejection. Further more, by studying the gene-gene interaction, we searched the association of the occurrence of SRAR with the appearance of AT1-AA.

2. Subjects and methods

2.1 Study patients and biopsies

A total 206 renal transplant recipients were included: 116 males and 90 females, mean age 29.6±10.2 years range 22–55 years transplanted at Department of Urology of Xi Jing hospital, 4th Military Medical University from January 1st, 2001, through December 31st, 2005. The transplants were first grafts in all cases. Serum samples obtained during rejection episodes were screened for donor specific anti-HLA antibodies and also agonistic antibodies targeting the AT1 receptor. This study was approved by the Ethics Committee of the Hospital, and all patients gave their oral informed consent while he or she was awaiting transplantation.

Allograft-biopsy specimens were processed by standard techniques and graded according to the Banff97 criteria. C4d staining on paraffin-embedded sections was made according to a protocol described previously [12, 13].

2.2 Immunosuppressive treatment

Initial immunosuppressive therapy consisted of a calcineurin inhibitor, mycophenolate mofetil, methylprednisolone, and antibody against interleukin- 2 receptor for induction. All the recipients were treated with high dose pulse of methylprednisolone for 3 days with the dose of 0.5g, 0.5g, 0.25g in each day after the operation and a dose of 0.75g methylprednisolone was used on the operation day. Cyclosporine A or tacrolimus were introduced when serum creatinine levels were below 300 μ mol/L. Anti-proliferative agents, mycophenolate mofetil (1.5 g/day) or azathioprine (1–2 mg/kg/ day) were started on the day of transplantation. Prednisolone was reduced to 20mg daily after 7 days. Daily doses of CsA and tacrolimus were adjusted according to peak and trough blood levels respectively. High dose of methylprednisolone was utilized when the subject developed acute rejection after renal transplantation.

Patients resistant to steroid were experienced further treatments. The further therapy includes protein A immunoadsorption (IA) and intravenous immune globulin. Patients who were positive for AT1-AA were added with angiotensin II Receptor Blockers (ARB). Patients initially treated with cyclosporine were switched to high dose tacrolimus when refractory rejection was detected.

2.3 DNA extraction, PCR analysis and genotyping

Genomic DNA prepared from blood cells using a standard column extraction technique. ACE I/D polymorphism in intron 16 of the ACE gene was determined as described previously [14]. In order to exclude mistyping of heterozygotes, all DD individuals were also examined using primers specific for the insertion variant. PCR products were resolved on a 2% agarose gel by ethidium bromide staining.

AGT M 235 T was determined by PCR amplification according to a method described previously [15].The 165 bp PCR product was digested with TthIII at 37°C for 3h and resolved on a 2.5% agarose gel by ethidium bromide staining.

For the analysis of the AT1R (A1166C) polymorphism [16], a 410bp PCR product was digested with DdeI enzyme at 37°Cfor 3h and separated by electrophoresis in 2% agarose gel.

CYP11B2 gene polymorphism was performed according to method described by Brand *et al* [17]. The PCR product was restricted with 5 U of the restriction endonuclease HaeIII over 2 h at 37°C and final product was electrophoresed in 2% agarose gel and visualized directly by ethidium bromide staining. The -344T allele lacks the HaeIII site that is present in the -344C allele and gives rise to a fragment of 273 bp rather than 202 bp.

2.4 Antibody assays

The detection of AT1-AA The peptides corresponding to the sequence of the second extracellular loop of the human AT1 receptor positions 165aa-191aa (I-H-R-N-V-F-F-I-E-N-T-N-I-T-V-C-A-F-HY- E-S-Q-N-S-T-L) were synthesized by a peptide synthesis system [18]. The peptide was evaluated by HPLC analysis on a Vydac C-18 column, and 95% purity was achieved. The ELISA assay of antibodies was performed according to the described previously [19].

2.5 Statistics

All statistical analyses were performed with the help of the SPSS 10.0 statistical software package. Categorical variables were assessed by the chi-square test. Survival curves for each group were calculated by the Kaplan-Meier method. Differences in genotype and allele distributions between groups were tested by the χ^2 test. To compare the prevalence of SRAR among the genotypes of each polymorphism, genotypic odds ratios (OR) and 95% confidence intervals (CI) for SRAR were estimated using logistic regression analysis. Data are given as means with SD. In all statistical analysis the significance was considered significant when level (P) values were lower than 0.05. Test of Hardy–Weinberg equilibrium was performed in the subjects.

3. Results

All patients were classified into three groups according to the occurrence of SRAR. Two hundred and six renal transplant recipients were concerned by this study. Posttransplant hypertension was found in 102 cases (49.5%) of all patients. According to the presence of SRAR, patients were classified into two groups: group I (G I), 19 patients (9.2%) underwent SRAR (10 men and 9 women), among them 14 had malignant hypertension. Group II (GII) was the rest 187 patients who did not suffer from SRAR (104 men and 83 women), 16 of them had malignant hypertension, the difference between the two groups is significant. And 150 normal people were set as control group (GIII). Baseline characteristics of the GI and GII were compared. No difference was observed in terms of age and sex in the donors. Moreover, no statistically significant differences were found between the GI and GII in terms of sex distribution, percentage of first kidney transplantation and cause of end-stage renal disease And there were no significant differences between the GI and GII for total number of HLA-mismatches, ischemia times (Table 1).

The DD genotype of ACE and CC genotype of AT1R were risk factors for the development and progression of the SRAR. The genotype distributions of four key genes ACE I/D, AGT M235T, AT1R A1166C and CYP11B2 -344C/T of the RAS polymorphisms exhibited a nonsignificant difference with that predicted by the Hardy–Weinberg equilibrium in all cases. The significant differences of gene frequencies between all patients and control group were not observed.

Differences between GI and GII and controls in genotype distributions were observed for both ACE gene polymorphisms with DD genotype and CC genotype of AT1R polymorphism being more prevalent in GI than in other two groups. Genotype distributions of other polymorphisms investigated in AGT and CYP11B2 genes did not differ between these three groups. The difference in allele distributions was only observed for AT1R A1166C with the C allele being more frequent in G I than G II and controls (42.1% v 29.9% and 30.1%) (Table 2). To test the association of ACE and AT1R gene polymorphisms with SRAR, genotypic ORs were calculated. Taking the II genotype of the ACE I/D polymorphism as a reference, the OR for SRAR associated with the ID genotype was 1.53

	Non-SRAR (n=187)	SRAR (n=19)
Age (years)	36.5±11.6	37.7±12.5
Male (%)	53	47
IgG	9.3±2	10.4±2.8
No. of HLA MM	3.6±1.2	3.2±1.8
PRA positive (%)	7.6±1.2	7.5±1.5
Duration of dialysis before NTx (mon)	20.3±16.2	23.6±18.6
CIT(h)	10.6±7.1	11.6±7.3
Cause of ESRD		
Chronic glomerulonephritis	56.9	50.6
Hereditary	16.1	17.6
High blood pressure	6.5	10.6
IgA nephropathy	3.2	4.5
Unknown	17.1	16.7

CIT = Cold ischemia time; NTx=renal transplantation; HLA MM = HLA mismatch

Table 1. Characteristics of patients involved in the study.

	Genotypes			Alleles
AGT M235T	*MM* (%)	*MT*(%)	*TT*(%)	*M*(%)
GI	6 (31.6)	9 (47.3)	4(21.1)	21(55.3)
GII	61 (32.6)	87(46.5)	39(20.9)	209(55.9)
GIII	44 (29.3)	70 (46.7)	36(24)	158(52.7)
ACE I/D +	*II* (%)	*ID* (%)	*DD* (%)	*D* (%)
GI	3 (15.8)	9 (47.3)	7 (36.8)	19 (50)
GII	55 (29.4)	108 (57.8)	24 (12.8)	156 (42.9)
GIII	43 (28.7)	85 (56.7)	22 (14.6)	129 (43)
*AT1R A1166C**	*AA* (%)	*AC* (%)	*CC* (%)	*C* (%)
GI	6 (31.6)	6 (31.6)	7 (36.8)	16 (42.1)
G II	92 (49.2)	82 (43.9)	13 (8.0)	112 (29.9)
G III	72 (48.0)	64 (42.7)	14 (9.3)	92 (30.1)
CYP11B2	*CC* (%)	*TC* (%)	*TT* (%)	*C* (%)
GI	3 (15.8)	8 (42.1)	8 (42.1)	14 (36.8)
GII	25 (13.3)	84 (44.9)	78 (41.8)	134 (35.8)
GIII	19 (12.7)	67 (44.7)	64 (42.6)	105 (35.0)

*: Significant difference in genotype and allele frequencies of GIversus both G II and G III ($P<0.01$);

+: Significant difference in genotype frequencies of G I versus both G II and G III ($P<0.01$).

Table 2. Distributions of genotype and allele frequencies in each group.

(95% confidence interval [CI] 0.40-5.86) and the OR associated with the DD genotype was 5.34 (95% CI 1.27-22.42), indicating a recessive effect of the D allele on risk (Table 3). A similar situation was observed for the A1166C polymorphism in the AT1R gene. Taking AA genotype as a reference, the OR for SRAR associated with the AC genotype was 1.15 (95% CI 0.36-3.70) and that associated with the CC genotype was 8.34 (95% CI 2.43-28.69).

The OR associated with the combination of DD and CC genotypes versus all other combinations was 5.92 (95% CI 2.85-12.37), that is, very similar to the one observed in the separate analyses of these two polymorphisms (Table 3).

		OR	95% CI
ACE *I/D*	*ID* versus *II*	1.53	0.40-5.86
	DD versus *II*	5.34	1.27-22.42*
AT1R *A1166C*	*CC* versus *AA*	8.34	2.43-28.69*
	AC versus *AA*	1.15	0.36-3.70
ACE *I/D* and AT1R *A1166C*	*DD+CC* versus all other genotypes on two loci	5.92	2.85-12.37*

CI = confidence interval; OR = odds ratio. *: $P<0.05$.

Table 3. Odds rations for the presence of SRAR by ACE *I/D* and AT1R *A1166C*.

Malignant hypertension was companied with the AT1-AA mediated SRAR. We performed univariate analysis of the factors affecting SRAR to the overall group. The factors significantly associated with graft transplant failure were HLA mismatch >1 ($P > 0.05$). Among the nineteen recipients suffered SRAR, fourteen patients occurred malignant hypertension. In the detection of AT1R antibodies and DSA, the former were invariably positive in the malignant hypertension recipients and the DSA negative in their peripheral blood. While the rest 4 cases of SRAR recipients have the peripheral DSA and 1 case with neither AT1-AA nor DSA.

The demographic data from the 14 patients who were positive for AT1-receptor antibodies were compared with those for the 4 patients with donor-specific anti-HLA antibodies. As shown in Table 4, patients with anti-HLA antibodies were more likely to have staining for C4d in their renal biopsy specimens and had less rapid allograft loss. Otherwise, there were no significant differences in clinical or demographic characteristics between the two groups.

The biopsy specimens from patients with malignant hypertension and refractory rejection who had no donor-specific anti-HLA antibodies (stained with hematoxylin and eosin) showed the evidence of tubulitis and intravascular inflammatory cells. Interlobular arteries were obstructed by swollen endothelial cells which underwent necrosis and vacuolation. The smooth muscle cells proliferated and the intima thickened greatly. Inflammatory cells can be seen inside the vascular and segmental veinlets. The atrophied glomcrulus were divided into subsections. Tubules were expanded with red cell cast inside it. The peritubular capillaries were aggregated with polymorph nuclear leukocytes. Interstitium was infiltrated with inflammatory cells. The renal shows multiple perfusion defects and cortical infarctions (Figure 1).

Characteristic	AT1-Receptor Antibodies (n=14)	Anti-HLA Antibodies (n=4)
Male sex (n)	8	2
Cold-ischemia (h)		
Median	6.7	6.5
Range	2.4-18.5	2.2-19.1
No. of HLA mismatches		
Median	3	3
Range	0-3	1-5
PRA at transplantation (%)		
Median	5	6
Range	0-7	0-9
Age at transplantation (yr)		
Median	36.5	37.2
Range	19-49	20-48
Time from transplantation to rejections(days)		
Median	3	6
Range	2-360	3-351
C4d-positive (No.)*	3	4

*: $P<0.01$.

Table 4. Characteristics of patients with AT1-Receptor antibodies and patients with donor-specific anti-HLA antibodies but without AT1R-Receptor antibodies.

AT1-AA mediated SRAR was markedly associated with the prognosis of the renal transplant recipients. The occurrence of SRAR was analyzed for an association with the susceptibility to worsening renal graft function. A stable renal function was more often observed in recipients who did not suffered from SRAR than in GI. There was a striking effect of the SRAR and long-term stable graft function (Figure 2A), with more patients suffering from worsening renal function with the occurrence of SRAR (Kaplan-Meier, $P<0.05$). The analysis also discovered that the occurrence of SRAR is strongly associated with the appearance of the antibodies of AT1R. The χ^2 analysis revealed that the positive of AT1-AA is strongly related to the appearance of SRAR. We also noticed that the frequency of the AT1R-C allele and ACE D-allele is comparable in SRAR group. Patients with anti-HLA antibodies had substantially better graft survival than did those who had malignant hypertension but did not have anti-HLA antibodies (Figure 2B).

Treatment consisting of protein A immunoadsorption (IA), intravenous immune globulin, and 100 mg of losartan daily in nine patients with AT1R antibodies resulted in significantly improved allograft survival, as compared with that in patients receiving standard anti-rejection treatment (Figure 2C). Serum from four patients with the longest rejection-free follow-up (who are still receiving losartan) became negative for AT1-receptor antibodies.

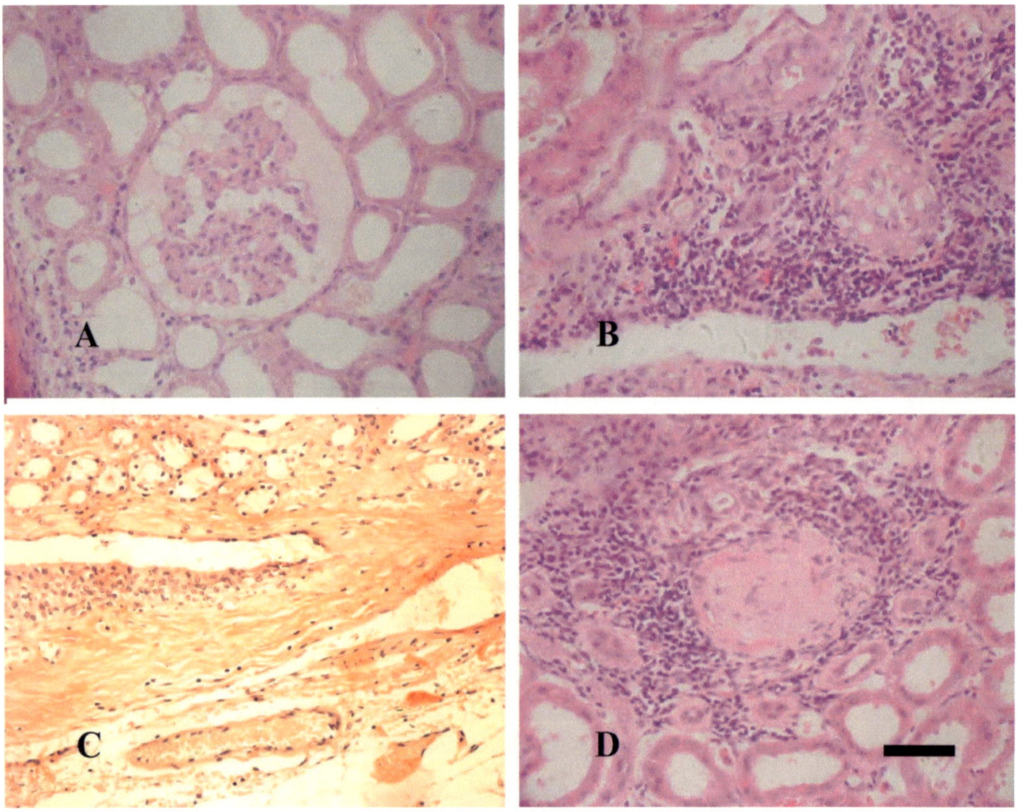

Fig. 1. Features of Refractory Rejection in Patients without Donor-Specific Anti-HLA Antibodies The biopsy specimens from representative patients showed the evidence of tubulitis and intravascular inflammatory cells. The atrophied glomcrulus were divided into subsections. Tubules were expanded with red cell cast inside it (Panel A). Inflammatory cells can be seen inside the vascular and segmental veinlets (Panel B). Interlobular arteries were obstructed by swollen endothelial cells which underwent necrosis and vacuolation. The smooth muscle cells proliferated and the intima thickened greatly. The peritubular capillaries were aggregated with polymorph nuclear leukocytes. Interstitium was infiltrated with inflammatory cells (Panel C and D).

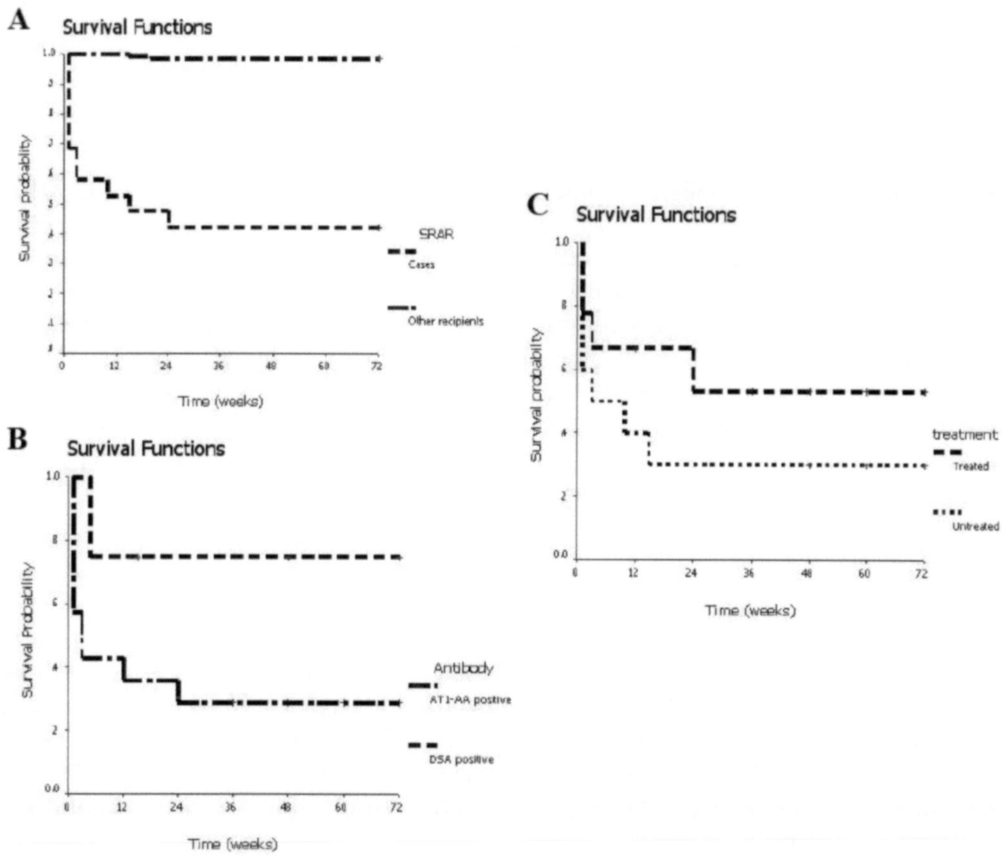

Fig. 2. Graft survival in the Kaplan–Meier analysis was significantly decreased in the patients with SRAR compared with those who did not suffered from it (Panel A). The graph in Panel B demonstrates accelerated allograft loss in patients who had refractory vascular rejection with non-HLA antibodies, compared with patients who had vascular rejection and donor-specific anti-HLA antibodies. Graft survival in the Kaplan–Meier analysis was significantly increased in the patients with AT1-receptor antibodies who received losartan and IA, as compared with those who received nonspecific treatment (Panel C).

4. Discussion

The factors leading to SRAR are not fully understood, but they consist of humoral immune response and genetic factors [20]. We studied the SNP of RAS and AT1R antibodies and DSA in patients, and tested C4d on their biopsy specimens. The findings of this study suggest an association of RAS polymorphism and the occurrence of SRAR in renal transplantation recipients. The single nucleotide polymorphism of RAS may be one of the non-immunologic mechanisms of the SRAR. Yet the appearance of autoantibody of AT1R may be one of the immunologic mechanisms of the occurrence of this type rejection. Our results support the hypothesis that there is an association between the occurrence of the SRAR and the appearance of the AT1-AA in recipients whose genotype of RAS performed certain polymorphism. The recipients with the DD genotype of ACE and CC genotype of AT1R may trend to suffer the AT1-AA mediated rejection. The process of the rejection may be improved by the application of ARB, coupled with protein A immunoadsorption and high dose intravenous immunoglobulin.

The outcome of the renal transplantation was improved obviously with the use of CsA and FK506. Methylprednisolone was widely used in preventing and treatment of acute rejection and most recipients benefit from it. But there are still some patients who are refractory to the steroid treatment. Most of them have the similar characteristics including anuria after transplantation, malignant hypertension and graft function loss. It has been proved that many diseases have their own genotype polymorphism backgrounds. Genes that affect blood pressure regulation, mesangial or vascular proliferation or aspects of inflammatory response may play important roles in this complex syndrome. Genes determining the activity of a recipient's renin–angiotensin system (RAS) may be alloantigen-independent factors that influence the kidney allograft function.

Investigation of the genetics, physiology, and pharmacotherapeutics of RAS and its regulators has made it one of the most intensely studied molecular pathways of human diseases. The RAS is implicated in the development of a variety of human disorders, including cardiovascular diseases [21]. Inhibition of this system has had proven benefits in reducing the risk of cardiovascular endpoints [22], diabetes, and end stage renal disease (ESRD) [23]. Genetic variability in the RAS may modify renal responses to injury and disease progression. It seems some differential group of recipients is destined to lose their grafts faster. Our study was designed to elucidate the relationship between genetic RAS polymorphisms namely ACE I/ D, AGT M235T, AT1R A1166C and CYP11B2 and SRAR in Chinese renal transplant recipients.

The angiotensin converting enzyme (ACE) gene displays an insertion/deletion polymorphism in intron 16, and homozygosity of the deletion allele is known to be associated with higher serum ACE levels [24]. The DD genotype of ACE gene is a risk factor for the progression of chronic renal failure in IgA nephropathy [25]. It has also been reported that patients with ACE (DD) and angiotensinogen AGT (TT) genotypes are linked to poorer long-term renal transplant function [26, 27]. Demonstrated survival benefits may be a result, in large measure, of the salutary effects of angiotensin converting enzyme (ACE) inhibition on the endothelium [28] and vascular smooth muscle cells [29]. A beneficial association of CAD progression in Caucasian pediatric renal transplant recipients with the II genotype and/or the presence of the I allele is also found [26, 30, 31]. Current evidence on the nature of the renal risk is associated with the D-allele, as also apparent from a large meta-analysis that addressed cardiovascular risk, indicates that the D-allele acts as a course-modifying gene rather than as a disease-inducing gene [32].

In the present study, the D allele of ACE is a risk factor for the development and progression of the SRAR while no significant relationship was found between ACE I/D polymorphism and CAD [33]. The result is in line with other studies that examined the effect of the ACE

I/D polymorphism on the progression of diabetic nephropathy [34], and the progression of chronic renal failure in immunoglobulin A nephropathy [35] and in adult polycystic kidney disease [36]. This effect of the D allele of ACE is also similar with the findings reported by Abdi *et al* [30] and Akc¸ay *et al.* [37] which found that ACE DD genotype was associated with poorer chronic transplant function and more rapid chronic progression. Some related results also have been reported by Barocci *et al.* [38] in pediatric transplant recipients and Gaciong *et al.* [39] in adult transplant recipients. Our data are consistent with these views. Thus, the presence of a D-allele does not appear to enhance renal risk in itself, but once a sequence of events leading to progressive renal function loss is initiated by whatever cause, its course is more rapid in presence of the D allele [40].

Angiotensin II has been proven to have growth factor-like and angiogenic activities [41] and these activities are mediated through the activation of the angiotensin type 1 receptor [42]. The AGT1R A1166C polymorphism was found to predict the systemic and renal response to angiotensin receptor antagonism and angiotensin II infusion in healthy subjects [43]. In the present study patients with the AGT1R C allele tended to have a worse preservation of graft function than patient homozygous for the A allele. Yet patients with the C allele exhibited a stronger response to losartan, showed a faster serum creatinine degression, and had a better response of the decent of the mean blood pressure compared with subjects homozygous for the AA allele, suggesting an increase in intrarenal angiotensin II activity with the AC/CC genotype. However, the treatment was neither randomly assigned nor blinded, and the numbers of patients are too small to permit us to draw firm conclusions. This would indicate that recipient AGT1R C allele may adversely affect renal outcome after kidney transplantation. Moreover, our data are in contrast with another report in which the C allele of AT1R dose not adversely affect renal response after transplantation [44]. However, we do not know the genotype of the donors because they were not genotyped. As the frequency of the A allele in the general population is high (71% in our patients), the probability of a recipient with the C allele receiving a kidney with the C allele is low. In the analysis of the results, the incidence of SRAR is very low (9.2%), the recipients with AT1-AA is even lower (6.8%). We suppose that the occurrence of SRAR may be based on the condition when the C recipient meets the C donor coincidently, and then the autoantibody of AT1-AA would be created in this group. Of course this is only an imagination need to be tested.

There are many polymorphisms in the AGT gene located on chromosome 1q42–q43. In exon 2, a nonsynonymous substitution of T by C in codon 235 of the AGT gene, leads to a change from Methionine to Threonine. In Caucasians, African and Japanese populations, the T235 variant of this M235T polymorphism of this gene has been consistently associated with higher levels of angiotensinogen in plasma and an increased risk for hypertension [45, 46, 47].

The primary regulation of aldosterone synthesis is via the renin-angiotensin system, which is responsive to the state of the electrolyte balance and plasma volume. The -344T/C polymorphism in the CYP11B2 promoter region, the steroidogenic factor-1 binding site, was reported to be associated with blood pressure or aldosterone secretion. Some investigators found a positive association between the -344T polymorphism in the CYP11B2 gene and essential hypertension. Our study suggests that the CYP11B2 gene promoter region polymorphism and AGT M235T is not directly associated with SRAR. Therefore, this polymorphism may not be a risk factor for the rejection or the malignant hypertension, at least not in the Chinese population. The lack of relationship between these two genotypes and early graft function in our study may indicate that other factors have major impacts in the setting of kidney transplantation.

We also examine the relationship between the given RAS polymorphism and the emergency of peripheral AT1-AA of the recipients. Draun *et al* reported that AT1-receptor–mediated pathway may contribute to refractory vascular rejection [48]. Our results revealed that the recipients with D allele of the ACE and the C allele of the AT1R are inclined to have the AT1-AA. This phenomenon can partly explain the fact that only small percent of recipients have SRAR.

Our report suggests that a SNP of the RAS component may contribute to the development of the steroid refractory acute rejection of kidney grafts. Individuals bearing D allele of ACE and C allele of AT1R may be sensitive to suffer steroid resistant acute rejection after renal transplantation. And the patients subjected to SRAR always produce AT1-AA. There is some statistical association between the appearance of AT1-AA and the D allele of ACE and C allele of AT1R. Patients with these types of antibodies have a less favorable prognosis, greater graft loss, and poorer long-term function as compared with patients with DSA alone. The treatment against such antibody mediated immune response is necessary and effective. We speculate the AT1-AA may have been produced when the subjects experienced preeclampsia or renal transplantation before or for other reasons. The importance of the detection of the genotype of ACE and AT1R and AT1-receptor antibodies in patients on a waiting list for a transplant might be comparable with the detection of PRA in identifying risk factors for refractory rejection.

5. Conflict of interest

The authors have declared that no conflict of interest exists.

6. Acknowledgments

We would like to give special thanks to Professor Yanfang Liu for his insightful pathological observations.

7. References

[1] Terasaki PI. Deduction of the fraction of immunologic and non-immunologic failure in cadaver donor transplants. *Clin Transp* 2003; 449-452

[2] H.Andreas Bock. 2001. Steroid-Resistant Kidney Transplant Rejection: Diagnosis and Treatment. *J Am Soc Nephrol*. 12: S48–S52

[3] Van Saase JL, van der Woude FJ, Thorogood J, van Saase JL, van der Woude FJ, Thorogood J, Hollander AA, van Es LA, Weening JJ, and van Bockel JH, *et al*. The relation between acute vascular and interstitial renal allograft rejection and subsequent chronic rejection. *Transplantation* 1995; 15:1280-1285.

[4] Opelz G, Wujciak T and Ritz E. Association of chronic kidney graft failure with recipient blood pressure. *Collaborative Transplant Study. Kidney Int* 1998; 53: 217-222.

[5] Mange KC, Cizman B, Joffe M and Feldman HI. Arterial hypertension and renal allograft survival. *JAMA* 2000; 283: 633-638

[6] Guidi E, Cozzi MG, Minetti E and Bianchi G. Donor and recipient family histories of hypertension influence renal impairment and blood pressure during acute rejections. *J Am Soc Nephrol* 1998; 9: 2102-2107

[7] Volpe M, Musumeci B, De Paolis P, Savoia C and Morganti A. Angiotensin II AT2 receptor subtype: an uprising frontier in cardiovascular disease? *J Hypertens* 2003; 21:1429–1443

[8] Fellstrom B. Nonimmune risk factor for chronic allograft dysfunction. *Transplantation* 2001; 71:10-16 [suppl.]

[9] Diez J, Laviades C, Orbe J, Zalba G, Lopez B, Gonzalez A, Mayor G, Paramo JA, and Beloqui O. The A1166C polymorphism of the AT1 receptor gene is associated with collagen type I synthesis and myocardial stiffness in hypertensives. *J Hypertens* 2003; 21:2085–2092.

[10] Dragun D, Bräsen JH, C. Schönemann, L. Fritsche, K. Budde, H.-H. Neumayer, F.C. Luft, and G. Wallukat. Patients with steroid refractory acute vascular rejection develop agonistic antibodies targeting angiotensin II type 1 receptor. *Transplant Proc* 2003;35:2104-2105

[11] Nataraj C, Oliverio M, Mannon RB, Mannon PJ, Audoly LP, Amuchastegui CS, Ruiz P, Smithies O, Coffman TM. Angiotensin II regulates cellular immune responses through a calcineurin-dependent pathway. *J Clin Invest* 1999; 104:1693-1701

[12] Bohmig GA, Exner M, Habicht A, Schillinger M, Lang U, Kletzmayr J, Saemann MD, Horl WH, Watschinger B, and Regele H. Capillary C4d deposition in kidney allografts: a specific marker of alloantibodydependent graft injury. *J Am Soc Nephrol* 2002; 13:1091-1099

[13] Regele H, Exner M, Watschinger B, Wenter C, Wahrmann M, Osterreicher C, Saemann MD, Mersich N, Horl WH, and Zlabinger GJ *et al.* Endothelial C4d deposition is associated with inferior kidney allograft outcome inden pendently of cellular rejection. *Nephrol Dial Transplan* 2001; 16: 2058-2066

[14] Rigat B, Hubert C, Corvol P and Soubrier F. PCR detection of the insertion/deletion polymorphism of the human angiotensin converting enzyme gene. *Nucleic Acids Res* 1992; 20:1433

[15] Lovati E, Richard A, Frey BM, Frey FJ, and Ferrari P. Genetic polymorphisms of the renin-angiotensin-aldosterone system in end-stage renal disease. *Kidney Int* 2001; 60: 46

[16] Nicod J, Richard A, Frey FJ and Ferrari P. Recipient RAS gene variants and renal allograft function. *Transplantation* 2002; 73:960-965

[17] Brand E, Chatelain N, Mulatero P, Fery I, Curnow K, Jeunemaitre X, Corvol P, Pascoe L, and Soubrier F. Structural analysis and evaluation of the aldosterone synthase gene in human hypertension. *Hypertension* 1998; 32:198– 204

[18] Matsui S, Fu M L, Katsuda S, Hayase M, Yamaguchi N, Teraoka K, Kurihara T, Takekoshi N, Murakami E, and Hoebeke J *et al.* Peptides derived from cardiovascular G-protein-coupled receptors induce morphological cardiomyopathic changes in immunized rabbits. *J Mol Cell Cardiol* 1997; 29: 641-655

[19] Liao YH, Wei YM, Wang M, Wang ZH, Yuan HT, and Cheng LX. Autoantibodies against AT1receptor and Alphal–adrenergic receptor in patients with hypertension. *Hypertens Res* 2002; 25: 641 - 646.

[20] Cai J and Terasaki PI. Humoral theory of transplantation: mechanism, prevention, and treatment. *Hum Immunol* 2005; 66: 334-342.

[21] Li DY, Zhang YC, Philips MI, Sawamura T, and Mehta. Upregulation of endothelial receptor for oxidized low-density lipoprotein (LOX-1) in cultured human coronary artery endothelial cells by angiotensin II type 1 receptor activation. *Circ Res* 1999; 84:1043–1049

[22] Kjeldsen SE and Julius S. 2004. Hypertension mega-trials with cardiovascular end points: effect of angiotensin-converting enzyme inhibitors and angiotensin receptor blockers. *Am Heart J.* 148:747–754

[23] Brenner BM, Cooper ME, de Zeeuw D, Keane WF, Mitch WE, Parving HH, Remuzzi G, Snapinn SM, Zhang Z, and Shahinfar S. 2001. Effects of losartan on renal and cardiovascular outcomes in patients with type 2 diabetes and nephropathy. *N Engl J Med*, 345:861–869

[24] Mondy A, Loh M, Liu P, LinZhu A, and Nagel M. 2005. Polymorphisms of the insertion/deletion ACE and M235T AGT genes and hypertension: surprising new findings and meta-analysis of data. *BMC Nephrol.* 6:1- 11

[25] Di Paolo S, Schena A, Stallone G, Curello G, D'Altri C, Gesualdo L, and Schena FP. Angiotensin converting enzyme gene polymorphism in renal transplant patients with IgA nephropathy: relationship with graft function and prevalence of hypertension. *Transplant Proc* 1999; 31: 869- 872

[26] Filler G, Yang F, Martin A, Stolpe J, Neumayer HH, and Hocher B. Renin angiotensin system gene polymorphism in pediatric renal transplant recipients. *Pediatr Transplant* 2001; 5:166 -173

[27] Viklicky O, Hubacek J, Pitha J, Lacha J, Teplan V, Heemann UW, Lacha J, Vitko S. ACE gene polymorphism and long term renal graft function. *Clin Biochem* 2001; 34: 87 - 90

[28] Nadar S, Blann AD and Lip GY. Antihypertensive therapy and endothelial function. *Curr Pharm Des* 2004; 10:3607–3614

[29] Jaffe IZ, and Mendelsohn ME. Angiotensin II and aldosterone regulate gene transcription via functional mineralocortocoid receptors in human coronary artery smooth muscle cells. *Circ Res* 2005; 96:643–650

[30] Abdi R, Tran TB, Zee R, Brenner BM, and Milford EL. Angiotensin gene polymorphism as a determinant of posttransplantation renal dysfunction and hypertension. *Transplantation* 2001; 72:726–732

[31] Nicod J, Richard A, Frey FJ, and Ferrari P. Recipient RAS gene variants and renal allograft function. *Transplantation* 2002; 73:960- 962

[32] Navis OJ, de long PE, and de Zeeuw D. Insertion/deletion polymorphism of the angiotensin converting enzyme gene: A clue to heterogeneity of renal prognosis and renal response to therapy? *Nephrol Dial Transplant* 1997; 12: 1097-1100.

[33] James B, Wetmore, Kirsten L. Johansen, Saunak Sen, Adriana M. Hung, and David H. Lovett. An angiotensin converting enzyme haplotype predicts survival in patients with end stage renal disease. *Hum Genet* 2006; 120:201–210

[34] Hadjadj S, Belloum R, Bouhanick B, Gallois Y, Guilloteau G, Chatellier G, Alhenc-Gelas F, Marre M. Pronostic value of angiotensin I-converting enzyme I/D polymorphism for nephropathy in type 1 Diabetes Mellitus: a prospective study. *J Am Soc Nephrol* 2001; 12:541–549

[35] Frimat L, Philippe C, Maghakian MN, Jouveaux P, Hurault de Ligny B, Guillemin F, Kessler M. Polymorphism of angiotensin converting enzyme, angiotensinogen and angiotensin II type 1 receptor genes and end-stage renal failure in IgA nephropathy: IGARAS—A study of274 men. *J Am Soc Nephrol* 2000; 11: 2062-2067

[36] Crisan D, and Carr J. Angiotensin I-converting enzyme genotype and disease associations. *J Mol Diagn* 2000; 2:105–115

[37] Akcay A, Sezer S, Ozdemir FN, Arat Z, Atac¸ FB, Verdi H, Colak T, Haberal M. Association of the genetic polymorphisms of the renin– angiotensin system and endothelial nitric oxide synthase with chronic renal transplant dysfunction. *Transplantation* 2004; 27: 892 –898

[38] Barocci S, Ginevri F, Valente U, Torre F, Gusmano R, and Nocera A. Correlation between angiotensin converting-enzyme gene insertion/deletion polymorphism and kidney graft long-term outcome in pediatric recipients. *Transplantation* 1999; 67: 534–542

[39] Gaciong ZA, Religa P, Placha G, Rell K, and Paczek L. Ace genotype and progression of IgA Nephropathy. *Lancet* 1995; 346:570– 572

[40] JAN BROEKROELOFS, COEN A., and STEGEMAN. Risk Factors for Long-Term Renal Survival after Renal Transplantation: A Role for Angiotensin-Converting Enzyme (Insertion/Deletion) Polymorphism? *J Am Soc Nephrol* 1998; 9: 2075-2081

[41] Greco S, Muscella A, Elia MG, Salvatore P, Storelli C, and Marsigliante S. Activation of angiotensin II type I receptor promotes protein kinase C translocation and cell proliferation in human cultured breast epithelial cells. *J Endocrinol* 2002; 174:205–214

[42] Greco S, Muscella A, Elia MG, Salvatore P, Storelli C, Mazzotta A, Manca C, and Marsigliante S. Angiotensin II activates extracellular signal regulated kinases via protein kinase C and epidermal growth factor receptor in breast cancer cells. *J Cell Physiol* 2003; 196: 370–377

[43] Miller JA, Thai K, and Scholey JW. Angiotensin II type 1 receptor gene polymorphism predicts response to losartan and angiotensin II. *Kidney Int* 1999; 56: 2173-2180

[44] Hilgers KF, Langenfeld MR, Schlaich M, Veelken R, and Schmieder RE. 1166 A/C polymorphism of the angiotensin II type 1 receptor gene and the response to short-term infusion of angiotensin II. *Circulation* 1999; 100(13): 1394-1399

[45] Celerier J, Cruz A, Lamande N, Gasc JM, and Corvol P. Angiotensinogen and its cleaved derivatives inhibit angiogenesis. *Hypertension* 2002; 39: 224–228

[46] Ward K, Hata A, Jeunemaitre X, Helin C, Nelson L, Namikawa C, Farrington PF, Ogasawara M, Suzumori K, and Tomoda S, *et al*. A molecular variant of angiotensinogen associated with preeclampsia. *Nat Genet* 1993; 4: 59–61

[47] Jeunemaitre X, Soubrier F, Kotelevtsev YV, Lifton RP, Williams CS, Charru A, Hunt SC, Hopkins PN, Williams RR, Lalouel JM, *et al.* Molecular basis of human hypertension: role of angiotensinogen. *Cell* 1992; 71:169–180

[48] Duska Dragun, Dominik N. Müller, Jan Hinrich Bräsen, Lutz Fritsche, Melina Nieminen-Kelhä, Ralf Dechend, Ulrich Kintscher, Birgit Rudolph, Johan Hoebeke, and Diana Eckert, *et al.* Angiotensin II type I–receptor activating antibodies in renal-allograft rejection. *N Engl J Med* 2005; 352: 558-569

8

Soluble CD30 and Acute Renal Allograft Rejection

Koosha Kamali[1], Mohammad Amin Abbasi[2], Ata Abbasi[3] and Alireza R. Rezaie[4]
[1]Hasheminezhad hospital, Department of urology, Tehran University of medical science, Tehran
[2]Department of Internal Medicine, Shahid Beheshti University of Medical Sciences, Tehran
[3]Pathology department, Faculty of Medicine, Tehran University of medical science, Tehran
[4]Department of Biochemistry and Molecular Biology, Saint Louis University School of Medicine, Saint Louis, MO
[1,2,3]Iran
[4]United States of America

1. Introduction

1.1 Renal transplantation

Renal transplantation is the treatment of choice for most patients with end-stage renal diseases (ESRD). Patients usually undergo transplantation after a variable period of dialysis.

Recently, due to development of standard surgical techniques and improvement in post transplantation care such as organ preservation, immunosuppressive and antimicrobial agents graft and patient outcome has significantly improved. The recognition of anti-donor-HLA antibodies in a renal allograft recipient's serum, at the time of or after transplantation, is usually correlated with specific antibody-mediated clinical syndromes which can be categorized into three groups such as hyperacute rejection, acute humoral rejection and chronic humoral rejection. Allograft rejection is caused by several component of the immune system; consist of antibody, complement, T cells and other cell types. The mechanisms of pathways of acute rejection are being determined and the consequences of immune rejection are identified by graft dysfunction and classified by histological features of allograft biopsy specimens (Solez et al., 2008).

1.2 Hyperacute rejection

Hyperacute rejection occurs within 24 hours of reperfusion and is characterized by immediate loss of graft function resulting abrupt cessation of urine flow. Hyperacute rejection might be either diagnosed clinically by the surgeon with mottling cyanosis and reduced turgor in the graft or by a histopathologic feature of interstitial hemorrhage, microthrombosis and inflammation (neutrophils and fibrin infiltration) of the failed allografts which might be qualitatively similar to those seen in acute antibody mediated rejection (AMR). Hyperacute rejection is generally considered to be mediated by humoral immutnity (Baid S e al., 2001). Immunofluorescence (IF) studies demonstrated IgG (but not IgM) in glomerular and peritubular capillaries The pathogenesis of hyperacute rejection depends on the activation of complement activated through any pathway (classical, alternative, or lectin) can initiate hyperacute rejection regardless of how complement is activated (Chang A.T and Platt J.L. 2009). Hyperacute rejection of clinical allografts is most often caused by anti-HLA antibodies which bind to blood vessels and activate the complement system in a newly transplanted organ. Hyperacute rejection is observed in up to 80% of the kidneys transplanted into recipients with cytotoxic antibodies detected by cytotoxic cross match (Patel R and Terasaki PI, 1969). Hyperacute rejection is more common in allogarfts with these antibodies compared with ABO-incompatible renal transplants. Hyperacute rejection can also occur independent of anti-donor antibodies and these cases may reflect activation of the alternative or lectin pathways as might occur with ischemic injury (Chang A.T and Platt J.L, 2009).

Hyperacute rejection may occur in some recipients appearing to lack anti-donor antibodies. In some cases antibody capable of binding to and injuring the graft may be present but is not detected by assays in which leukocytes are used as the target. Fortunately, with the serologic technologies and expertise now available, hyperacute rejection has become an extremely rare occurrence.

1.3 Acute rejection

Acute rejection episodes (ARE) typically develop after transplantation at any time after organ transplantation and are divided histopathologically in to two categories: interstitial and vascular (Fig 1). A key clinical sign of acute rejection is a baseline rise in serum creatinine of 25% in the asymptomatic patient with no other apparent explanation. Novel immunosuppressive drugs and regimens have decreased the incidence of acute rejection occurrence, however, acute rejection (AR) is still a major risk of early graft dysfunction and late kidney graft loss (kamali et al., 2009). Despite the introduction of successful immunosuppressive drug therapies, acute renal allograft rejection still occurs in 10–20% of patients after cadaveric renal transplantation and causes graft loss in up to 6% in the first year after transplantation (Magee, Pascual., 2004). The early phase of diagnosis of acute allograft rejection might help clinicians to perform required procedures to prevent undesirable posttransplant complications (kamali et al., 2009).

1.3.1 Acute interstitial allograft rejection

Also termed acute cellular rejection or acute reversible rejection is characterized by an infiltration of inflammatory cells (mainly of CD8 T lymphocytes) in the interstitium, and tubular epithelium involvement named tubulitis (Racusen LC et al. 1999). Tubulitis has been regarded as a reliable marker for acute rejection even though it can be seen in other forms of interstitial nephritis (Colvin., 1996). The infiltrate is more concentrated in the cortex than in the renal medulla. Rejection that is predominantly cellular is considered to be readily reversible with therapy.

1.3.2 Acute vascular rejection

Acute vascular rejection is called as acute humoral rejection contains the most severe changes in the small arteries, veins, and arterioles. Humoral antibodies may cause tissue injury or organ dysfunction by themselves or in collaboration with immunocompotent cells (Fig2) (Lederer S.R et al, 2001). The diagnostic criteria for acute humoral rejection are given in Table 1.

1. Morphologic evidence of acute tissue injury acute tubular injury neutrophils and/or mononuclear cells in PTC and/or glomeruli and/or capillary thrombosis fibrinoid necrosis/intramural or transmural inflammation in arteries
2. Immunopathologic evidence for antibody action C4d and/or (rarely) immunoglobulin in PTC Ig and complement in arterial fibrinoid necrosis
3. Serologic evidence of circulating antibodies to donor HLA or other anti-donor endothelial antigen

*Cases that meet only two of the three numbered criteria are considered suspicious for acute humeral rejection (AHR). Acute cellular rejection may also be present.

Table 1. Diagnostic criteria for acute antibody-mediated rejection (adapted from Lorraine et al., 2006)*

It is emphasized that humoral immune reactions soon after transplantation had a much stronger impact than alloreactivity during later periods. Occurrence of delayed graft function (DGF) was assumed as long-term consequences of alloreactivity events early after transplantation (Ojo et a.l, 1997). Humoral reactions late after transplantation that are clearly detectable in serum and biopsy samples obviously do not significantly reduce graft survival (Lederer et al., 2001). In renal allograft recipients who experienced acute humoral rejection, donor-specific circulating alloantibody showed a sensitivity and specificity of 95% and 96% respectively (Feucht HE et al, 1991). Crespo and colleagues reported an acute rejection prevalence of 6.3% among 232 transplanted patients, two thirds of whom were steroid resistant (Crespo et a.l, 1999). Acute humoral rejection refractory to steroids and polyclonal antibodies leads to a 70% to 80% rate of graft loss (Watschinger B, Pascual M, 2002). The earliest morphologic characteristics of acute vascular rejection are swelling and vacuolization of the endothelial cells with areas of ulceration. Graft survival among patients with acute humoral rejection and without specific therapy is poor but novel treatment modalities of acute humoral rejection has saved some grafts (Watschinger B, Pascual M, 2002). Acute humoral rejection therapy seeks to remove circulating antibodies through plasmapheresis or immunabsorption and to inhibit B-cell proliferation using mycophenolate. Acute humoral rejection requires different therapy than cell-mediated rejection. Therapy for Acute humoral rejection is plasmapheresis and intravenous Ig combined with intense immunosuppression (typically tacrolimus and mycophenolate mofetil). In analysis of 113 renal allograft recipients by Péfaur J. et al, the recipients received high doses of IVIG (2 g/kg in five doses; two also received plasmapheresis or thymoglobulin). Mycophenolate, tacrolimus, and steroids were used as maintenance immunosuppressive therapy. Patient and graft survivals were 100% (abapted from Péfaur J. et al, 2008).

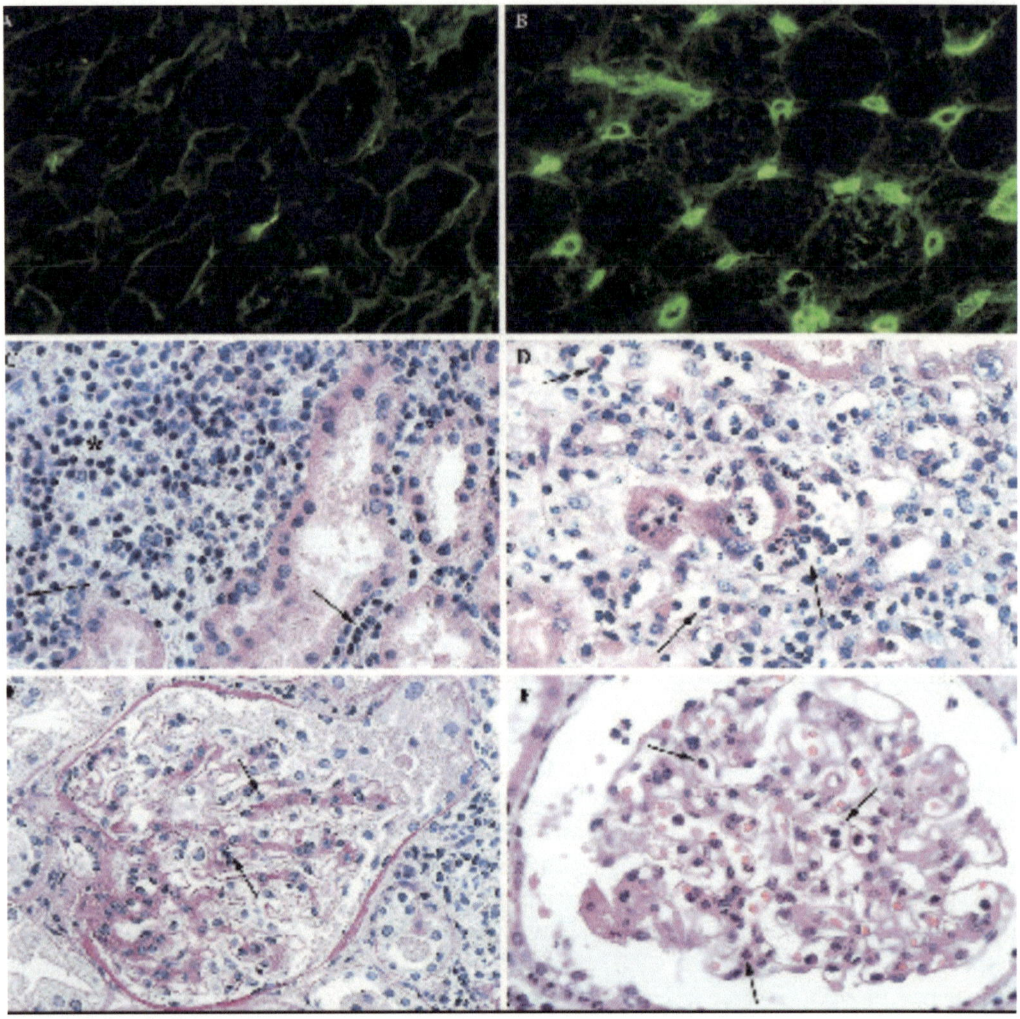

Fig. 1. (A) Acute cellular rejection (ACR): no staining for C4d is seen in peritubular capillaries. (B) Acute humoral rejection (AHR): widespread and bright staining for C4d is present in the peritubular capillaries that are interspersed in between the silhouettes of tubules. (C) ACR: mononuclear cells are present in the interstitium (*) and in peritubular capillaries (arrows). (D) AHR: abundant neutrophils are present in dilated peritubular capillaries (arrows). (E) ACR: scattered mononuclear cells are present in glomerular capillaries (arrows). (F) AHR: neutrophils are present in glomerular capillaries (arrows). Staining: C4d-FITC in A and B; Hematoxylin and eosin (H&E) in C, D, and F; and periodic acid-Schiff (PAS) in E. Magnifications: _400 in A through D; _450 in E and F. (adapted from Saadi et al. 2004)

1.4 Antibody-mediated rejection

As novel immunosuppressive protocols had effective control of T cell mediated acute rejection, antibody-mediated rejection (AMR) of renal allograft has re-emerged as an important post-transplant complication.The complement system plays an important role in antibody mediated rejection (AMR) via classical pathway activation. Antibody-mediated rejection is characterized pathologically by focal ischemia, severe injury to the endothelial cells lining blood vessels in the graft and diffuse intravascular coagulation .

Expression of anticoagulant molecules (thrombomodulin and heparan sulfate) from normal endothelial cells inhibit coagulation process (Miyata Y and Platt JL). Activated endothelial cells promote coagulation and inflammation which induce expression of cell adhesion molecules and cytokines (Saadi et al. 2004)

1.5 Delayed graft function (DGF)

Delayed graft function (DGF) and acute rejection are the two main early adverse events in renal transplantation. Historically, DGF was defined by the requirement for dialysis within the first week of renal transplantation. The rate of DGF varies between among different centers from 20 to 40% (Koning OH et al ,1997). The incidence of DGF was 20% to 29% among deceased donor kidneys and 6% among living donor kidneys (Halloran and Hunsicker, 2001). Investigation of 689 allograft renal transplants form HLA-mismatched unrelated living donors revealed the incidence of DGF was 7.7%, which was higher than reports with HLA-matched living related donors (Ghods AJ et al, 2007). Many pathological findings are associated with DGF, the most common being acute tubular necrosis. Typical histological findings of DGF are dilatation of tubules, loss of proximal epithelial cell brush border, epithelial cell necrosis/apoptosis, and cellular casts (Smith KD et al , 2003). The impact of DGF on long-term graft survival is controversial. Some, though not all, evidence suggests that DGF may increase the frequency of acute rejection and thus reduce long-term survival. Univariate and multivariate analyses showed that DGF significantly reduced the survival rate and half-life of renal grafts. Troppmann et al. Found that only if DGF and early acute rejection co-existed would DGF be one of the risk factors that reduced the long-term survival rate of recipient kidney (Troppmann C et al. 1996). The early inflammatory response is initiated by ischemia/reperfusion, activation of innate immunity and subsequent alloantigen-primed T cell recruitment, activation and proliferative expansion. DGF is also thought to up regulate MHC class II antigens, thus predisposing the transplanted graft to an increased incidence of acute rejection, which can be recognized histologically by the presence of tubulitis and infiltration of leukocytes into the tubular epithelium (Daily P et al, 2005). However, there are also reports showing that DGF played a greater role as a risk factor than acute rejection and HLA mismatch, and that DGF affected renal graft survival by increasing acute rejection and the chronic rejection rate, and decreased the survival rate of renal graft independent of acute rejection (Geddes CC et al. 2002). Aquino-Dias and associations have extended the diagnostic accuracy of mRNA profiles in recipients with DGF (Aquino-Dias EC. et al, 2008). Peripheral blood cell levels of TIM-3 mRNA are suspected to predict acute rejection in renal allograft recipients with DGF with a sensitivity of 100% and a specificity of 100% (Manfro RC et al, 2008). The main modality in management of DGF is to support the patient with dialysis and to monitor for rejection with serial biopsies.

At engraftment, ischemia-reperfusion injury occurs with activation of Toll-like receptors of the innate immune system and subsequent cytokine release. These pro-inflammatory mediators induce tubular epithelial cells to attract neutrophils and T cells by production of

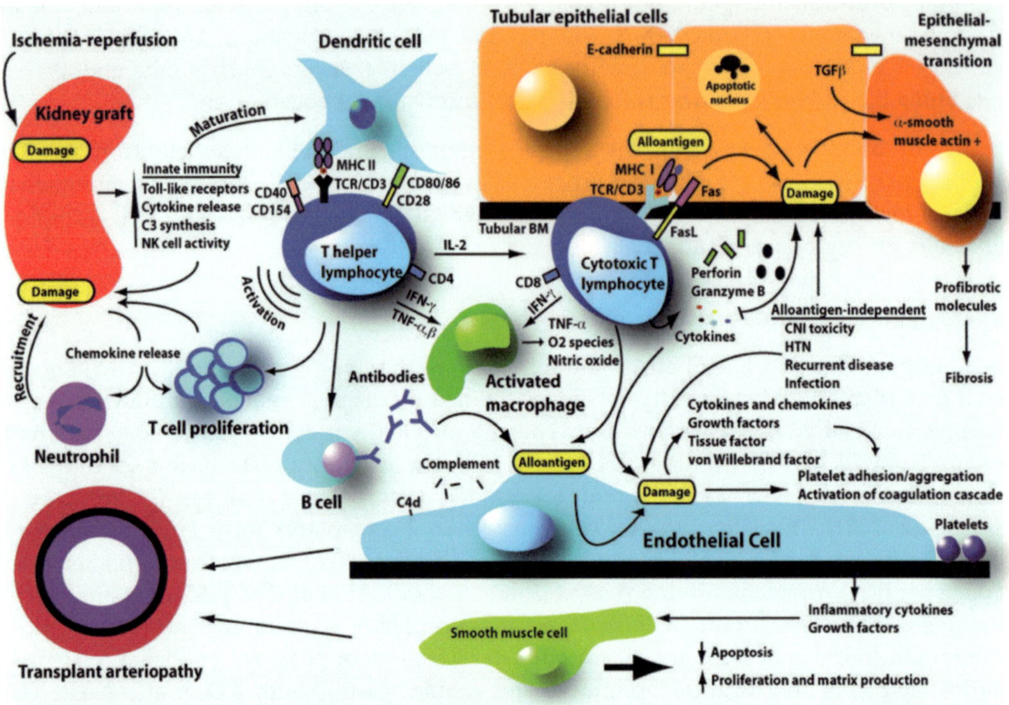

Fig. 2. Diagram of postulated events leading to graft damage during kidney transplantation (Adapted from Womer K.L. and Kaplan B, 2009).

chemokines. Innate immune system activation induces maturation of dendritic cells, leading the transition to the adaptive or antigen-specific phase of transplantation immunity. Dendritic cells activate CD4+ T helper cells through presentation of alloantigen in the context of major histocompatibility complex (MHC) molecules and ligation of appropriate T cell surface costimulatory molecules. After activation, CD4+ T helper cells induce further T cell proliferation, the production of alloantibodies from B cells, activation of macrophages, and differentiation of naïve CD8+ T cells into cytotoxic T lymphocytes. Mononuclear cells, especially cytotoxic T lymphocytes, enter between tubular cells and induce apoptosis by releasing cytolytic granules containing perforin and granzyme or by exposure to FasL on the T cell surface. Tubular cells chronically exposed to transforming growth factor β (TGFβ) may undergo epithelial-mesenchymal transition, an aberrant phenotype evidenced by epithelial cell expression of α-smooth muscle actin and loss of E-cadherin expression. These cells then may migrate to the interstitium and contribute to fibrosis. Both T cells and antibody likely recognize alloantigen on target endothelium. While T cells may cause cytotoxicity directly, alloantibody is usually directed against the MHC molecule, followed by activation of complement. Antigen recognition leads to endothelial secretion of factors that activate the immune and coagulation systems. These activities promote rejection and chronic changes of the endothelium and underlying smooth muscle layer, resulting in the characteristic histopathologic findings of transplant arteriopathy. Alloantigen-independent factors also contribute to tubular and endothelial cell damage.

2. HLA matching

The human leukocyte antigen system (HLA) is the name of the major histocompatibility complex (MHC) which contains a large number of genes related to immune system function in humans. This group of genes resides on chromosome 6 and encodes cell-surface antigen-presenting proteins and many other proteins. HLA antigens on the cell membrane play an important role in the immune response to foreign tissue (Muczynski KA et al. 2003). HLA complex is highly polymorphous (Marsh SG et al. 2002). Thus it is difficult to identify none-mismatched donors with only limited samples. In order to increase the matching rates, HLA typing has been recommended supported by the public epitope theory. MHC molecules are divided into 2 main classes: HLA class I antigens (HLA-A, HLA-B, HLA-C) are presented on the surface of all nucleated cells and platelets and HLA class II antigens (HLA-DR, HLA-DQ, HLA-DP, HLA-DM, HLA-DO) are expressed on professional antigen-presenting cells, but also on the surface of endothelial vascular cells and renal tubular epithelial cells (Muczynski KA et al. 2003). Human capillary endothelial cells, in contrast to rodents, express both human lymphocyte antigen (HLA) class I and class II molecules with high density even under normal physiological conditions (McDouall RM. et al, 1997). Cytotoxic antibodies (anti-HLA) are not detectable normally but after the blood/plasma transfusion, in pregnancy or after a previous transplant. When these antibodies are directed against HLA system of transplanted organ, their targets are represented by the graft endothelial cells which is followed by activation of complement, coagulation cascade and other inflammation factors. This mechanism mediated by anti-HLA antibodies is called humoral rejection (hyperacute rejection) that results in severe injury of endothelial cells and dysfunction of the transplanted organ (Moise A et al 2010). The first clinical importance of anti-HLA antibodies was demonstrated in 1969 (Patel R and Terasaki PI. 1969). Now it is known that the recipients who present preformed cytotoxic antibodies have a high rate of graft rejection. Production of antibodies after transplantation remains the main factor of acute and chronic rejections. Sometimes, antibody-mediated rejection (AMR) is still inevitable in human leukocyte antigen (HLA)-identical donor-recipient transplants (Zou Y and Stastny P, 2009). Antibody sensitization to alloantigens of the HLA system is one of the greatest barriers in successful renal transplantation (Zou YZ et al. 2007). Moise and colleagues reported that in both, compatible and incompatible subjects, post-renal transplantation could develop de novo anti-HLA antibodies especially those had an HLA mismatch with donor predictable for acute graft rejection (Moise A et al 2010). HLA-I antigens can be identified on nucleated cells, including on the endothelia of small renal vessels. Anti-HLA-I Ig G antibodies can injure the small vascular endothelia of the graft and induce serious rejections such as HR (Halloran PF et al 1990, 1992). HLA-II antigens are mainly expressed by immune cells. It is previously accepted that HLA-II antibodies have a relatively minor impact on the early graft outcome, despite a few cases reported with a higher rejection rate and humoral rejections occurrence due to HLA-II antibodies. A large-scale multi-center clinical study illustrated that graft survival rate at two or three years was decreased in recipients with both HLA-I and HLA-II antibodies, this was lower in recipients with more than three mismatched HLA alleles (Susal C and Opelz G. 2004). However, no significant difference was found in recipients with HLA-II antibodies compared with unsensitized patients. It is suggested that ELISA detected development of HLA antibodies, especially HLA-I antibodies, in the post-transplant period may provide a good predictor of acute rejection and of graft survival. Besides according to tissue inflammation and repair mechanisms inflicted by anti-HLA antibodies results in exposure of self antigens which lead to post-transplant autoimmunity. Detection of immune responses to self-antigens will provide new strategies to monitor and prevent development of late graft dysfunction (Natha DS. et al, 2010).

3. Immunologic factors in renal transplantation

A major challenge for the field of transplantation is the lack of understanding of molecular mechanisms of immune response early after transplantation. The association between the presence of donor specific antibodies (DSA) and acute rejection has been noted in the late 1970s (Hartono C et al. 2010). Complement proteins have been described to play a significant role in organ damage following transplantation both in the process of ischemia reperfusion and in modulating the activation of the adaptive immune response. Based on the knowledge alloreactive T cells are key mediators of transplant injury (Dinavahi R. et al, 2008). It has become clear that the type of specific immune response to offending agents is largely dependent on the preferential activation of peculiar CD41 T helper (Th) cells able to secrete defined patterns of cytokines. Two distinct CD41 T helper cell subsets, coded as Th_1 and Th_2, showing distinct and mutually exclusive patterns of cytokine secretion, have been identified in both mice and humans (Romagnani S. et al, 1995). Significant efforts have been carried out to demonstrate methodologies that reliably measure cellular alloimmunity, and in determining the utility of these approaches as biomarkers for acute rejection, biopsy proven fibrosis and impaired allograft function. Traditional methods of measuring T cell alloreactivity include proliferation and cytotoxicity assays, performed either on bulk cultures (mixed lymphocyte responses) or as limiting dilution assays. While these methods are accepted as useful research tools, their intensive labor requirements and limited reproducibility have prevented them from becoming standardized clinical tests (Dinavahi R. et al, 2008).

4. Serum markers of allograft dysfunction

Identification of serum markers or parameters before and after transplantation of recipients assuming increased risk of allograft rejection helps clinicians for a successful performance in individualization of immunosuppression therapeutic regimens and ensures a more adequate follow-up of these patients (Rouschop KM et al, 2005). High dose immunosuppression should be avoided at least for low-risk recipients due to the massive side effects such as cancer development, infection and toxicity. For example, Aggressive immunosuppression may reactivate polyoma BK virus, which is usually latent in the urinary tract. Few biologic assays that might be potentially useful for monitoring the immune status of renal graft recipients have been reported (Susal C et al. 2003). Some reports have elucidated that a number of acute-phase reactants, such as C-reactive protein (Oyen O et al, 2001) and pro-inflammatory cytokinesn (IL-6), have been associated with allograft rejection (Waiser J et al, 1997), although their usefulness also has been debated (Cueto-Manzano et al, 2005). It is noted that IL-17 may be involved early alloimmune response during the course of acute rejection. IL-17 may play the role of an early initiator of the T cell-dependent inflammatory reaction. Human IL-17, a new cytokine secreted from CD4+ activated memory T cells, can stimulate the production of proinflammatory and haematopoietic cytokines by macrophages and stromal cells (Fossiez F et al, 1996). Immunofluorescence has shown the expression of IL-17 in kidney biopsies from patients suffering from graft rejection, while pretransplant biopsies and normal kidneys were negative. Recently, monocyte-associated IL-18 has been suggested to be a pertinent biomarker in keeping with growing interest in monocyte infiltration during rejection. Striz *et al.* also observed a significant increase in serum IL-18 levels in patients with acute renal allograft rejection, compared with patients with uncomplicated transplantation, and further showed that IL-18 mRNA was released in response to increased TNF-_ and IFN-_ production (Striz I et al, 2005). Another complement component which has important role in organ transplantation is CD55, which is also called Decay Accelerating Factor (DAF). This molecule is present on the cell surface e where it accelerates the decay of C3 and C5 convertases from the classic and alternative pathway of complement to prevent their amplification and self-damaging effect on cells (Medof ME. et al, 1984). Early post-transplant acute rejection and infection are major causes of morbidity and mortality, whereas, lack of full rehabilitation, drug toxicity, chronic rejection and malignancies constitute debilitating the long-term complications. All problems described above may be (directly or indirectly) related to the lack of easy and feasible immunological tests for predicting the risk of rejection and recognizing ongoing rejections after transplantation as early as possible. (Truong DQ. et al, 2007). It has long been a goal of transplant immunologists to develop tests for assessing the pretransplant risk of patients for immunologic rejection and for recognizing impending rejections after transplantation as early as possible (Susal C. al, 2004).

5. Soluble CD30 (sCD30)

In addition to cytokines, other relevant proteins have been studied. Soluble CD30 (sCD30), a member of the TNF receptor superfamily that is a 120 kD membrane glycoprotein and expressed on Th2 cells, may be useful. (Serum levels of sCD30 are associated with disease activity of Th2-type cells and with disease remission in Th1-mediated disease states. Although the role of Th1 versus Th2 responses in allograft rejection has been strongly debated, CD30_ T cells are implicated in the alloimmune response (Martinez OM et al, 1998).

Recent reports have proposed sCD30 as a noninvasive serological marker to predict immunological risk and graft failure among kidney transplant recipients (Pelzl S. et al, 2003). Both CD4 and CD8 T cells expressed CD30 after primary alloantigenic stimulation (Martinez OM. et al, 1998). Th_1 cytokines including IL-2, TNF-α, and IFN-γ mediate cellular immune responses and are pro-inflammatory, whereas, Th2-type cytokines IL-4 and IL-10 have been shown to inhibit the development and function of Th1-cells, to suppress inflammation, and to enhance humoral pathways of the immune response (Warle Mc. et al, 2001). Some studies suggested that CD30 may serve as a marker for human T lymphocytes that produce Th_2 cytokines (Manetti R. et al, 2007), while others demonstrated a strict association between CD30 expression and Th_1 cytokine production (Martinez OM. et al, 1998). However, Pellegrini et al. found that CD30 may be an important co-stimulatory molecule and marker for the physiological balance between Th_1/Th_2 immune response (Pellegrini P. et al, 2003). After activation of CD30+ T cells, a soluble form of CD30 (sCD30) is released proteolytically, however, the biological significance of this process is still not clearly defined (Dong W. et al, 2006). Th_1-cytokines are mainly involved in allograft rejection, while Th2-type immune response may be graft protective by blocking the graft damaging Th1-type anti-donor response (Reding R. et al, 2006). A soluble form of CD30 (sCD30) is released into the bloodstream after activation of CD30+ T cells (Romagnani S. et al, 1995).

5.1 Pre transplant CD30

Several reports from the Collaborative Transplant Study (CTS) have suggested that elevated pre and post-transplantation levels of the soluble CD30 (sCD30) molecule might be predictive for an increased incidence of rejection and worse kidney graft prognosis (Sengul S et al 2006).

Many reports have supported a role for sCD30 in the immune response associated with renal allograft rejection. The presence of increased pretransplantation concentrations of sCD30 has been associated with the development of acute rejection (Langan LL et al. 2007) and with humoral rejection and graft loss. While some reports demonstrated that T-cell activation marker soluble CD30 (sCD30) was an independent predictor of immunologic risk in renal transplant recipients without preformed alloantibodies (Vaidya S et al. 2006). It was reported that high sCD30 levels measured before transplantation, which might be a sign of activation of Th2 responses and, consequently, antibody production, could correlate with the risk of vascular rejection and production of DSA (Weimer R. et al, 2006). However lower levels of sCD30 was determined to be a helpful marker to distinguish patients with a low risk for development of DSA and antibody-mediated rejection (Slavcev A. et al, 2007). Study by Vaidya et al. recognized that estimation of sCD30 before transplantation might be a better predictive factor than PRA for the evaluation of the risk for occurrence of DSA and development of vascular rejection (Vaidya S et al. 2006). Some authors described an increased sCD30 level only during a rejection episode of the vascular type, while the more common tubulointerstitial type showed decreased sCD30 levels even lower than those of healthy volunteers (Rajakariar R. et al, 2005). According to some studies the sCD30 concentration was also high in both groups of patients before transplantation and levels of sCD30 decreased during the first 3 to 5 posttransplant days, increasing significantly between 5 and 15 days following transplantation among recipients who developed acute rejection episodes (Ayed K et al. 2006). Measurements of serial changes in soluble CD30 levels after transplantation have revealed a decrease of sCD30 in stable transplant recipients (Sengul S et al 2006). Kamali and colleagues have measured Pre and post-operative sCD30 levels of 3 groups (acute rejection, delayed graft function, and uncomplicated course group). It has been described significant decreases in sCD30 plasma levels on 14th day after transplant. Despite a significant decrease, groups of patients with acute rejection had higher CD30 concentrations on the 14th day after the transplants, compared with delayed graft function and uncomplicated course groups (Kamali K. et al, 2009). Based on published results pre-transplant sCD30 serum levels higher than 100 U/ml have been classified as a risk factor for the survival of kidney allografts (Cinti P. et al, 2005). In a large series of nearly 3900 kidney transplants performed at 29 centers in 15 countries, it was demonstrated that pretransplant determination of the Th2-type activation marker sCD30 is a powerful indicator for estimating the risk of graft rejection not only in presensitized but also in nonsensitized recipients (Susal et al. 2002). Patients with history of renal transplantation had higher levels of s CD30 than first kidney graft recipients (Susal et al. 2002). Investigation of pretransplant serum sCD30 content in 2998 recipients with a low sCD30 of <100 U/ml demonstrated a higher a 5-yr graft survival rate compared with 901 recipients with a high sCD30 of >100 U/ml. Determination of the sensitivity and specifity sCD30 testing based on positive (≥100U/ml) and negative (<100 U/ml) levels has revealed that with a specificity of sCD30 >80%, negative sCD30 levels might be a useful marker for identifying patients with a low risk for development of donor specific antibody (DSA) and antibody-mediated rejection

(Slavcev A. et al, 2007). Spiridon C and associates found no statistically significant difference among patients with 3–6 HLA-A, B, DR mismatches and 0–2 HLA-A, B, DR mismatches when pre-transplant level of sCD30 was below 90 U/mL. It is indicated that the effect of HLA mismatches can only be seen among patients with high level of sCD30 (Spiridon C. et al, 2008). Correlation between serum levels of sCD30 and Neopterin, which is a known activation marker of the T-cell/monocyte system and plays an important role in the chronic allograft nephropathy (CAN) process, demonstrated that up-regulation of 1-year sCD30 levels was associated with decreased 2-year GFR (. It was observed that increased 1-year sCD30 as well as Neopterin/CR are significantly associated with impaired 2-year graft function and serve as indicators of graft deterioration by chronic allograft nephropathy (Weimer R. et al, 2006). Association of sCD30 levels and immunosuppressive regimen has also been investigated. Pretransplant sCD30 assessment may serve as a useful parameter because high pretransplant sCD30 levels were shown to be associated with impaired kidney graft survival in Cyclosporine-A treated recipients (Susal C. et al, 2002). The current prospective randomized study shows that both cyclosporine-A and Tacrolimus based immunosuppressive regimens, used either in combination with Azathioprine or mycophenolate mofetil (CellCept), were associated with down-regulation of pretransplant sCD30 levels 4 months post-transplant, without a further significant change from 4 months to 1 and 2 years. It was demonstrated that Tacrolimus based regimens are more effective in suppressing sCD30 levels and thus might be the appropriate treatment in patients with pretransplant elevated sCD30. It was found an association between CD4 helper function and sCD30 2 years post-transplant, both in Cyclosporine-A and Tacrolimus treated patients, which might be the result of diminished suppression of CD4 helper activity due to reduced Calcineurin inhibitor drug exposure (Weimer R. et al, 2000). This evidence suggests that the measurement of sCD30 levels offers relevant clinical information regarding rejection risk and can contribute to the selection of the appropriate immunosuppressive regimen in high-risk recipients for the prevention of acute rejection and chronic allograft nephropathy (Kim MS et al. 2006).

5.2 Post transplant CD30

To prevent irreversible graft damage, it is important to diagnose and treat acute rejection in its earliest phase. Serial measurement of sCD30 levels after transplantation could become a feasible and non invasive method to predict acute graft rejection and might allow identifying patients prone to acute rejection during the first days after transplantation; before an acute rejection was occurred and diagnosed by conventional methods. Importantly, at this early time point, detection of acute rejection in the kidney with DGF is made difficult because conventional noninvasive rejection parameters, such as rising serum creatinine and oliguria cannot be used to make the diagnosis, however, sCD30 allowed a differentiation of group acute rejection from group DGF patients (Dong W. et al, 2006). In contrast to patients with an uncomplicated course or acute tubular necrosis (ATN) in the absence of rejection, plasma sCD30 levels remained high during the first 3 to 5 posttransplant days in recipients who subsequently developed acute allograft rejection (Susal C. et al, 2004). Now it is clear that the sCD30 levels decrease significantly after renal transplantation. It was reported that even in patients developed kidney rejection sCD30 levels decreased up to 55% at day 7 post-transplantation (Truong DQ. et al, 2007). In a similar study, showed that an important decrease of sCD30 was detected 2 weeks after renal transplantation and patients without rejection had lower sCD30 value compared to patient who experienced rejection episodes (Slavcev A. et al, 2005). Comparison of CD30 concentrations on the 14th day after transplantation, within acute rejection, delayed graft function (DGF) and uncomplicated course groups revealed that a higher soluble CD30 concentration on day 14 after transplant is associated with acute rejection (Kamali K. et al, 2009). In sera of 231 patients average sCD30 level before transplantation was much higher than that of healthy individuals. Most important, the decrease of sCD30 levels after transplantation varied in different groups. Compared with Group UC and DGF, patients of Group acute rejection had higher sCD30 levels on day 5 posttransplantation. Data also show that there was no association between rejection time and sCD30 levels (Dong W. et al, 2007). It is demonstrated that patients free of rejection in the first month post-transplant had lower sCD30 concentrations 2 weeks after transplantation compared to rejecting patients (Slavcev A. et al, 2005). Thus, an integration of the individualized evaluation of posttransplant sCD30 serum level as one biomarker, together with accompanying diseases which affect the immunological reactivity post-transplantation, may be a feasible approach for the non-invasive post-transplant prediction of acute kidney allograft rejection.

6. Panel-reactive antibody (PRA)

Renal transplantation in sensitized patients remains a highly significant challenge worldwide. However, highly sensitized candidates should not be eliminated from transplant waiting lists, as post-transplant survival rate and life quality can be greatly improved with transplantation, despite the risks. The level of sensitization in a kidney transplant recipient can be monitored before and after renal transplantation via PRA (panel-reactive antibody) test. Highly sensitized recipients usually refer to those with antibodies against HLA, who are defined as panel reactive antibody (PRA) >10%, or >20%. The humoral immune system is an important determinant of outcome: hypersensitized patients show reduced long term graft survival and 10% panel reactive antibodies (PRA) is a risk factor (Davis CL, 2004 and Opelz G, 2001). Thus elevated panel reactive antibody (PRA) levels, produced against HLA and induced by transfusions, pregnancies and prior transplants for HLA allo-immunization are linked to hyper-acute rejections, delayed graft functions and poor graft survival rates. Measurement of anti-HLA antibodies before and after transplantation is important, as their presence increases the risk and severity of rejection episodes and is a significant risk factor for allograft loss (Zhou YC. et al, 1996). During past years, transplant surgeons usually focused on the results of PRA levels and lymphocyte toxicity test in the treatment of sensitized patients, but sometimes serious antibody mediated rejections also happened in HLA-identical donor-recipient transplants. Although we have not yet confirmed whether there are any anti-HLA antibodies not well detected with existing technologies, the concept of non-HLA antibodies bring the transplant surgeons and researchers with great inspiration. Following the more recent development of ELISA methodology for detecting HLA antibodies, several reports showed that patients with pretransplant HLA-I antibodies (>10% PRA) had greater risk for acute or chronic rejection, or an increase in post-transplant reactivity (Van Kampen CA. et al, 2001). It was observed a higher incidence of post-transplant donor specific HLA antibodies in patients having 3–50% PRA compared with patients having 0% PRA at the time of transplantation (Supon P. et al, 2001). The determination of panel reactive antibodies, which at present are exclusively used as indicators for an increased risk of graft rejection, is currently being critically discussed. It is illustrated that combination of positive PRA and elevated sCD30 levels have an additional diagnostic value, as well as independent factors, to predict acute rejection risk and subsequent graft outcome (Langan L L. et al, 2007). For this reason novel markers are recommended for proper monitoring of pre- and post-transplant risks. Using the modalities described, immunosuppressive therapies in transplant recipients can now be selected on the basis of individual demand, with anti-B-cell directed immunosuppression being most promising during the early postoperative period.

7. Immunosuppressive therapy

The influence of immunosuppressive regimens on sCD30 levels was provoked in many studies. Presensitized (PRA >5%) patients had a higher serum sCD30 content than nonsensitized (5% >PRA) patients. whereas, as shown in Figure 3, the effects of the two parameters on graft outcome were additive. Therefore presensitized patients are preferentially transplanted with HLA well-matched kidneys and receive stronger posttransplant immunosuppression, including prophylactic treatment with antilymphocyte antibodies (susal et at. 2002). Immunosuppressive treatment in recipients usually contains either with a triple drug regimen (Cyclosporine, Steroids and Azathioprine) or, in Presensitized patients with immunologic risk factors (presence of panel-reactive antibodies or history of graft rejection), a quadruple regimen, including polyvalent or monoclonal antilymphocyte antibodies. When patients were divided into well-matched group (with three or less mismatches) and poor-matched group (with more than three mismatches), no significant difference of sCD30 levels was shown between two groups. Soluble CD30 levels

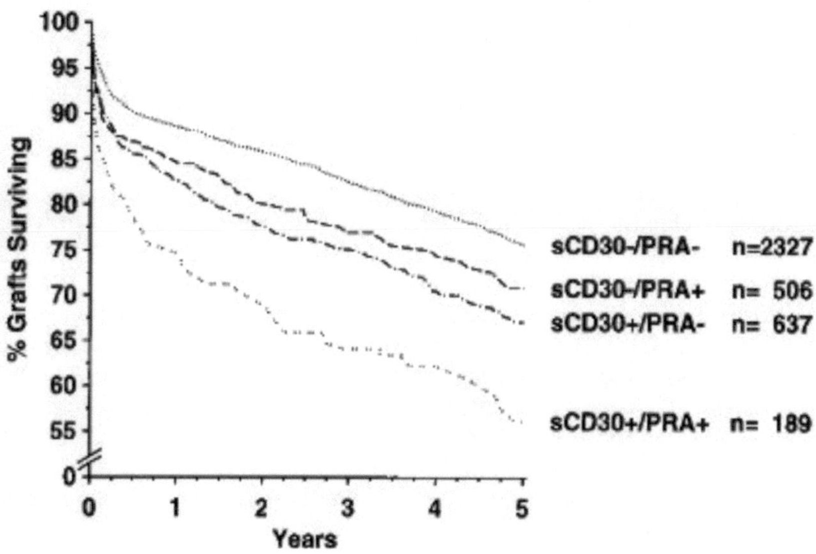

(Adapted from susal et at. 2002)

Fig. 3. Combined effect of serum sCD30 content and lymphocytotoxic panel reactivity (PRA) on kidney graft survival. sCD30- positive and PRA-positive recipients (sCD30+/PRA+) had a significantly impaired graft outcome, compared with sCD30-negative and PRA-negative (sCD30_/PRA_), sCD30-negative and PRA-positive (sCD30_/PRA+), or sCD30-positive and PRA negative recipients (sCD30+/PRA_) ($P < 0.0001$, $P = 0.0003$, and $P = 0.0048$, respectively).

were also independently evaluated in patients receiving cyclosporine A and FK506. There was also no significant difference of sCD30 levels between two groups. Significant difference of sCD30 levels was only observed between patients with acute rejection episodes and those without acute rejection on day 5 post-transplantation (Dong W. et al, 2006). Antithymocyte globulin (ATG) is recommended for desensitization of kidney transplant recipients with high panel-reactive antibody (PRA) and ABO-incompatibility as main modality for the treatment of AMR (Akalin E. et al, 2003 and Gloor JM. et al, 2003). But antilymphocyte antibodies did not improve graft outcome in patients with high sCD30. Graft survival of recipients with a high pretransplant sCD30 treated with prophylactic antilymphocyte antibodies (ATG, ALG, or OKT3), was significantly worse than the rate in recipients with low sCD30 levels. It is suggested that a single dose of Rituximab (50 mg/m^2 BSA) is as effective as higher doses (150 and 375 mg/m^2 BSA) in depleting Bcells and reducing PRA levels, While the standard dose of Rituximab in AMR is 375 mg/m2 BSA (Vieira CA. et al, 2004). Thus, to improve graft outcome in patients with high sCD30 levels, other strategies seem to be necessary, possibly immunosuppressive regimens that specifically inhibit CD30$^+$ T cells.

8. Conclusion

It is illustrated that combination of positive PRA and elevated sCD30 levels have an additional diagnostic value, as well as independent factors, to predict acute rejection risk and subsequent graft outcome. For this reason novel markers are recommended for proper monitoring of pre- and post-transplant risks. This evidence suggests that the measurement of sCD30 levels offers relevant clinical information regarding rejection risk and can contribute to the selection of the appropriate immunosuppressive regimen in high-risk recipients for the prevention of acute rejection and also chronic allograft nephropathy.

9. References

Akalin E, Ames S, Sehgal V, et al. (2003). Intravenous immunoglobulin and thymoglobulin facilitate transplantation in complementdependent cytotoxicity B-cell and flow cytometry T or B-cell crossmatch positive patients. *Transplantation*, 76: 1444-7.

Altermann W, Schlaf G, Rothhoff A and Seliger B. (2007). High variation of individual soluble serum CD30 levels of pre-transplantation patients: sCD30 a feasible marker for prediction of kidney allograft rejection? *Nephrol Dial Transplant*, 22, 2795–2799

Ayed K, Abdallah T.B, Bardi R, Abderrahim E, and Kheder A. (2006). Plasma Levels of Soluble CD30 in Kidney Graft Recipients as Predictors of Acute Allograft Rejection. *Transplantation Proceedings*, 38, 2300–2302.

Baid S, Saidman S L, Tolkoff-Rubin N. et al. (2001). Managing the highly sensitized transplant recipient and B cell tolerance. *Current Opinion in Immunology*, 13:577–581.

Chang A.T and Platt J.L. (2009). The Role of Antibodies in Transplantation. *Transplant Rev*, 23(4): 191–198.

Cinti P, Pretagostini R, Arpino A et al.(2005). Evaluation of pretransplant immunologic status in kidney-transplant recipients by panel reactive antibody and soluble CD30 determinations. *Transplantation*, 79: 1154–1156

Collins AB, Schneeberger E, Pascual M, et al. (1999). Complement activation in acute humoral renal allograft rejection: Diagnostic significance of C4d deposits in peritubular capillaries. *J Am Soc Nephrol*, 10:2208,

Colvin RB. (1996). The renal allograft biopsy. *Kidney Int*, 50: 1069-1082.

Colvin RB, Nickeleit V. (2006). Renal transplant pathology. In: *Heptinstall's Pathology of the Kidney*, 6th Ed., edited by Jennette JC, Olson JL, Schwartz MM, Silva FG, Philadelphia, Lippincott-Raven, , 1347–1490.

Cueto-Manzano AM, Morales-Buenrostro LE, Gonzalez- Espinoza L, et al.(2005). Markers of inflammation before and after renal transplantation. *Transplantation* 80: 47–51,

Daly PJ, Power RE, Healy DA, Hickey DP, Fitzpatrick JM, Watson RW. (2005) Delayedgraft function: a dilemma in renal transplantation. *BJU Int*, 96(4):498-501.

Davis CL, (2004). Transplant immunology and treatment of rejection. *Am J Kidney Dis*,43:1116

Dinavahi R and Heeger PS. (2008). T cell Immune Monitoring in Organ Transplantation.*Curr Opin Organ Transplant*, 13(4): 419–424.

Dong W, Shunliang Y, Weizhen W, et al. (2006). Prediction of acute renal allograftrejection in early post-transplantation period by soluble CD30. *TransplantImmunology*, 16 41–45

Feucht HE, Felber E, Gokeel MJ, et al. (1991).Vascular deposition of complement–splitproduct in kidney allografts with cell Imediated rejection. *Clin Exp Immunol*, 86:464,

Fossiez F, Djossou O, Chomarat P, et al. (1996). T-cell interleukin-17 induces stromal cellsto produce proinflammatory and hematopoietic cytokines. *J Exp Med*, 183: 2593–603.

Geddes CC, Woo YM, Jardine AG. (2002). The impact of delayed graft function on thelong-term outcome of renal transplantation. *J Nephrol*, 15: 17-21.

Ghods AJ., Savaj S., Abbasi MA., Heidari H. and Rokhsatyazdi H. (2007).The Incidenceand Risk Factors of Delayed Graft Function in 689 Consecutive Living UnrelatedDonor Renal Transplantation. *Transplantation Proceedings*, 39, 846–847

Gloor JM, Lager DJ, Moore SB, et al. ABO-incompatible kidney transplantation usingboth A2 and non-A2 living donors. *Transplantation* 2003;75:971-7.

Halloran PF, Hunsicker LG: (2001).Delayed graft function: State of art. *Am J Transplant* 1:115-20

Halloran PF, Wadgymar A, Ritchie S, Falk J, Solez K, Srinivasa NS. The significance ofthe anti-class I antibody response. I. Clinical and pathologic features of anti-class Idiated rejection. Transplantation 1990; 49: 85-91.

Halloran PF, Schlaut J, Solez K, Srinivasa NS. (1992).The significance of the anti-class I response.II. Clinical and pathologic features of renal transplants with anti-class I-likeantibody. *Transplantation*; 53: 550-555.

Hartono C, Muthukumar T, and Suthanthiran M. (2010). Noninvasive Diagnosis of AcuteRejection of Renal Allografts. *Curr Opin Organ Transplant*.; 15(1): 35–41.

Kamali K. Abbasi M.A , Farokhi B. et al. Posttransplant Soluble CD30 as a Predictor ofAcute Renal Allograft Rejection. *Experimental and Clinical Transplantation* (2009) 4:237-240

Kim MS, Kim HJ, Kim SI, et al. (2006). Pretransplant soluble CD30 level has limited effecton acute rejection, but affects graft function in living donor kidney transplantation.*Transplantation*; 82: 1602-5

Koning OH, Ploeg RJ, van Bockel JH, et al. (1997). Risk factors for delayed graft functionin cadaveric kidney transplantation. A prospective study of renal function and graftsurvival after preservation with University of Wisconsin solution in multi-organdonors. European Multicenter Study Group. *Transplantation*; 63 : 1620–8

Lagan LL, Park LP, Hughes TL, et al. (2007). Posttransplant HLA class II antibodies andhigh soluble CD30 levels are independently associated with poor kidney graftsurvival. *Am J Transplant*, 7:847,.

Lederer S.R, Kluth-Pepper B, Schneeberger H, et al. (2001). Impact of humoralalloreactivity early after transplantation on the long-term survival of renal allografts.*Kidney International*, 59. 334–341

Lorraine C. Racusen and Mark Haas. (2006). Antibody-Mediated Rejection in Renal Allografts: Lessonsbfrom Pathology. *Clin J Am Soc Nephrol* 1: 415–420

Magee CC, Pascual M. (2004). Update in renal transplantation. *Arch Intern Med*, 164:1373–1388.

Manetti R, Annunziato F, Biagiotti R, Giudizi MG, Piccinni MP, Giannarini L. (1994).CD30 expression by CD8+ T cells producing type 2 helper cytokines: evidence forlarge numbers of CD8+CD30+ T cells clones in human immunodeficiency virusinfection. *J Exp Med*, 180: 2007–11.

Manfro RC, Aquino-Dias EC, Joelsons G, et al. (2008). Noninvasive Tim-3 messengerRNA evaluation in renal transplant recipients with graft dysfunction.*Transplantation;* 86:1869-74

Mannon RB. and Kirk AD. (2006). Beyond Histology: Novel Tools to Diagnose AllograftDysfunction. *Clin J Am Soc Nephrol*, 1: 358–366

Marsh SG, Albert ED, Bodmer WF, et al. (2002). Nomenclature for factors of the HLAsystem, 2002. *Hum Immunol;* 63: 1213-1268.

Martinez OM, Villanueva J, Abtahi S, Beatty PR, Esquivel CO, Krams SM. (1998). CD30expression identifies a functional alloreactive human T-lymphocyte subset.*Transplantation*.65: 1240–1247,

Mauiyyedi S, Crespo M and Collins A.B et al. (2002). Acute Humoral Rejection in KidneyTransplantation: II. Morphology, Immunopathology, and Pathologic Classification. *JAm Soc Nephrol*, 13: 779–787

McDouall RM, Batten P, McCormack A, Yacoub MH, Rose ML. (1997). MHC class IIexpression on human heart microvascular endothelial cells: exquisite sensitivity tointerferon-gamma and natural killer cells. *Transplantation*,27;64(8):1175-80.

Medof ME, Kinoshita T, Nussenzweig V. (1984). Inhibition of complement activation onthe surface of cells after incorporation of decay-accelerating factor (DAF) into theirmembranes. *J Exp Med*, 160 (5):1558–78.

Miyata Y, Platt JL. (2002). The role of complement in acute vascular rejection: lessonsfrom the inhibition of C1rs activity. *Transplantation;* 73:675.

Moise A, Nedelcu D, Toader A, et al. (2010). Cytotoxic antibodies--valuable prognosticfactor for long term kidney allograft survival. *J Med Life*, 3(4):390-5.

Muczynski KA, Ekle DM, Coder DM, Anderson SK. (2003). Normal human kidney HLAR-expressing renal microvascular endothelial cells: characterization, isolation, andregulation of MHC class II expression. *J Am Soc Nephrol*, 14: 1336–48.

Natha DS, Ilias Basha H and T Mohanakumar. (2010). Anti-Human Leukocyte AntigenAntibody Induced Autoimmunity: Role In Chronic Rejection. *Curr Opin OrganTransplant*, 15(1): 16–20.

Newstead CG, Lamb WR, Brenchley PE, Short CD: Serum and urine IL-6 and TNF-alphain renal transplant recipients with graft dysfunction. *Transplantation* 56: 831–835,1993

Ojo AO, Wolfe RA, Held PJ, et al. (1997). Delayed graft function: Risk factors andimplications for renal allograft survival. *Transplantation* 63:968–974,.

Opelz G: (2001). Collaborative transplant study. Investigation of the relationship between maintenance dose of cyclosporine and nephrotoxicity or hypertension. *Transplant Proc*, 33(7-8):3351-4

Oyen O, Wergeland R, Bentdal O, Hartmann A, Brekke IB, Stokke O. (2001). Serialultrasensitive CRP measurements may be useful in rejection diagnosis after kidneytransplantation. *Transplant Proc* 33: 2481–2483,

Patel R, Terasaki PI. (1969). Significance of the positive crossmatch test in kidney transplantation. *N Engl J Med*, 280: 735-9.

Péfaur J., Diaz P., Panace R. (2008). Early and Late Humoral Rejection: AClinicopathologic Entity in Two Times. *Transplantation Proceedings*, 40, 3229–3236

Pellegrini P, Berghella AM, Contasta I, Adorno D. (2003). CD30 antigen: not aphysiological marker for TH2 cells but an important costimulator molecule in theregulation of the balance between TH1/TH2 response. *Transpl Immunol*,12:49–61

Pelzl S, Opelz G, Daniel V, et al. (2003). Evaluation of posttransplantation soluble CD30for diagnosis of acute renal allograft rejection. *Transplantation*, 75:421,

Pollinger HS, Stegall MD, Gloor JM, Moore SB, Degoey SR, Ploeger NA. (2007). Kidneytransplantation in patients with antibodies against donor HLA class II. *Am JTransplant*, 7: 857-863

Racusen L C. and Haas M. (2006). Antibody-Mediated Rejection in Renal Allografts:Lessons from Pathology. *Clin J Am Soc Nephrol* 1: 415–420

Racusen LC, Solez K, Colvin RB et al. (1999). The Banff 97 working classification of renalallograft pathology. *Kidney Int*, 55: 713–723.

Rajakariar R, Jivanji N, Varagunam M, Rafiq M, Gupta A, Sheaff M, et al.(2005). Highpre-transplant soluble CD30 levels are predictive of the grade of rejection. *Am JTransplant*, 5(8):1922–5.

Reding R, Gras J, Truong DQ, Wieers G, Latinne D. (2006). The immunologicalmonitoring of alloreactive responses in liver transplant recipients: a review. *LiverTranspl*, 12:373–83.

Romagnani S, Del Prete G, Maggi E, Chilosi M, Caligaris-Cappio F, Pizzolo G. (1995).CD30 and type 2 T helper (Th2) responses. *J Leukoc Biol*, 57:726–30.

Rouschop KM, Roelofs JJ, Rowshani AT, et al. (2005). Pre-transplant plasma and cellularlevels of CD44 correlate with acute renal allograft rejection. *Nephrol Dial Transplant*,20(10):2248-54.

Sengul S, Keven K, Gormez U, et al. (2006). Identification of patients at risk of acuterejection by pretransplantation and posttransplantation monitoring of soluble CD30levels in kidney transplantation. *Transplantation* 81:1216

Slavcev A, Honsova E, Lodererova A, et al. (2007). Soluble CD30 in patients withantibody-mediated rejection of the kidney allograft. *Transplant Immunology*, 18 22–27

Slavcev A, Lacha J, Honsova E, et al. (2005). Soluble CD30 and HLA antibodies aspotential risk factors for kidney transplant rejection. *Transplant Immunol* ,14(2):11721

Smith KD, Wrenshall LE, Nicosia RF, et al. (2003). Delayed graft function and castnephropathy associated with tacrolimus plus rapamycin use. *J Am Soc Nephro*, 14:1037–45

Solez K, Colvin RB, Racusen LC, et al. (2008). Banff 07 classification of renal allograftpathology: updates and future directions. *Am J Transplant*, 8:753.

Spiridon C, Nikaein A, Lerman M, Hunt J, Dickerman R, Mack M. (2008). CD30, a markerto detect the high-risk kidney transplant recipients. *Clin Transplant*, 22: 765–769.

Striz I, Eliska K, Eva H, et al. (2005). Interleukin 18 (IL-18) upregulation in acute rejectionof kidney allograft. *Immunol Lett* , 99: 30–35

Striz I, Krasna E, Honsova E, et al. (2005). Interleukin 18 (IL-18) upregulation in acuterejection of kidney allograft. *Immunol Lett*, 99:30.

Supon P, Constantino D, Hao P et al. (2001). Prevalence of donorspecific anti-HLAantibodies during episodes of renal allograft rejection. *Transplantation*, 71: 577–580

Susal C, Pelzl S, Dohler B and Opelz G. (2002). Identification of Highly ResponsiveKidney Transplant Recipients Using Pretransplant Soluble CD30. *J Am Soc Nephrol*13: 1650–1656

Susal C, Pelzl S, Opelz G. (2003). Strong human leukocyte antigen matching effect innonsensitized kidney recipients with high pretransplant soluble CD30.*Transplantation*, 76:1231.

Susal C, Opelz G. (2004). Good kidney transplant outcome in recipients withpresensitization against HLA class II but not HLA class I. *Hum Immunol*; 65: 810-816.

Susal C, Pelzl S, Simon T and Opelz G. (2004). Advances in Pre- and PosttransplantImmunologic Testing in Kidney Transplantation. *Transplantation Proceedings*, 36,29_34

Troppmann C, Gillingham KJ, Gruessner RWG, Dunn DL, Payne WD, Najarian JS.(1996). Delayed graft function in the absence of rejection has no long-term impact. Astudy of cadaver kidney recipients with good graft function at 1 year aftertransplantation. *Transplantation*; 61: 1331-1337

Truong DQ, Darwish AA, Gras J, et al. (2007). Immunological monitoring after organtransplantation: Potential role of soluble CD30 Blood level measurement. *TranspIImmunol*, 17(4):283-7

Vaidya S, Partlow D, Barnes T, Gugliuzza K. (2006). Pretransplant soluble CD30 is abetter predictor of post-transplantation development of donor-specific antibodiesand acute vascular rejection than panel reactive antibodies. *Transplantation*;82: 1606

Vaidya S, Partlow D, Barnes T, Thomas P, Gugliuzza K.(2006). Soluble CD30concentrations in ESRD patients with and without panel reactive HLA antibodies.*Clin Transplant*, 20(4):461–4.

Van Kampen CA, Maarschalk MFJV, Roelen DL, TenBerge IJM, Claas FHJ. (2001).Rejection of a kidney transplant does not always lead to priming of cytotoxic T cellsagainst mismatched donor HLA class I antigens. *Transplantation*; 71: 869–874

Vieira CA, Agarwal A, Book BK, et al. (2004). Rituximab for reduction of anti-HLAantibodies in patients awaiting renal transplantation: 1. Safety, pharmacodynamicsand pharmacokinetics. *Transplantation*; 77:542-8.

Waiser J, Budde K, Katalinic A, Kuerzdorfer M, Riess R, Neumayer HH.(1997).Interleukin-6 expression after renal transplantation. *Nephrol Dial Transplant* 12: 753759

Watschinger B, Pascual M. (2002). Capillary C4d deposition as a marker of humoralimmunity in renal allograft rejection. *J Am Soc Nephrol* 13:1420

Weimer R, Melk A, Daniel V, Friemann S, Padberg W, Opelz G. (2000). Switch fromcyclosporine A to tacrolimus in renal transplant recipients: Impact on Th1, Th2, andmonokine responses. *Hum Immunol*; 61: 884–897

Weimer R, Susal C,Yildiz S, Staak A, Pelzl S, Renner F, et al. (2006). Post-transplantsCD30 and neopterin as predictors of chronic allograft nephropathy: impact ofdifferent immunosuppressive regimens. *Am J Transplant*, 6 (8):1865–74.

Yao QC, Wang W, Li XB, Yin H, Zhang XD. (2011). Expression characteristics of majorhistocompatibility complex class I-related chain A antibodies andimmunoadsorption effect in sensitized recipients of kidney transplantation. *ChinMed J (Engl)*, 124(5):669-73.

Zhou YC, Cecka JM. (1991). Sensitization in renal transplantation. *Clin Transplant*, 5:313323.

Zou Y, Stastny P. (2009). The role of major histocompatibility complex class I chainrelated gene A antibodies in organ transplantation. *Curr Opin Organ Transplant*, 14:414-418.

Zou YZ, Stastny P, Süsal C, Opelz G. (2007). Antibodies against MICA antigens andkidney-transplant rejection. *N Engl J Med*, 357: 1293-1300.

9

Role of Cytomegalovirus Reinfection in Acute Rejection and CMV Disease After Renal Transplantation

Kei Ishibashi and Tatsuo Suzutani
Fukushima Medical University
Japan

1. Introduction

Renal transplantation is a most valuable treatment for patients with end-stage renal disease as it offers improved survival and quality-of-life benefits compared with dialysis (Evans, Manninen et al. 1985; Port, Wolfe et al. 1993). However, there has been no satisfactory increase in long-term graft survival despite significant advances in the field of renal transplantation (Meier-Kriesche, Schold et al. 2004). Long-term graft failure is generally due to death despite a functioning graft, chronic rejection, or recurrent kidney disease (Valente, Hariharan et al. 1997). Among these, chronic rejection is the most important cause of long-term graft failure (Jindal and Hariharan 1999). Graft failure owing to chronic rejection is a common reason for retransplantation, and the most important predictor of chronic rejection is a previous episode of acute rejection (Almond, Matas et al. 1993; Hariharan, Alexander et al. 1996; Cosio, Pelletier et al. 1997). Clinical acute rejection within the first year after transplantation has been reported to have a detrimental effect on long-term graft survival (Hariharan, Johnson et al. 2000). The projected half-life for cadaveric transplants in patients who did not have an episode of clinical acute rejection in the first year after transplantation was 17.9 years in 1995, compared with that of 8.8 years for patients who had an episode of clinical acute rejection (Hariharan, Johnson et al. 2000). This reduction in the relative risk of graft failure was significant among patients without acute rejection, whereas no reduction in the relative risk of graft failure was observed among those with acute rejection. Thus, the main issue asociated with renal transplantation is the suppression of allograft rejection.

Cytomegalovirus (CMV) infection, which is the most common infection following renal transplanation, continues to be a potential contributor to graft loss and a cause of severe mortality and morbidity. Several studies have suggested that CMV infection can lead to allograft rejection (Lautenschlager, Soots et al. 1997; Humar, Gillingham et al. 1999; McLaughlin, Wu et al. 2002; Meier-Kriesche, Schold et al. 2004; Nett, Heisey et al. 2004). Although the role of CMV infection in acute rejection after renal transplantation remains controversial, many reports have demonstrated that CMV serostatus, as defined by conventional classifications, influences clinical outcome in renal transplantation (Humar, Gillingham et al. 1999; McLaughlin, Wu et al. 2002). The combination of CMV-seronegative recipients (R-) with CMV-seropositive donors (D+) led to the highest risk of CMV disease.

Historically, concern has focused on avoiding CMV infection in D+/R- settings. However, some transplant recipients in the D+/R+ group experience severe CMV disease and/or acute rejection despite their pre-existing immunity. For example, in D+R+ cases, approximately 20% of recipients experienced CMV disease in the absence of any prophylaxis (Sagedal, Nordal et al. 2000). Analysis of the data from the United States Renal Data System and United Network of Organ Sharing revealed that the D+/R+, not the D+/R- group, had the worst graft and patient survival by 3 years (Schnitzler, Woodward et al. 1997; Schnitzler, Woodward et al. 1997). This may reflect the prevalence of multiple CMV virotypes, and that D+/R+ recipients may have double exposure to different CMV strains.

This article addresses the impact of CMV reinfection with different CMV strains on the clinical course after renal transplantation.

2. Background

2.1 Cytomegalovirus virology

CMV is the fifth member of the 8 known human herpes viruses (HHVs). HHVs are classified into three subgroups, alpha herpesvirinae, beta herpesvirinae and gamma herpesvirinae. CMV, a member of the beta herpes virus family together with HHV-6 and HHV-7, is a widespread opportunistic pathogen. Primary CMV infection usually occurs during the first decades of life. CMV is transmitted via salvia, body fluids, cells and tissues (Egli, Binggeli et al. 2007). Primary infection is followed by a latent infection that can persist throughout the entire life of the host. The principal reservoirs of latent CMV are the white blood cells and CD13-positive cells (Larsson, Soderberg-Naucler et al. 1998) and the latent virus has been detected in most tissues in the body. CMV can infect most renal cell types, including glomerular, tubular, and endothelial cells (Heieren, Kim et al. 1988; Heieren, van der Woude et al. 1988; Ustinov, Loginov et al. 1991).

CMV is a DNA virus containing 230-kb double-strand DNA. CMV has a typical herpes virion structure consisting of viral DNA, capsid, tegument and envelope. The envelope contains structural proteins including glycoproteins. The glycoproteins are used for cellular entry by the virus. CMV initially tethers itself to cell-surface heparan sulfate proteoglycans (HSPGs) via viral envelope glycoproteins (Kari and Gehrz 1992; Compton, Nowlin et al. 1993), although HSPGs alone are not sufficient to mediate viral entry. The ability of CMV to enter a wide variety of cell types indicates multiple receptors for entry, and many cell-surface components have been identified as virus receptors. It is reported that CMV uses epidermal growth factor receptor (EGFR), platelet-derived growth factor-α receptor (PDGFR-α) and cellular integrins for cellular entry (Wang, Huong et al. 2003; Feire, Koss et al. 2004; Soroceanu, Akhavan et al. 2008), although these findings remain controversial (Isaacson, Feire et al. 2007). The entry of CMV into host cells requires interactions between cellular and viral molecules, and glycoproteins. Pretreatment of CMV with glycoprotein-specific antibodies could disrupt interaction between CMV and cellular molecules (Wang, Huang et al. 2005; Soroceanu, Akhavan et al. 2008).

The complete genome of the laboratory strain of CMV AD169 has been sequenced (Chee, Bankier et al. 1990), however, genetic differences among CMV strains have been observed in multiple genes. Those polymorphisms may be implicated in immunopathogenesis as well as CMV strain-specific behavior and cell tropism.

2.2 Glycoproteins of Cytomegalovirus

The initial events associated with CMV infection require interactions between the host cell-surface molecules and the CMV envelope. The early steps of virion attachment, fusion and penetration of the host cell have been assumed to be functions of the viral envelope glycoproteins. To date, at least 57 potential glycoproteins are known to be encoded by the laboratory strain of CMV (AD169), and several envelope glycoproteins have been characterized (Chee, Bankier et al. 1990; Britt and Mach 1996; Cha, Tom et al. 1996). These glycoproteins associate in high molecular weight complexes and the mature complexes are referred to as glycoprotein complex I (gC-I), glycoprotein complex II (gC-II) and glycoprotein complex III (gC-III). The genes encoding glycoproteins often show genetic polymorphism. Because the envelope glycoproteins elicit strong host immune responses, including the production of neutralizing antibodies, understanding of the genetic polymorphism of the glycoproteins will have an impact on strategies to protect against CMV infection as well as clinical studies.

2.2.1 Glycoprotein H (gH)

The disulphide-bond tripartite gC-III envelope complex consists of gH, gL and gO (Huber and Compton 1999). Glycoprotein H is one of the immunologically dominant glycoproteins in the CMV envelope, and is encoded by open reading frame (ORF) unique long (UL) region 75 (Pachl, Probert et al. 1989). The gH gene of the AD169 strain is 2,229 nucleotides long and that of the Towne strain is 2,226 in length. The gH product of AD169 UL75 comprises 743 amino acids (aa) and that of Towne is 742 aa, with a deletion of proline 36 (Pachl, Probert et al. 1989; Britt and Mach 1996). Although the UL75 is highly conserved among multiple CMV strains, sequence variations were found in the first 37 aa (Chou 1992). Based on the sequence analysis of UL75 from multiple strains, it was estimated that CMV gH has two genotypes (Chou 1992). gH mediates viral/host cell membrane fusion in the initial step of infectivity, and monoclonal anti-gH antibodies can inhibit virus infectivity (Keay and Baldwin 1991). Antibodies against gH can be detected after natural infection with CMV (Rasmussen, Matkin et al. 1991). Anti-CMV gH antibodies exhibit virus neutralizing activity and gH is considered a major antigen for the humoral immune response (Urban, Klein et al. 1996). A linear antibody binding site is located within the amino-terminal region of gH (aa 34-43), which shows sequence heterogeneity between the AD169 and Towne strains (Urban, Britt et al. 1992). This heterogeneity is characterized by the deletion of a proline residue at position 36 and the substitution of lysine for histidine at position 37 in the Towne strain as compared with the AD169 strain. This antibody binding site is recognized as strain-specific epitope(Urban, Britt et al. 1992), and the heterogeneity influences CMV susceptibility to host neutralizing antibodies. A recent report on congenital CMV infection has provided clear evidence that exposure to CMV with a different genotype causes congenital infection, even in seropositive mothers (Boppana, Rivera et al. 2001).

2.2.2 Glycoprotein B (gB)

Glycoprotein B, a component of the envelope complex gC-I, is the most abundant glycoprotein in the CMV envelope. gB is one of the most highly conserved components among all members of the herpesvirus family. It is encoded by UL55 and exhibits genetic polymorphism. The 906 aa polypeptide of the AD169 strain gB is cleaved at position 460 by a cellular endoprotease. Nucleotide and peptide sequence analysis revealed that variations were most frequent between positions 448 and 480, which includes the cleavage site (Chou and Dennison 1991). Restriction enzyme analysis has identified four main gB groups (gB-1, gB-2, gB-3 and gB-4). While variations were found in gB, substantial conservation of the peptide sequence is observed in this region. The closely regulated variations in gB may suggest its important role in the viral life cycle (Chou and Dennison 1991). Although little is known of the effect of gB variations on biologic function, genetic variations have been used for epidemiologic purpose.

gB has a role in binding to cell surface receptors, and neutralizing gB-specific antibodies can inhibit the binding (Ohizumi, Suzuki et al. 1992). CMV interacts with cellular integrins, EGFR and PDGFR-α through gB, and these compounds are considered as potential cellular receptors of CMV (Wang, Huong et al. 2003; Feire, Koss et al. 2004; Soroceanu, Akhavan et al. 2008).

The antigenicity of gB has been well studied and linear neutralizing and non-neutralizing antibody-binding sites have been defined (Britt and Mach 1996). The antigen domain 1 (AD1), which is located between positions 560 and 640 of gB, is a major neutralizing epitope (Schoppel, Hassfurther et al. 1996) and is the most highly conserved region among viral strains. The second antibody binding site on gB is the antigen domain 2 (AD2), which is located between aa 28 and 84 of gB (Meyer, Sundqvist et al. 1992). Within the AD2 domain, two antigenic sites have been identified. Site I is located between aa 68 and 77, and this region is conserved among CMV wild-type strains and is the target of neutralizing antibodies. Site II, another binding sequence in the AD2, is located between aa 50 and 54. Site II binds non-neutralizing antibodies and is strain-specific (Meyer, Sundqvist et al. 1992).

2.2.3 Glycoprotein N (gN)

Glycoprotein N is a component of the envelope complex gC-II (Mach, Kropff et al. 2000; Dal Monte, Pignatelli et al. 2001). gN has been identified as one of the major antigens together with gH and gB (Shimamura, Mach et al. 2006). It is encoded by the ORF UL73, and antibodies against gN neutralize virus infectivity. The immunogenic gC-II is also the major heparin binding complex (Kari and Gehrz 1992).

UL73 has four main genomic variants, denoted gN-1, gN-2, gN-3 and gN-4 (Pignatelli, Dal Monte et al. 2001). The worldwide geographical distribution of identified variants of the gN was investigated and it was found that the variants do not necessarily exhibit the same frequency distribution (Pignatelli, Dal Monte et al. 2003). The gN genomic variants are related to the immunopathogenesis of CMV in immunocompromised hosts and in congenitally infected infants (Pignatelli, Dal Monte et al. 2003; Pignatelli, Rossini et al. 2003).

2.2.4 Other Glycoproteins

Other than gH, gB and gN, the large CMV genome encodes many additional glycoproteins. UL100 encodes glycoprotein M (gM), which, together with gN, is a component of gC-II. gM is essential for viral replication (Hobom, Brune et al. 2000), and seems to be highly conserved (Lehner, Stamminger et al. 1991). It was shown that most sera failed to react with either gM or gN alone (Mach, Kropff et al. 2000). Virus neutralizing antibodies were shown to be directed at the gN component of the gM–gN complex.

In addition to gH, the gC-III envelope complex contains glycoprotein O (gO) and glycoprotein L (gL) (Huber and Compton 1999). gO is encoded by the UL74 ORF. The sequence analysis of UL74 showed a high degree of variability at the N-terminal end (Paterson, Dyer et al. 2002). The analysis of clinical isolates identified four major phylogenetic groups, denoted gO-1, gO-2, gO-3 and gO-4 (Mattick, Dewin et al. 2004). gL is encoded by the UL115 ORF. Four major phylogenetic groups were again identified and denoted gL-1, gL-2, gL-3 and gL-4 (Rasmussen, Geissler et al. 2002). gL is essential for the transport of the gH glycoprotein to the cell surface (Kaye, Gompels et al. 1992; Spaete, Perot et al. 1993).

The large number of gH-gO-gL combinations suggests that gC-III has an immunological potential, and has implications for viral tropism and spread (Rasmussen, Geissler et al. 2002).

2.3 CMV genpotype and renal transplantation

Transplantation in a D+/R+ setting is usually accompanied by multiple CMV strains in recipients after transplantation (Manuel, Pang et al. 2009), with mixtures of gB and gH genptypes were commonly observed in organ transplant recipients (Zhou, Fan et al. 2007). As CMV displays genetic polymorphism among glycoproteins thought to be implicated in tissue tropism and immunopathogenesis, an association betweenf glycoprotein genotype with CMV infection in organ transplantation has been reported (Woo, Lo et al. 1997) (Humar, Kumar et al. 2003; Retiere, Lesimple et al. 2003; Coaquette, Bourgeois et al. 2004; Rossini, Pignatelli et al. 2005; Zhou, Fan et al. 2007; Manuel, Asberg et al. 2009). It is known that gB plays an important role in virus entry and is also a target of neutralizing antibodies (Cranage, Kouzarides et al. 1986; Ohizumi, Suzuki et al. 1992; Navarro, Paz et al. 1993; Hopkins, Fiander et al. 1996; Lantto, Fletcher et al. 2003). Therefore, many studies have attempted to find a correlation between gB genotype and the occurrence of CMV infection or disease in organ transplant recipients. In a study involving 50 transplant recipients, the gB genotype was found not to effect viral load or clinical response to therapy (Humar, Kumar et al. 2003). Although another study also found no significant differences among gB genotypes with regard to the development of symptomatic disease, acute graft rejection, or CMV load, immunocompromised patients infected with multiple gB genotypes showed a progression to CMV disease, had an increased rate of graft rejection and had higher CMV loads (Coaquette, Bourgeois et al. 2004). Recent large, prospective cohort studies of organ transplantation have shown mixed infection to be associated with higher viral loads and delayed virologic clearance according on the basis of gB distribution analysis (Manuel, Asberg et al. 2009). Mixed genotype infection was more likely when both donor and recipient were CMV seropositive.

In addition to gB, associations between gN genotype and clinical features in organ transplant recipients were investigated (Rossini, Pignatelli et al. 2005). This study involving 74 solid organ transplant recipients showed a difference in virulance between those with the gN-1 and gN-4 strains. The gN-4 strain was associated with higher levels of antigenemia-positive cells. However, in this study, no mixed gentype infection was found and only 19 of the 74 recipients underwent kidney transplantation. Thus the influence of infection with multiple gN genotypes in cases of renal transplantation remains unclear.

These studies of glycoprotein genotypes may have some implications for the immunity of recipients as well as viral pathogenesis. gB has been implicated in host cell entry, cell-to-cell transmission of virus and fusion of infected cells, and is an important target for humoral and cellular immune responses (Cranage, Kouzarides et al. 1986; Navarro, Paz et al. 1993; Hopkins, Fiander et al. 1996; Lantto, Fletcher et al. 2003). Although polymorphisms in the cleavage site of the gB gene allow classification into of 4 distinct genotypes, the sequence of the antigenic site is well conserved (Roy, Grundy et al. 1993). The linear antibody binding sites include AD-1 and AD-2, which induce neutralizing antibodies and are highly conserved (Roy, Grundy et al. 1993). It seems that gB genotypes based on the cleavage site don't affect CMV infection in transplant recipients (Humar, Kumar et al. 2003). However, mixed gB genotype infections are associated with severe clinical manifestations (Coaquette, Bourgeois et al. 2004; Manuel, Asberg et al. 2009). In contrast to gB, the linear neutralizing antibody binding sites on gH and gN exhibit variations and form strain-specific epitopes (Urban, Britt et al. 1992; Burkhardt, Himmelein et al. 2009). These variations in the antibody binding epitopes of glycoproteins influence viral infection as they allow the virus to evade humoral immune responses.

3. CMV gH strain-specific antibody epidemiology of cytomegalovirus

3.1 ELISA for glycoproteins

The induction of an effective antibody response against CMV is an important defense mechanism as it is capable of neutralizing infectious viruses. An analysis of transplant patients revealed that during primary infection strain-specific and strain-common antibodies are produced asynchronously (Klein, Schoppel et al. 1999). The strain-specific neutralizing antibodies are induced during infection with CMV. Because CMV can persist throughout the entire life of the host after primary infection, we hypothesized that detection of strain-specific antibodies can be used to identify the CMV strain latent in the host. To evaluate CMV glycoprotein strain-specific antibodies, we analyzed for strain-specific immunoglobulin G (IgG) antibodies against the polymorphic epitopes on the envelope gH glycoproteins of CMV by means of an enzyme-linked immunosorbent assay (ELISA) method (Ishibashi, Tokumoto et al. 2007; Ishibashi, Tokumoto et al. 2008).

CMV strain-specific antibody responses were determined on the basis of polymorphisms in the antibody binding epitopes within gH between the 2 prototypical laboratory strains of CMV, AD169 and Towne. In addition to gH, we employed AD2 site I, which is conserved among CMV isolates and is the target of neutralizing antibodies, as well as AD2 site II, which binds non-neutralizing antibodies and is strain specific, for the detection of antibodies against gB (Figure 1).

3.2 Strain-specific seroepidemiology of CMV

The prevalence of CMV seropositivity varies around the world with seroprevalence ranging from 45 to 100% (Cannon, Schmid et al. 2010). For example, the CMV seroprevalence is

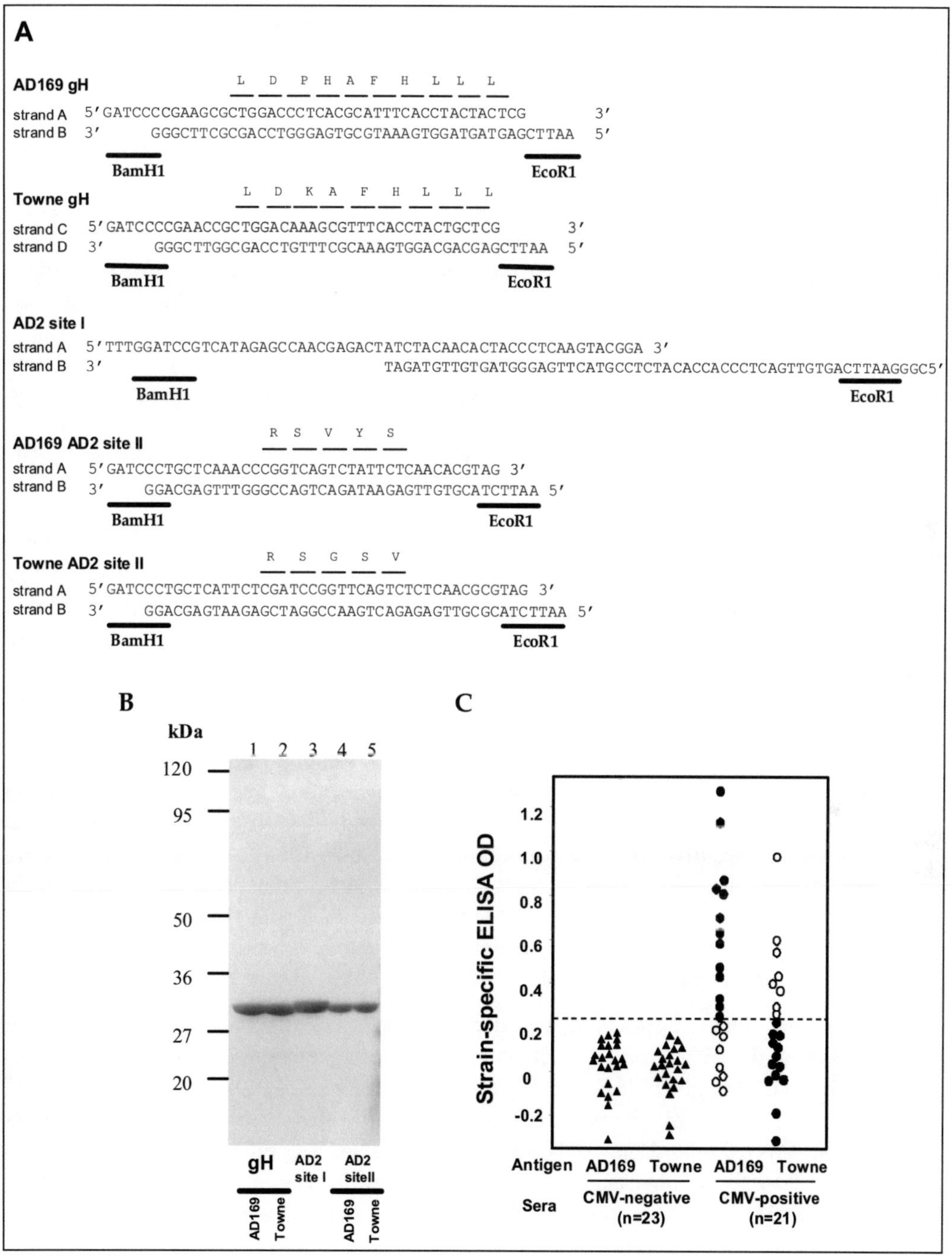

Fig. 1. Cloning and expression of recombinant antigens of CMV glycoproteins for ELISA. **A**, Oligonucleotides containing CMV gH epitopes, gB AD2 site I and site II from the AD169 and Towne strains, were used for the expression of gH epitopes as GST fusion proteins. DNA fragments encoding the epitopes were prepared by annealing two synthetic oligonucleotides. The DNA strand for the AD2 site I region was synthesized by Taq DNA

polymerase after annealing the two oligonucleotides. Each cassette has BamHI and EcoRI sites at the ends for cloning. These DNA cassettes were cloned into the *EcoRI* and *BamHI* sites of expression vector pGEX-5x. **B**, SDS-PAGE of the purified GST fusion proteins containing the AD169-gH (lane 1), Towne-gH (lane 2), AD2 site I epitope (lane 3), AD169-AD2 site II (lane 4) and Towne-AD2 site II epitopes (lane 5). Each epitope was expressed in *E. coli* strain DH5α as a fusion protein with GST, and purified using GSTrap FF (Amersham Bioscience). Size standards are shown on the left side of the gel. **C**, ELISA using purified GST fusion proteins containing AD169- and Towne-specific gH epitopes. Reactivity of CMV-seronegative sera (closed triangles) and CMV-seropositive sera reacting with the gH epitopes specific to AD169 (closed circles) and Towne (open circles) were plotted. A dashed horizontal line indicates the cut-off OD. Optical density (OD) values specific to each strain-specific gH antigen were obtained by subtracting the OD values for GST. An arbitrary cutoff for the ELISA (OD=0.25) was defined as the mean plus two standard deviations (SD) of OD values obtained from a panel of 23 healthy CMV seronegative volunteers. Figures were modified from our recent papers (Ishibashi, Tokumoto et al. 2007; Ishibashi, Tokumoto et al. 2008).

93.8% in Japan, 86.7% in Chile (Lagasse, Dhooge et al. 2000), 82.5% in the United States (Fowler, Stagno et al. 2003) and 49.5% in France (Lepage, Leroyer et al. 2011). CMV antibodies reflect prior exposure and existing immunity. However, it has been reported that the protection conferred by pre-existing immunity is limited because of the strain-dependence of the immune responses(Boppana, Rivera et al. 2001). CMV exists as a variety of different strains according to the genotype of its envelope glycoproteins. The analysis of CMV reinfection or of mixed infections has become increasingly important. Reinfection may occur when a subsequent CMV infection evades the pre-existing humoral immunity of the host. In this study, which was approved by the institutional ethics committee, blood samples were obtained from a total of 352 subjects (aged 15 to 75), consisting of healthy volunteers and consecutive potential donors and recipients for renal transplantation. We employed ELISA using GST-fusion proteins containing the strain-specific gH epitopes from AD169 and Towne strains as well as gB AD2 site I and AD2 site II to detect preexisting strain-specific antibodies in transplant recipients and healthy blood donors. The distribution of antibody responses against glycoproteins is summarized in Figure 2.

A panel of sera obtained from 352 blood donors was evaluated using the GST fusion proteins. Among the 255 serum samples with antibodies against gH and/or gB, 207(81.2%) were reactive with the gH ELISA and 178(69.8%) with the gB AD2 site I ELISA, with 132 samples reactive with both gB and gH. The CMV seropositive rate was lower in subjects aged in their teens (50%) and 20s (62%), and the rate increased significantly with increases in age, reaching 80-90% in subjects aged 30 years or over. Strain-specific antibody responses among the 207 gH seropositive samples showed that 44 samples were reactive with the gH of both AD169 and Towne. Of the 44 donors whose serum contained antibodies against both AD169 and Towne, 27 (61%) were aged 50 years or over (Figure 2B). This dual-positive rate was significantly higher than that for donors under 50 years ($p<0.01$). This result indicates that organ transplantation from older donors to younger recipients; for example, from a father or mother to one of their children, as is common in living-related transplantation, can increase the risk of reinfection with CMV.

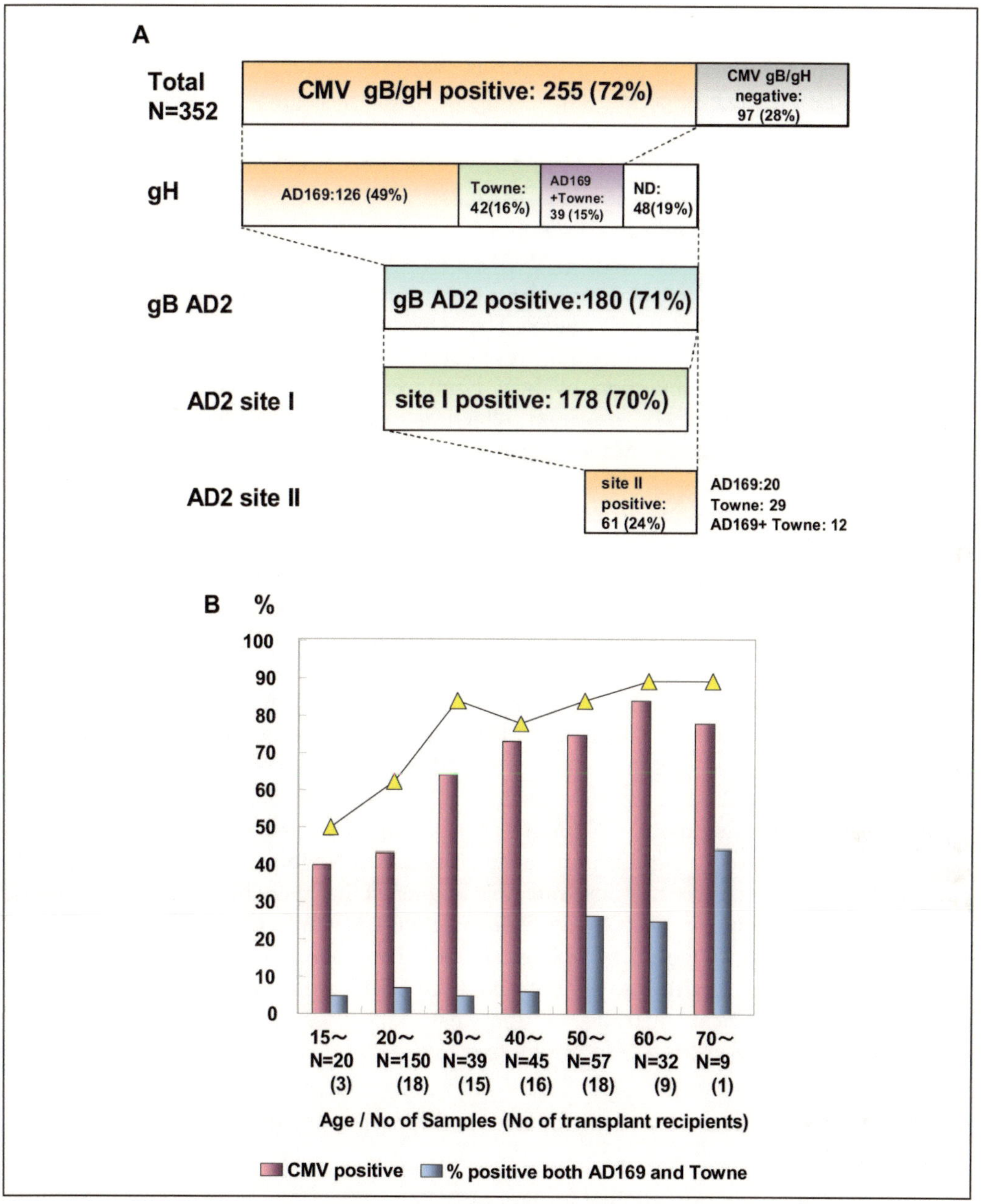

Fig. 2. Distribution of gH and gB-specific antibodies and their seroprevalence.
A: Summary of the number and distribution of serum samples according to antibody responses against gH epitopes and gB AD2.
B: Seroprevalence of CMV. Closed yellow triangles indicate CMV serostatus analyzed using a conventional ELISA kit. Rate of positive antibodies against gH and rate of positive strain-specific antibodies against both AD169 and Towne strains according to age. Age group and number of serum samples are shown on the horizontal axis. Figures were modified from our recent paper (Ishibashi, Tokumoto et al. 2008).

3.3 Association of HLA-DR with strain-specific antibodies

Several reports have described the association between the occurrence of viral infection and disease and the presence of certain HLA antigens in the host (Stewart, Kelsall et al. 1981; Baldwin, Claas et al. 1983; Roenhorst, Tegzess et al. 1985; Kraat, Christiaans et al. 1994; Varga, Rajczy et al. 2008). Many HLA antigens, including HLA-A2, HLA-A24, HLA-A32, HLA-B52, HLA-Bw4, HLA-DR6, HLA-DR11, HLA-DR15 and HLA-DQ3, were reported to increase the risk of CMV infection (Roenhorst, Tegzess et al. 1985; Chen, Rocha et al. 2001; Hodge, Boivin et al. 2004; Fan, Meng et al. 2006), although there were some conflict among the results (Gomez, Aguado et al. 1993). Major histocompatibility complex (MHC) molecules are critical for the presentation of antigens. The association between HLA alleles and CMV infection may be due to the differential presentation of CMV peptides by HLA molecules and/or the differential recognition by host lymphocytes. Studies in animals showed a genetic susceptibility to CMV infection which is controlled by the MHC (Chalmer, Mackenzie et al. 1977; Grundy, Mackenzie et al. 1981). Although the immune responses to CMV infection could be linked to CMV infection, polymorphism of CMV antigenic proteins may constitute an immune evasion mechanism. The differential presentation of polymorphic gB or Immediate Early-1 peptide by HLA molecules was suggested by the data from renal transplant recipients (Retiere, Lesimple et al. 2003). Another possible association between HLA and CMV infection is in the production of antibodies. It has been reported that deficiencies in the production of neutralizing antibodies against CMV gB in certain HLA types may lead to increased susceptibility (Wada, Mizuno et al. 1997). In this report, subjects with HLA-DR9 had a higher positive rate against CMV gB and subjects with HLA-DR15 had a lower positive rate against gB. Production of antibodies against another major epitope of CMV, gH, may correlate with certain HLA types. We investigated HLA-DR type and strain-specific antibody responses against gH in potential donors and recipients for renal transplantation (Ishibashi, Tokumoto et al. 2009). Our results showed that subjects with HLA-DR10 showed a significantly lower response rate against CMV gH and subjects with HLA-DR11 had a lower response rate. It is of interest that there have been some reports that HLA-DR11 alleles are more susceptible to active CMV infection in the case of solid organ transplantation (Retiere, Lesimple et al. 2003; Fan, Meng et al. 2006). However, the percentages of subjects with HLA-DR10 and HLA-DR11 were very small in our study population. Geographical analysis of the distribution of antibodies against CMV glycoproteins and HLA types would be of interest.

4. Differences in adverse events between CMV primary infections and reinfections

4.1 Pattern of infection and clinical impact of CMV

CMV infection and disease are crucial causes of morbidity and mortality among transplant recipients. The term "CMV infection" applies to a condition in which there is evidence of CMV replication whether or not symptoms are present. There are three main patterns of CMV infection, primary infection, reactivation and reinfection (Ljungman, Griffiths et al. 2002). Primary infection is defined as a new-onset infection in recipients who had been found to be seronegative. The recipients acquire CMV from their donors for the first time. If the latent infected recipient's original CMV is reactivated in recipients who were seropositive, it is understood as reactivation. Reinfection is defined as infection of new CMV strain in recipients who were previously seropositive. Reinfection is diagnosed if the detected CMV strain was different from that of their donor's by using a variety of molecular techniques or inferred if the recipients acquire new antibodies against strain-specific epitopes.

CMV infections in solid organ transplant recipients induce serious direct and indirect consequences. The direct clinical effects of CMV include CMV infection, CMV disease and end-organ diseases; *i.e.,* gastrointestinal disease, hepatitis, retinitis, nephritis, cystitis, myocarditis, encephalitis and pancreatitis. In addition to the directly effects, CMV is associated with graft rejection, allograft dysfunction and failure, cardiovascular complications, and fungal, viral or bacterial superinfection, all of which are known as the "indirect effects" of CMV (Ljungman, Griffiths et al. 2002).

Classically, because of its high rate of CMV primary infection, concern was mainly focused on CMV in D+/R- settings. However, in D+/R+ transplantation, the presence of antibodies against matched CMV gH epitopes influence the outcome of transplantation. More adverse events were observed in the case of reinfection with different CMV strains.

4.2 Classification of transplant pairings according to CMV strain-specific antibody responses

To identify potential CMV reinfections before renal transplantation, genotypes of the CMVs latently infecting donors and recipients should be detected. One of the methods considered for the genotyping of CMV is the detection of CMV DNA directly from blood donors using PCR. However, CMV DNA during the latency phase is seldom detected in healthy blood donors with validated PCR (Roback, Drew et al. 2003). The low copy number of latency infected cells is a major limitation to PCR. It is estimated that 0.004 to 0.12 percent of CMV-positive peripheral blood mononuclear cells harbor 2 to 13 genomes per cell (Slobedman and Mocarski 1999; Soderberg-Naucler, Streblow et al. 2001). The highest detection rate obtained with PCR to date was approximately 39% (Pignatelli, Dal Monte et al. 2006).

Instead of PCR methods, we employed a serologic assay using *E. coli*-expressed strain-specific epitopes (Ishibashi, Tokumoto et al. 2007). This serologic assay can estimate the CMV strain previously and latently infecting the blood donors. From the combination of antibody responses against the strain-specific gH epitopes, the conventional CMV D+/R+ pairings can be classified into two groups. When a recipient receives an organ graft from a donor who has the same strain-specific gH antibody of CMV as the recipient, the pairing is classified as a "matched gH" pairing. The pairings in which the recipients do not have strain-specific gH antibodies matching their donor's are classified as "mismatched gH" pairings. The "mismatched gH" pairings indicate that the recipients can not neutralize the CMV from donors. It is considered that this pairing in a D+/R+ setting can cause CMV reinfection. We distinguished 114 renal transplantation pairings according to the strain-specific responses and analyzed the data (Figure 3). We found differences in the clinical course after transplantation among the D+/R-, matched gH and mismatched gH pairings.

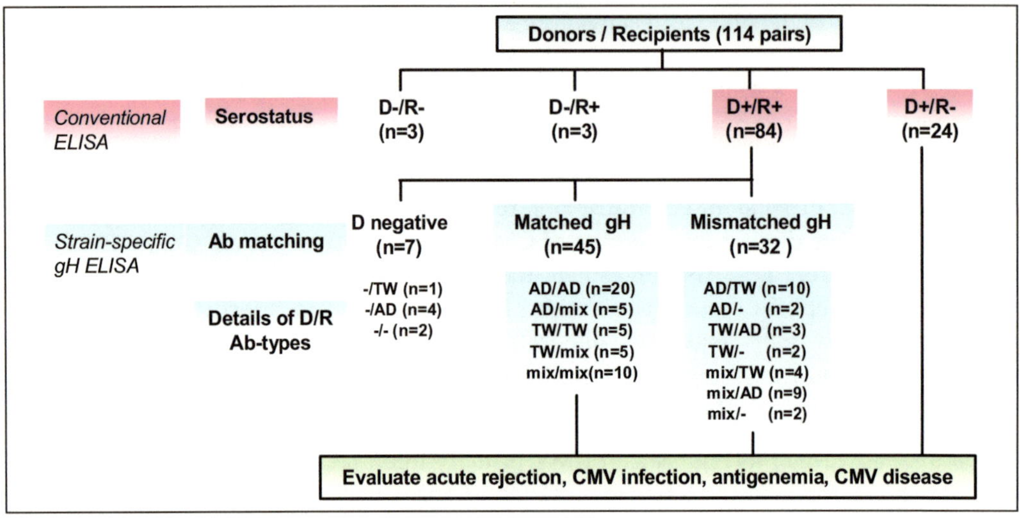

Fig. 3. Classification of transplant pairings according to strain-specific gH antibody responses. Classifications of the donors (D) and recipients (R) according to the conventional CMV serostatus (+ or -) and CMV strain-specific antibodies (Ab) against gH epitopes. Details of the combinations based on strain-specific Ab against gH epitopes (AD: AD169, TW: Towne, mix: both AD169 and Towne, and -: undetectable) are also shown. The 84 D+/R+ pairs were classified into three subgroups, "matched gH", "mismatched gH" and "D-negative". As antibodies against gH were undetectable in 7 donors, they were excluded from the analysis. The figure was slightly modified from our recent paper (Ishibashi, Tokumoto et al. 2007).

4.3 Acute rejection after renal transplantation

In this study, which was approved by the institutional ethics committee, 114 pairs of consecutive donors and recipients undergoing living-related renal transplantation were included. Immunosuppression for recipients consisted of triple-drug therapy (tacrolimus or cyclosporine, mycophenolate mofetile, and predonisolone). Among the 114 transplants, cyclosporin was used in 7 recipients who had chest pain or hyperglycemia. Rejection was suspected when serum creatinine level increased more than 25% from the basal level in the absence of urinary tract obstruction or renal graft artery stenosis. During the follow up after transplantation, the first rejection episode was confirmed histologically by biopsy samples from the grafts.

Five recipients (21%) among the 24 D+/R- pairs and 31 recipients (37%) among the 84 D+/R+ pairs experienced biopsy-proven acute rejection. There was no statistically significant difference in the acute rejection rate between the D+/R- and D+/R+ settings (p=0.14). Among the 27 D+/R+ patients with acute rejection whose matching of strain-specific gH antibodies were known, 17 (53%) did not have matched strain-specific antibodies and was categorized as "mismatched gH"(Figure 4). The rate of acute rejection after renal transplantation was significantly higher in recipients in "mismatched gH" groups than in those of "matched gH" groups (22%; p=0.0051) and of the D+/R- groups (21%;, p=0.014). The average number of days after transplantation to diagnosis of acute rejection was 25 days for all cases with acute rejection, and there were no statistical differences in incubation period for acute rejection among the three groups.

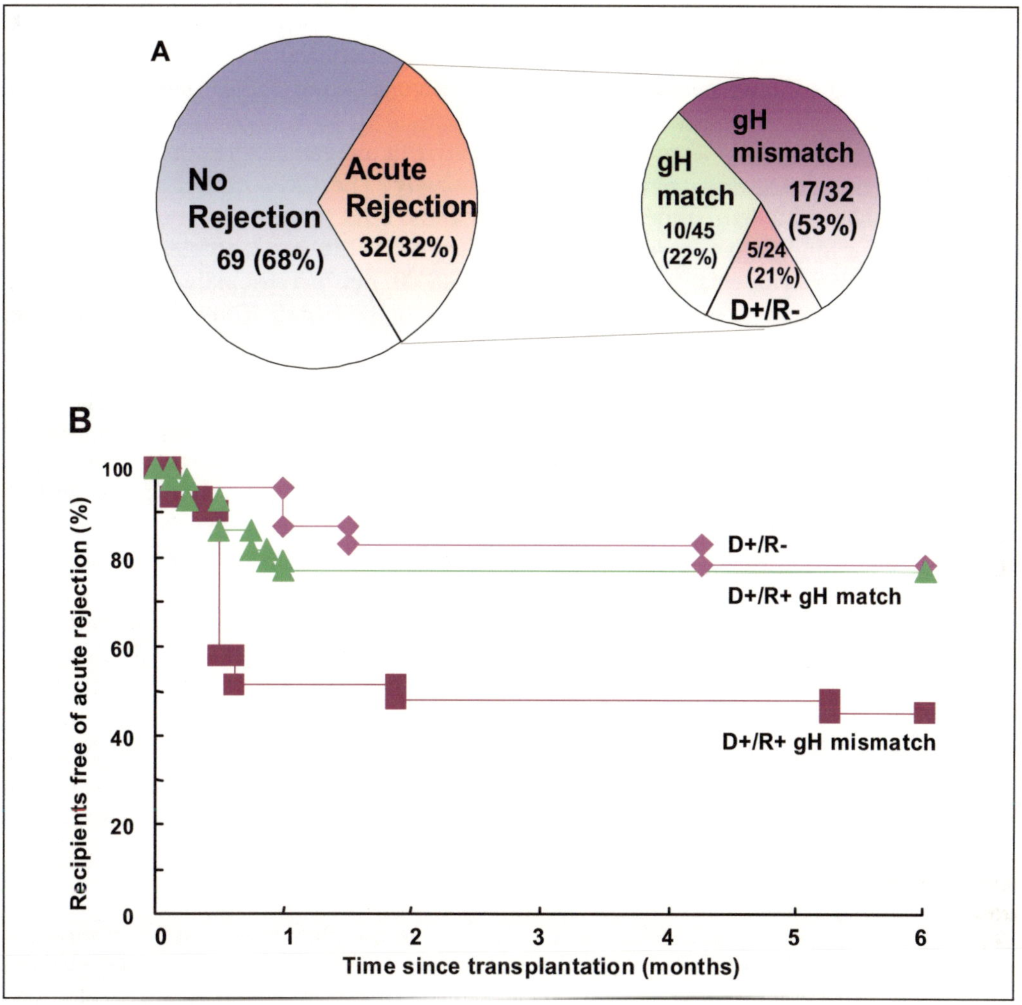

Fig. 4. Incidences of acute rejection.
A, Among the 101 transplant recipients with the three types of settings, the D+/R- (n=24), D+/R+ matched gH (n=45) and D+/R+ mismatched gH (n=32) groups, 32 (32%) experienced biopsy-proven acute rejection after transplantation. The acute rejection rate in the gH mismatch group was significantly higher than those of the D+/R- (p=0.0051) and gH match (p=0.014) groups.
B, Kaplan-Meier curves for the cumulative probability of freedom from biopsy-proven acute rejection. The incidence of acute rejection in the gH mismatched group was significantly higher than those in the D+/R- and gH matched groups (p=0.002). Figures were modified from our recent paper (Ishibashi, Tokumoto et al. 2007).

4.4 CMV infection and disease in gH mismatch settings

Incidences of CMV infection and CMV disease were monitored in the D+/R-, gH matched and gH mismatched groups of transplant recipients (Figure 5). Antigenemia using pp65 antibodies was routinely evaluated weekly for six months after transplantation. CMV infection was defined as the occurence of antigenemia (> 1 pp65-positive cells/300,000 leukocytes) during the monitoring period irrespective of clinical manifestations. Patients with a low level of antigenemia (1 to 9 pp65-positive cells per $3.0x10^5$ leukocytes) were monitored frequently and preemptive therapy was initiated once 10 or more pp65-positive cells per $3.0x10^5$ leukocytes were detected. Irrespective of antigenemia results, patients with CMV-related manifestations were treated immediately. The CMV-related manifestations include unexplained fever (temperature $\geq$ 38°C with no other source to account for it) for 2 or more days, arthralgia, leucopenia (leukocyte count of $\leq$ 4000/mm^3), atypical lymphocytes of $\geq$ 3% or thrombocytopenia (platelet count of $\leq$ 100,000/mm^3), a rise in liver enzyme level, gastrointestinal ulceration or hemorrhage, and pneumonitis (Singh, Yu et al. 1994; Tanabe, Tokumoto et al. 1997).

Sixteen of 24 recipients (67%) among the D+/R- group had CMV infection, and 13 (54%) of them developed CMV disease (Figure 5A). Among the 84 D+/R+ transplant pairings, 77 pairings were classified as gH-matched pairings or gH-mismatched pairings. During the 6-month follow up after renal transplantation, 37 (48%) of the 77 recipients in the D+/R+ group were found to be positive for CMV infection by the pp65-antigenemia assay, and 13 recipients (17%) were diagnosed with CMV disease. The incidence of CMV disease in the recipients in the D+/R- group was statistically higher than in those in the D+/R+ group ($p=0.0003$). When the 13 recipients in the D+/R+ group who experienced CMV disease were classified by antibody response against CMV gH, 9 (9/32, 28%) were in the gH mismatch group and 4 were in the gH matched group (4/45, 9% Figure 5 B). Consequently, CMV disease was significantly more prevalent in the gH mismatched group than in the gH matched group. The proportion of cases with CMV infection that progressed to CMV disease in the gH mismatched and gH match groups were 64% and 17%, respectively ($p=0.0038$, Figure 5 C).

4.5 CMV pp65 antigenemia and antibodies against gB and gH matching

We performed antigenemia assays weekly during the 6-month follow up. The medians (ranges) of the maximum number of positive cells in the recipients from the D+/R+ gH mismatched and gH matched groups were 38 (1-818) and 2 (1-142), respectively. The maximum number of pp65-positive cells differed significantly between these two groups. The medians (ranges) of the maximum number of positive cells in the recipients from the D+/R- group was 113 (1-3128), and there was no significant difference between the D+/R- group and the gH mismatched group (Ishibashi, Tokumoto et al. 2007). These results reflect the incidence of CMV disease among each group. Matching of antibody responses against strain-specific CMV gH could reduce the risk of CMV disease. The gH sequences of the CMV strains from the recipients who showed the highest level of antigenemia after transplantation were found to match the antibodies present in their donors (Ishibashi, Tokumoto et al. 2008).

In addition to gH, gB is considered to be one of the major target molecules for neutralizing antibodies as well as for cellular immune response (Gyulai, Endresz et al. 2000). We also evaluated the correlation between the maximum number of pp65-positive cells during the 6 months after transplantation and antibody responses against the gB AD2 site I epitope, as well as the matching of antibodies against gH. Seventy-seven recipients in the D+/R+ matched gH or mismatched gH groups, were classified into 4 subgroups based on the

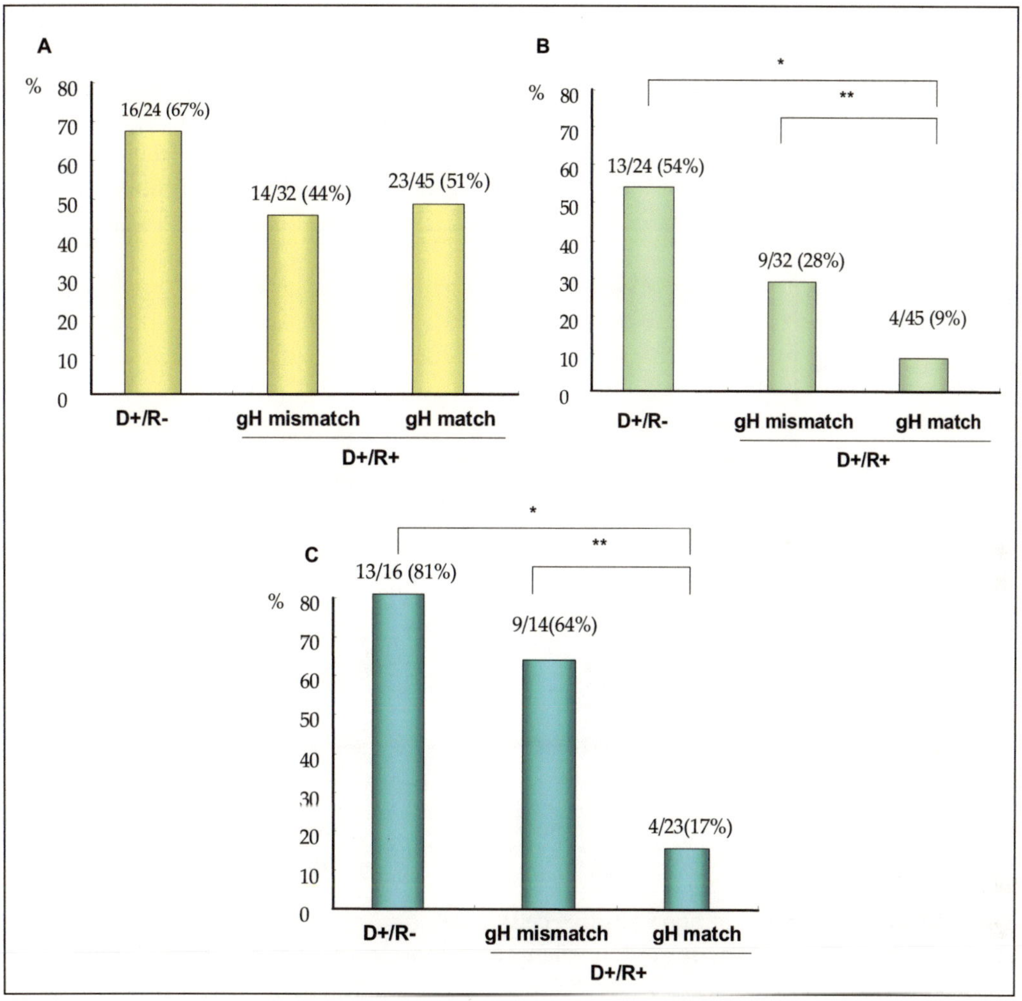

Fig. 5. CMV infection and CMV disease after renal transplantation.
A, The rate of recipients diagnosed with CMV infection. If recipients showed at least 1 pp65-positive cell during the follow up, they were diagnosed with CMV infection. There was no significant difference among the groups. B, The rate of CMV disease among the three groups. In the D+/R+ gH matched group, the rate of CMV disease was significantly lower than those in the other groups (*p=0.006, **p=0.013). C, The rate of recipients with CMV infection who progressed to CMV disease. Among the 53 recipients diagnosed with CMV infection, 26 patients progressed to CMV disease. Among them, 13 were D+/R- and 9 were gH mismatched. These rates were significantly higher than that in the gH matched group (*p=0.0001, **p=0.0038). Figures were modified from our recent paper (Ishibashi, Tokumoto et al. 2007).

combinations of antibody responses against both gH and gB (matched gH/gB-, matched gH/gB+, mismatched gH/gB-, mismatched gH/gB+). Significant differences in the maximum numbers of pp65-positive cells obtained during the 6 months in the patients with CMV infection were observed. The medians of the maximum number of positive cells were

1 (range, 1–9), 20 (range, 1-142), 26 (range 1-254), and 45 (range 2-818) for the matched gH/gB-, matched gH/gB+, mismatched gH/gB- and mismatched gH/gB+ groups, respectively (Figure 6). These differences resulted from differences in the number of patients who diagnosed with CMV disease and given preemptive therapy. Consequently, the introduction of preemptive therapy was significantly more prevalent in the subgroups lacking antibodies against gH and/or gB than in the matched gH/gB+ subgroup.

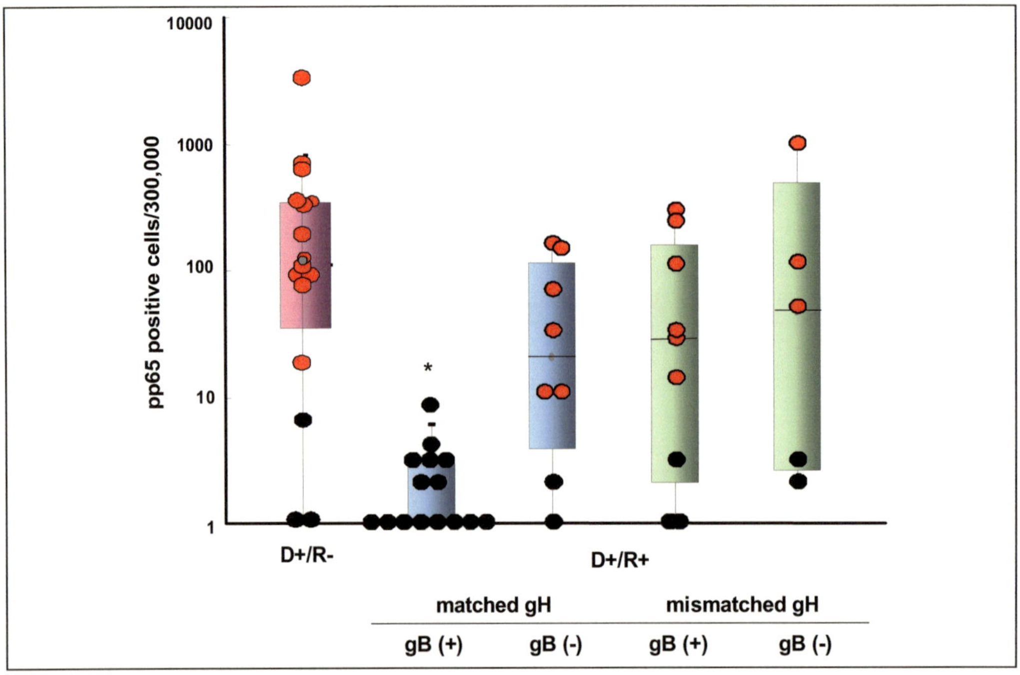

Fig. 6. Maximum number of pp65-positive cells.
Antigenemia in the 5 subgroups of transplant recipients classified based on seroimmunity against the particular epitopes of CMV gH and gB. The maximum number of pp65-positive cells during the monitoring period for each recipient with CMV infection was plotted. Each closed circle indicates one recipient. The broken bars in the box plot indicate the median of pp65-positive cells. Closed red circles indicate recipients who had given preemptive therapy for CMV disease. Figures were modified from our recent paper (Ishibashi, Tokumoto et al. 2011).

Previous studies have demonstrated that the antibody titers against AD2 measured in ELISA had a good correlation with neutralizing antibody titers (Rothe, Pepperl-Klindworth et al. 2001). However, the role of neutralizing antibodies in the control of CMV infection in transplantation recipients has been a matter of discussion (Schoppel, Schmidt et al. 1998; Volpi, Pica et al. 1999; Munoz, Gutierrez et al. 2001). Alternatively, positive anti-gB AD2 antibodies may indicate the presence of sufficient anti-CMV cellular immune responses as a consequence of the natural course of CMV infection. Among the viral proteins in CMV, gB has been identified as a potential target for CMV-specific CD8+ and CD4+ T-cell immunity (Gyulai, Endresz et al. 2000; Elkington, Walker et al. 2003). Deficiencies in the response of cytotoxic T lymphocytes specific for CMV are important in the pathogenesis of CMV disease in immunocompromised recipients (Reusser, Riddell et al. 1991). It would be interesting to see whether the CMV specific T-cell activity against CMV-gB correlates with the outcome of our ELISA against gB AD2.

However, CMV infection was not completely prevented in spite of the presence of antibodies against matched gH and gB. A recent report on bacterial artificial chromosome-derived recombinant viruses that differed only in the expression of the gN genotype on the background of the AD169 strain showed that 30% of human sera showed strain-specific neutralization (Burkhardt, Himmelein et al. 2009). It suggested that gN constituted a major determinant for the induction of strain-specific neutralizing antibodies as well as gH and gB. The antigenic variations in a single envelope protein of CMV were shown to be sufficient to escape neutralization. It would be interesting to see the matching of antibodies against strain-specific gN in addition to the matching of gH

5. Association of CMV reinfection and acute rejection

Many reports indicate a relationship between CMV infection and allograft rejection in renal transplantation (Lautenschlager, Soots et al. 1997; Humar, Gillingham et al. 1999; McLaughlin, Wu et al. 2002; Sagedal, Nordal et al. 2002; Nett, Heisey et al. 2004). According to a prospective study of 477 consecutive renal transplant patients, CMV infection and disease are independent risk factors for clinical acute rejection (Sagedal, Nordal et al. 2002). In another study of 106 consecutive renal transplants, CMV disease, but not asymptomatic infection, was shown to be an independent risk factor for biopsy-proven acute rejection (Reischig, Jindra et al. 2006). Control of CMV infection has the potential to reduce the prevalence of acute rejection. Even one episode of acute rejection of renal allografts substantially shortens overall graft survival (Ferguson 1994), and prophylaxis could offer greater benefits compared with pre-emptive therapy. Patients provided with prophylaxis showed a significantly lower incidence of biopsy-proven acute rejection compared with those undergoing pre-emptive therapy (Reischig, Jindra et al. 2008). Prophylaxis has been shown to improve long-term graft survival in renal transplant patients (Pachl, Probert et al. 1989; Kliem, Fricke et al. 2008).

In our study, which applied pre-emptive therapy, acute rejection was observed in 32 (32%) of 101 renal transplant recipients. Among them, patients in the mismatched gH group, which indicates reinfection with a different gH strain of CMV, showed a higher rate of acute rejection (Figure 4). It is unclear why reinfection with CMV increased the risk of acute rejection while there were no significant differences in the incidence of CMV infection or disease from those in patients with a D+/R- setting (Figure 5). Considered from the perspective of immunity against CMV, escape from humoral responses, especially from antibodies against gH and/or gB, can induce a local inflammatory response through Toll-like receptors (TLRs). Inflammatory cytokine stimulation by CMV is mediated by interaction between the glycoproteins and TLR2 (Compton, Kurt-Jones et al. 2003). Neutralizing antibodies against gB and gH inhibit inflammatory cytokine responses of TLR2 to CMV infection (Boehme, Guerrero et al. 2006). However, this lack of efficient neutralizing antibodies against glycoproteins is shared by patients in a mismatched gH setting and those in a D+/R- setting. Differences in immunity against CMV between the mismatched gH and D+/R- groups could be due to the presence of memory T cells. Abate *et al.* reported that R+ recipients treated with preemptive therapy displayed a steady and constant CMV-specific immune reconstitution with a highly heterogeneous pattern 60–360 days after transplantation, when evaluated by interferon (IFN)-γ enzyme-linked immunospot (ELISPOT) assay (Abate, Saldan et al. 2010). Indeed, the R- recipients treated with prophylaxis presented a very different scenario of immune reconstitution: none of the recipients analyzed showed evident immune reconstitution up to day 180 after transplantation. In this report, which analyzed 85 renal transplant recipients, 10 (IA:7, IB:3) of 70 R+ patients(14%) and 1 (IA) of 13 R- patients (8%) experienced acute rejection (Abate, Saldan et al. 2010). Another report indicated that there were no differences in the frequency of CMV-specific T-cell frequencies between patients with and without acute rejection (Nickel, Bold et al. 2009). In cardiac transplantation, recipients with early detectable levels of CMV-specific CD4 T-cells were protected from high viral loads and acute rejection (Tu, Potena et al. 2006). To date, CMV-specific cellular responses seem to be favorable to prevent adverse events after transplantation. However, IFN-γ is a proinflammatory Th1 type 1 that regulates cell-mediated responses and favors allograft rejection (Crispim, Wastowski et al. 2010; Sementilli and Franco 2010; Tellides and Pober 2007). The excessive reconstitution of IFN-γ–secreting effector cells might contribute to allograft rejection because circulating virus-specific T cells synthesize type 1 cytokines such as IFN-γ. In addition, the correlation of viral load with the development of CMV-specific T-cell responses remains unclear. We speculate that in a mismatched gH setting, a high viral load and IFN-γ from prompt cell-mediated responses induce acute rejection, whereas recipients in a matched gH setting were protected from high viral loads and those in a D+/R-setting lacked prompt cellular immune responses.

6. Conclusion

We would like to propose a working hypothesis that the mismatch of gH types, probably due to reinfection with a strain different from the original strain, is the major risk factor for CMV disease and acute rejection after renal transplantation. Pre-existing immunity against CMV glycoproteins has a critical role in the prevention of CMV infection, and it might allow recipients to avoid acute rejection. Measuring antibodies against CMV glycoproteins for both transplant donors and recipients can provide crucial information on CMV infection, particularly CMV reinfection, and the possibility of acute rejection after transplantation.

7. References

Abate, D., A. Saldan, et al. (2010). "Evaluation of cytomegalovirus (CMV)-specific T cell immune reconstitution revealed that baseline antiviral immunity, prophylaxis, or preemptive therapy but not antithymocyte globulin treatment contribute to CMV-specific T cell reconstitution in kidney transplant recipients." *J Infect Dis* 202(4): 585-94.

Almond, P. S., A. Matas, et al. (1993). "Risk factors for chronic rejection in renal allograft recipients." *Transplantation* 55(4): 752-6; discussion 756-7.

Baldwin, W. M., 3rd, F. H. Claas, et al. (1983). "Renal graft dysfunction during infection with cytomegalovirus: association with IgM lymphocytotoxins and HLA-DR3 and DR7." *Br Med J (Clin Res Ed)* 287(6402): 1332-4.

Boehme, K. W., M. Guerrero, et al. (2006). "Human cytomegalovirus envelope glycoproteins B and H are necessary for TLR2 activation in permissive cells." *J Immunol* 177(10): 7094-102.

Boppana, S. B., L. B. Rivera, et al. (2001). "Intrauterine transmission of cytomegalovirus to infants of women with preconceptional immunity." *N Engl J Med* 344(18): 1366-71.

Britt, W. J. and M. Mach (1996). "Human cytomegalovirus glycoproteins." *Intervirology* 39(5-6): 401-12.

Burkhardt, C., S. Himmelein, et al. (2009). "Glycoprotein N subtypes of human cytomegalovirus induce a strain-specific antibody response during natural infection." *J Gen Virol* 90(Pt 8): 1951-61.

Cannon, M. J., D. S. Schmid, et al. (2010). "Review of cytomegalovirus seroprevalence and demographic characteristics associated with infection." *Rev Med Virol* 20(4): 202-13.

Cha, T. A., E. Tom, et al. (1996). "Human cytomegalovirus clinical isolates carry at least 19 genes not found in laboratory strains." *J Virol* 70(1): 78-83.

Chalmer, J. E., J. S. Mackenzie, et al. (1977). "Resistance to murine cytomegalovirus linked to the major histocompatibility complex of the mouse." *J Gen Virol* 37(1): 107-14.

Chee, M. S., A. T. Bankier, et al. (1990). "Analysis of the protein-coding content of the sequence of human cytomegalovirus strain AD169." *Curr Top Microbiol Immunol* 154: 125-69.

Chen, Y., V. Rocha, et al. (2001). "Relationship between HLA alleles and cytomegalovirus infection after allogenic hematopoietic stem cell transplant." *Blood* 98(2): 500-1.

Chou, S. (1992). "Molecular epidemiology of envelope glycoprotein H of human cytomegalovirus." *J Infect Dis* 166(3): 604-7.

Chou, S. W. and K. M. Dennison (1991). "Analysis of interstrain variation in cytomegalovirus glycoprotein B sequences encoding neutralization-related epitopes." *J Infect Dis* 163(6): 1229-34.

Coaquette, A., A. Bourgeois, et al. (2004). "Mixed cytomegalovirus glycoprotein B genotypes in immunocompromised patients." *Clin Infect Dis* 39(2): 155-61.

Compton, T., E. A. Kurt-Jones, et al. (2003). "Human cytomegalovirus activates inflammatory cytokine responses via CD14 and Toll-like receptor 2." *J Virol* 77(8): 4588-96.

Compton, T., D. M. Nowlin, et al. (1993). "Initiation of human cytomegalovirus infection requires initial interaction with cell surface heparan sulfate." *Virology* 193(2): 834-41.

Cosio, F. G., R. P. Pelletier, et al. (1997). "Impact of acute rejection and early allograft function on renal allograft survival." *Transplantation* 63(11): 1611-5.

Cranage, M. P., T. Kouzarides, et al. (1986). "Identification of the human cytomegalovirus glycoprotein B gene and induction of neutralizing antibodies via its expression in recombinant vaccinia virus." *Embo J* 5(11): 3057-63.

Crispim, J. C., I. J. Wastowski, et al. (2010). "Interferon-gamma +874 polymorphism in the first intron of the human interferon-gamma gene and kidney allograft outcome." *Transplant Proc* 42(10): 4505-8.

Dal Monte, P., S. Pignatelli, et al. (2001). "The product of human cytomegalovirus UL73 is a new polymorphic structural glycoprotein (gpUL73)." *J Hum Virol* 4(1): 26-34.

Egli, A., S. Binggeli, et al. (2007). "Cytomegalovirus and polyomavirus BK posttransplant." *Nephrol Dial Transplant* 22 Suppl 8: viii72-viii82.

Elkington, R., S. Walker, et al. (2003). "Ex vivo profiling of CD8+-T-cell responses to human cytomegalovirus reveals broad and multispecific reactivities in healthy virus carriers." *J Virol* 77(9): 5226-40.

Evans, R. W., D. L. Manninen, et al. (1985). "The quality of life of patients with end-stage renal disease." *N Engl J Med* 312(9): 553-9.

Fan, J., X. Q. Meng, et al. (2006). "Association of cytomegalovirus infection with human leukocyte antigen genotypes in recipients after allogeneic liver transplantation." *Hepatobiliary Pancreat Dis Int* 5(1): 34-8.

Feire, A. L., H. Koss, et al. (2004). "Cellular integrins function as entry receptors for human cytomegalovirus via a highly conserved disintegrin-like domain." *Proc Natl Acad Sci U S A* 101(43): 15470-5.

Ferguson, R. (1994). "Acute rejection episodes--best predictor of long-term primary cadaveric renal transplant survival." *Clin Transplant* 8(3 Pt 2): 328-31.

Fowler, K. B., S. Stagno, et al. (2003). "Maternal immunity and prevention of congenital cytomegalovirus infection." *Jama* 289(8): 1008-11.

Gomez, E., S. Aguado, et al. (1993). "Absence of association between HLA-DR7 and cytomegalovirus infection in renal transplant patients." *Lancet* 341(8858): 1480-1.

Grundy, J. E., J. S. Mackenzie, et al. (1981). "Influence of H-2 and non-H-2 genes on resistance to murine cytomegalovirus infection." *Infect Immun* 32(1): 277-86.

Gyulai, Z., V. Endresz, et al. (2000). "Cytotoxic T lymphocyte (CTL) responses to human cytomegalovirus pp65, IE1-Exon4, gB, pp150, and pp28 in healthy individuals: reevaluation of prevalence of IE1-specific CTLs." *J Infect Dis* 181(5): 1537-46.

Hariharan, S., J. W. Alexander, et al. (1996). "Impact of first acute rejection episode and severity of rejection on cadaveric renal allograft survival." *Clin Transplant* 10(6 Pt 1): 538-41.

Hariharan, S., C. P. Johnson, et al. (2000). "Improved graft survival after renal transplantation in the United States, 1988 to 1996." *N Engl J Med* 342(9): 605-12.

Heieren, M. H., Y. K. Kim, et al. (1988). "Human cytomegalovirus infection of kidney glomerular visceral epithelial and tubular epithelial cells in culture." *Transplantation* 46(3): 426-32.

Heieren, M. H., F. J. van der Woude, et al. (1988). "Cytomegalovirus replicates efficiently in human kidney mesangial cells." *Proc Natl Acad Sci U S A* 85(5): 1642-6.

Hobom, U., W. Brune, et al. (2000). "Fast screening procedures for random transposon libraries of cloned herpesvirus genomes: mutational analysis of human cytomegalovirus envelope glycoprotein genes." *J Virol* 74(17): 7720-9.

Hodge, W. G., J. F. Boivin, et al. (2004). "Laboratory-based risk factors for cytomegalovirus retinitis." *Can J Ophthalmol* 39(7): 733-45.

Hopkins, J. I., A. N. Fiander, et al. (1996). "Cytotoxic T cell immunity to human cytomegalovirus glycoprotein B." *J Med Virol* 49(2): 124-31.

Huber, M. T. and T. Compton (1999). "Intracellular formation and processing of the heterotrimeric gH-gL-gO (gCIII) glycoprotein envelope complex of human cytomegalovirus." *J Virol* 73(5): 3886-92.

Humar, A., K. J. Gillingham, et al. (1999). "Association between cytomegalovirus disease and chronic rejection in kidney transplant recipients." *Transplantation* 68(12): 1879-83.

Humar, A., D. Kumar, et al. (2003). "Cytomegalovirus (CMV) glycoprotein B genotypes and response to antiviral therapy, in solid-organ-transplant recipients with CMV disease." *J Infect Dis* 188(4): 581-4.

Isaacson, M. K., A. L. Feire, et al. (2007). "Epidermal growth factor receptor is not required for human cytomegalovirus entry or signaling." *J Virol* 81(12): 6241-7.

Ishibashi, K., T. Tokumoto, et al. (2011). "Lack of antibodies against the antigen domain 2 epitope of cytomegalovirus (CMV) glycoprotein B is associated with CMV disease after renal transplantation in recipients having the same glycoprotein H serotypes as their donors." *Transpl Infect Dis* 13(3): 318-23.

Ishibashi, K., T. Tokumoto, et al. (2008). "Strain-specific seroepidemiology and reinfection of cytomegalovirus." *Microbes Infect* 10(12-13): 1363-9.

Ishibashi, K., T. Tokumoto, et al. (2009). "Association between antibody response against cytomegalovirus strain-specific glycoprotein H epitopes and HLA-DR." *Microbiol Immunol* 53(7): 412-6.

Ishibashi, K., T. Tokumoto, et al. (2007). "Association of the outcome of renal transplantation with antibody response to cytomegalovirus strain-specific glycoprotein H epitopes." *Clin Infect Dis* 45(1): 60-7.

Jindal, R. M. and S. Hariharan (1999). "Chronic rejection in kidney transplants. An in-depth review." *Nephron* 83(1): 13-24.

Kari, B. and R. Gehrz (1992). "A human cytomegalovirus glycoprotein complex designated gC-II is a major heparin-binding component of the envelope." *J Virol* 66(3): 1761-4.

Kaye, J. F., U. A. Gompels, et al. (1992). "Glycoprotein H of human cytomegalovirus (HCMV) forms a stable complex with the HCMV UL115 gene product." *J Gen Virol* 73 (Pt 10): 2693-8.

Keay, S. and B. Baldwin (1991). "Anti-idiotype antibodies that mimic gp86 of human cytomegalovirus inhibit viral fusion but not attachment." *J Virol* 65(9): 5124-8.

Klein, M., K. Schoppel, et al. (1999). "Strain-specific neutralization of human cytomegalovirus isolates by human sera." *J Virol* 73(2): 878-86.

Kliem, V., L. Fricke, et al. (2008). "Improvement in long-term renal graft survival due to CMV prophylaxis with oral ganciclovir: results of a randomized clinical trial." *Am J Transplant* 8(5): 975-83.

Kraat, Y. J., M. H. Christiaans, et al. (1994). "Risk factors for cytomegalovirus infection and disease in renal transplant recipients: HLA-DR7 and triple therapy." *Transpl Int* 7(5): 362-7.

Lagasse, N., I. Dhooge, et al. (2000). "Congenital CMV-infection and hearing loss." *Acta Otorhinolaryngol Belg* 54(4): 431-6.

Lantto, J., J. M. Fletcher, et al. (2003). "Binding characteristics determine the neutralizing potential of antibody fragments specific for antigenic domain 2 on glycoprotein B of human cytomegalovirus." *Virology* 305(1): 201-9.

Larsson, S., C. Soderberg-Naucler, et al. (1998). "Productive cytomegalovirus (CMV) infection exclusively in CD13-positive peripheral blood mononuclear cells from CMV-infected individuals: implications for prevention of CMV transmission." *Transplantation* 65(3): 411-5.

Lautenschlager, I., A. Soots, et al. (1997). "Effect of cytomegalovirus on an experimental model of chronic renal allograft rejection under triple-drug treatment in the rat." *Transplantation* 64(3): 391-8.

Lehner, R., T. Stamminger, et al. (1991). "Comparative sequence analysis of human cytomegalovirus strains." *J Clin Microbiol* 29(11): 2494-502.

Lepage, N., A. Leroyer, et al. (2011). "Cytomegalovirus seroprevalence in exposed and unexposed populations of hospital employees." *Eur J Clin Microbiol Infect Dis* 30(1): 65-70.

Ljungman, P., P. Griffiths, et al. (2002). "Definitions of cytomegalovirus infection and disease in transplant recipients." *Clin Infect Dis* 34(8): 1094-7.

Mach, M., B. Kropff, et al. (2000). "Complex formation by human cytomegalovirus glycoproteins M (gpUL100) and N (gpUL73)." *J Virol* 74(24): 11881-92.

Manuel, O., A. Asberg, et al. (2009). "Impact of genetic polymorphisms in cytomegalovirus glycoprotein B on outcomes in solid-organ transplant recipients with cytomegalovirus disease." *Clin Infect Dis* 49(8): 1160-6.

Manuel, O., X. L. Pang, et al. (2009). "An assessment of donor-to-recipient transmission patterns of human cytomegalovirus by analysis of viral genomic variants." *J Infect Dis* 199(11): 1621-8.

Mattick, C., D. Dewin, et al. (2004). "Linkage of human cytomegalovirus glycoprotein gO variant groups identified from worldwide clinical isolates with gN genotypes, implications for disease associations and evidence for N-terminal sites of positive selection." *Virology* 318(2): 582-97.

McLaughlin, K., C. Wu, et al. (2002). "Cytomegalovirus seromismatching increases the risk of acute renal allograft rejection." *Transplantation* 74(6): 813-6.

Meier-Kriesche, H. U., J. D. Schold, et al. (2004). "Lack of improvement in renal allograft survival despite a marked decrease in acute rejection rates over the most recent era." *Am J Transplant* 4(3): 378-83.

Meyer, H., V. A. Sundqvist, et al. (1992). "Glycoprotein gp116 of human cytomegalovirus contains epitopes for strain-common and strain-specific antibodies." *J Gen Virol* 73 (Pt 9): 2375-83.

Munoz, I., A. Gutierrez, et al. (2001). "Lack of association between the kinetics of human cytomegalovirus (HCMV) glycoprotein B (gB)-specific and neutralizing serum antibodies and development or recovery from HCMV active infection in patients undergoing allogeneic stem cell transplant." *J Med Virol* 65(1): 77-84.

Navarro, D., P. Paz, et al. (1993). "Glycoprotein B of human cytomegalovirus promotes virion penetration into cells, transmission of infection from cell to cell, and fusion of infected cells." *Virology* 197(1): 143-58.

Nett, P. C., D. M. Heisey, et al. (2004). "Association of cytomegalovirus disease and acute rejection with graft loss in kidney transplantation." *Transplantation* 78(7): 1036-41.

Nickel, P., G. Bold, et al. (2009). "High levels of CMV-IE-1-specific memory T cells are associated with less alloimmunity and improved renal allograft function." *Transpl Immunol* 20(4): 238-42.

Ohizumi, Y., H. Suzuki, et al. (1992). "Neutralizing mechanisms of two human monoclonal antibodies against human cytomegalovirus glycoprotein 130/55." *J Gen Virol* 73 (Pt 10): 2705-7.

Pachl, C., W. S. Probert, et al. (1989). "The human cytomegalovirus strain Towne glycoprotein H gene encodes glycoprotein p86." *Virology* 169(2): 418-26.

Paterson, D. A., A. P. Dyer, et al. (2002). "A role for human cytomegalovirus glycoprotein O (gO) in cell fusion and a new hypervariable locus." *Virology* 293(2): 281-94.

Pignatelli, S., P. Dal Monte, et al. (2001). "gpUL73 (gN) genomic variants of human cytomegalovirus isolates are clustered into four distinct genotypes." *J Gen Virol* 82(Pt 11): 2777-84.

Pignatelli, S., P. Dal Monte, et al. (2006). "Latency-associated human cytomegalovirus glycoprotein N genotypes in monocytes from healthy blood donors." *Transfusion* 46(10): 1754-62.

Pignatelli, S., P. Dal Monte, et al. (2003). "Intrauterine cytomegalovirus infection and glycoprotein N (gN) genotypes." *J Clin Virol* 28(1): 38-43.

Pignatelli, S., G. Rossini, et al. (2003). "Human cytomegalovirus glycoprotein N genotypes in AIDS patients." *Aids* 17(5): 761-3.

Port, F. K., R. A. Wolfe, et al. (1993). "Comparison of survival probabilities for dialysis patients vs cadaveric renal transplant recipients." *Jama* 270(11): 1339-43.

Rasmussen, L., A. Geissler, et al. (2002). "The genes encoding the gCIII complex of human cytomegalovirus exist in highly diverse combinations in clinical isolates." *J Virol* 76(21): 10841-8.

Rasmussen, L., C. Matkin, et al. (1991). "Antibody response to human cytomegalovirus glycoproteins gB and gH after natural infection in humans." *J Infect Dis* 164(5): 835-42.

Reischig, T., P. Jindra, et al. (2008). "Valacyclovir prophylaxis versus preemptive valganciclovir therapy to prevent cytomegalovirus disease after renal transplantation." *Am J Transplant* 8(1): 69-77.

Reischig, T., P. Jindra, et al. (2006). "The impact of cytomegalovirus disease and asymptomatic infection on acute renal allograft rejection." *J Clin Virol* 36(2): 146-51.

Retiere, C., B. Lesimple, et al. (2003). "Association of glycoprotein B and immediate early-1 genotypes with human leukocyte antigen alleles in renal transplant recipients with cytomegalovirus infection." *Transplantation* 75(1): 161-5.

Reusser, P., S. R. Riddell, et al. (1991). "Cytotoxic T-lymphocyte response to cytomegalovirus after human allogeneic bone marrow transplantation: pattern of recovery and correlation with cytomegalovirus infection and disease." *Blood* 78(5): 1373-80.

Roback, J. D., W. L. Drew, et al. (2003). "CMV DNA is rarely detected in healthy blood donors using validated PCR assays." *Transfusion* 43(3): 314-21.

Roenhorst, H. W., A. M. Tegzess, et al. (1985). "HLA-DRw6 as a risk factor for active cytomegalovirus but not for herpes simplex virus infection after renal allograft transplantation." *Br Med J (Clin Res Ed)* 291(6496): 619-22.

Rossini, G., S. Pignatelli, et al. (2005). "Monitoring for human cytomegalovirus infection in solid organ transplant recipients through antigenemia and glycoprotein N (gN) variants: evidence of correlation and potential prognostic value of gN genotypes." *Microbes Infect* 7(5-6): 890-6.

Rothe, M., S. Pepperl-Klindworth, et al. (2001). "An antigen fragment encompassing the AD2 domains of glycoprotein B from two different strains is sufficient for differentiation of primary vs. recurrent human cytomegalovirus infection by ELISA." *J Med Virol* 65(4): 719-29.

Roy, D. M., J. E. Grundy, et al. (1993). "Sequence variation within neutralizing epitopes of the envelope glycoprotein B of human cytomegalovirus: comparison of isolates from renal transplant recipients and AIDS patients." *J Gen Virol* 74 (Pt 11): 2499-505.

Sagedal, S., K. P. Nordal, et al. (2000). "A prospective study of the natural course of cytomegalovirus infection and disease in renal allograft recipients." *Transplantation* 70(8): 1166-74.

Sagedal, S., K. P. Nordal, et al. (2002). "The impact of cytomegalovirus infection and disease on rejection episodes in renal allograft recipients." *Am J Transplant* 2(9): 850-6.

Schnitzler, M. A., R. S. Woodward, et al. (1997). "The effects of cytomegalovirus serology on graft and recipient survival in cadaveric renal transplantation: implications for organ allocation." *Am J Kidney Dis* 29(3): 428-34.

Schnitzler, M. A., R. S. Woodward, et al. (1997). "Impact of cytomegalovirus serology on graft survival in living related kidney transplantation: implications for donor selection." *Surgery* 121(5): 563-8.

Schoppel, K., E. Hassfurther, et al. (1996). "Antibodies specific for the antigenic domain 1 of glycoprotein B (gpUL55) of human cytomegalovirus bind to different substructures." *Virology* 216(1): 133-45.

Schoppel, K., C. Schmidt, et al. (1998). "Kinetics of the antibody response against human cytomegalovirus-specific proteins in allogeneic bone marrow transplant recipients." *J Infect Dis* 178(5): 1233-43.

Sementilli, A. and M. Franco (2010). "Renal acute cellular rejection: correlation between the immunophenotype and cytokine expression of the inflammatory cells in acute glomerulitis, arterial intimitis, and tubulointerstitial nephritis." *Transplant Proc* 42(5): 1671-6.

Shimamura, M., M. Mach, et al. (2006). "Human cytomegalovirus infection elicits a glycoprotein M (gM)/gN-specific virus-neutralizing antibody response." *J Virol* 80(9): 4591-600.

Singh, N., V. L. Yu, et al. (1994). "High-dose acyclovir compared with short-course preemptive ganciclovir therapy to prevent cytomegalovirus disease in liver transplant recipients. A randomized trial." *Ann Intern Med* 120(5): 375-81.

Slobedman, B. and E. S. Mocarski (1999). "Quantitative analysis of latent human cytomegalovirus." *J Virol* 73(6): 4806-12.

Soderberg-Naucler, C., D. N. Streblow, et al. (2001). "Reactivation of latent human cytomegalovirus in CD14(+) monocytes is differentiation dependent." *J Virol* 75(16): 7543-54.

Soroceanu, L., A. Akhavan, et al. (2008). "Platelet-derived growth factor-alpha receptor activation is required for human cytomegalovirus infection." *Nature* 455(7211): 391-5.

Spaete, R. R., K. Perot, et al. (1993). "Coexpression of truncated human cytomegalovirus gH with the UL115 gene product or the truncated human fibroblast growth factor receptor results in transport of gH to the cell surface." *Virology* 193(2): 853-61.

Stewart, G. J., B. L. Kelsall, et al. (1981). "The role of HLA-DR determinants in monocyte-macrophage presentation of herpes simplex virus antigen to human T cells." *Cell Immunol* 61(1): 11-21.

Tanabe, K., T. Tokumoto, et al. (1997). "Comparative study of cytomegalovirus (CMV) antigenemia assay, polymerase chain reaction, serology, and shell vial assay in the early diagnosis and monitoring of CMV infection after renal transplantation." *Transplantation* 64(12): 1721-5.

Tellides, G. and J. S. Pober (2007). "Interferon-gamma axis in graft arteriosclerosis." *Circ Res* 100(5): 622-32.

Tu, W., L. Potena, et al. (2006). "T-cell immunity to subclinical cytomegalovirus infection reduces cardiac allograft disease." *Circulation* 114(15): 1608-15.

Urban, M., W. Britt, et al. (1992). "The dominant linear neutralizing antibody-binding site of glycoprotein gp86 of human cytomegalovirus is strain specific." *J Virol* 66(3): 1303-11.

Urban, M., M. Klein, et al. (1996). "Glycoprotein H of human cytomegalovirus is a major antigen for the neutralizing humoral immune response." *J Gen Virol* 77 (Pt 7): 1537-47.

Ustinov, J. A., R. J. Loginov, et al. (1991). "Cytomegalovirus infection of human kidney cells in vitro." *Kidney Int* 40(5): 954-60.

Valente, J. F., S. Hariharan, et al. (1997). "Causes of renal allograft loss in black vs. white transplant recipients in the cyclosporine era." *Clin Transplant* 11(3): 231-6.

Varga, M., K. Rajczy, et al. (2008). "HLA-DQ3 is a probable risk factor for CMV infection in high-risk kidney transplant patients." *Nephrol Dial Transplant* 23(8): 2673-8.

Volpi, A., F. Pica, et al. (1999). "Neutralizing antibody response against human cytomegalovirus in allogeneic bone marrow-transplant recipients." *J Infect Dis* 180(5): 1747-8.

Wada, K., S. Mizuno, et al. (1997). "Immune response to neutralizing epitope on human cytomegalovirus gylcoprotein B in Japanese: correlation of serologic response with HLA-type." *Microbiol Immunol* 41(10): 841-5.

Wang, X., D. Y. Huang, et al. (2005). "Integrin alphavbeta3 is a coreceptor for human cytomegalovirus." *Nat Med* 11(5): 515-21.

Wang, X., S. M. Huong, et al. (2003). "Epidermal growth factor receptor is a cellular receptor for human cytomegalovirus." *Nature* 424(6947): 456-61.

Woo, P. C., C. Y. Lo, et al. (1997). "Distinct genotypic distributions of cytomegalovirus (CMV) envelope glycoprotein in bone marrow and renal transplant recipients with CMV disease." *Clin Diagn Lab Immunol* 4(5): 515-8.

Zhou, L., J. Fan, et al. (2007). "Genetic variation within the glycoprotein B and H genes of human cytomegalovirus in solid organ transplant recipients." *Transpl Infect Dis* 9(1): 73-7.

10

Pharmacogenetics of Immunosuppressive Drugs in Renal Transplantation

María Galiana, María José Herrero**, Virginia Bosó, Sergio Bea, Elia Ros, Jaime Sánchez-Plumed, Jose Luis Poveda and Salvador F. Aliño*

1. Introduction

Facing the demand of obtaining the best cost-efficacy treatments, we are always searching for new alternatives to the existing therapies. The incorporation of new diagnostic techniques and screening, along with the continued development of safer and more effective drugs has improved considerably the expectations and the quality of life of patients.

Still, there is no ideal solution to many of the diseases faced by health professionals in daily clinical practice, so we still have to look for alternatives to the established treatments. The idea of a targeted and personalized therapy to achieve therapeutic success is a goal that is getting more and more important every day. In this context there arises the concept of personalized medicine which is related in our case to the genetic variability associated with different individual response to the same treatment. That is, there is a difference in the response to the same drug in different patients that appears to be related to the different versions of each patient's genes coding for transport proteins, for enzymes involved in metabolism and those genes responsible for the drug mechanism of action, all necessary for the drug to perform its therapeutic effect. This kind of research is developed by two disciplines: pharmacogenetics and pharmacogenomics. These two terms are often mixed and difficult to distinguish, so the international regulatory organizations have tried to fix the proper definitions of both terms. The European Medicines Agency shows the definitions on its web site (www.ema.europa.eu, EMEA/CHMP/ICH/437986/2006) where according to the the International Conference on Harmonisation (ICH), Pharmacogenomics is defined as the study of variations of DNA and RNA characteristics as related to drug response, while Pharmacogenetics is a subset of pharmacogenomics and is defined as the study of variations in DNA sequence as related to drug response.

So, in practice Pharmacogenetics studies the influence of genetic factors in transport, metabolism and drug action. The examples of pharmacogenetic tests employed in the clinical practice are increasing day by day, as for instance when establishing first treatment

* *Servicio de Farmacia e Instituto de Investigación Sanitaria del Hospital Universitario y Politécnico La Fe de Valencia, Servicio de Nefrología, Unidad de Trasplante Renal, Hospital La Fe de Valencia, Dpto. Farmacología, Facultad de Medicina, Universidad deValencia Spain*

** Corresponding Author

in HIV patients, before employing Cetuximab in colorectal cancer and before Warfarin treatment. In these cases, where it has been demonstrated that it exists a correlation between some known genetic variants and low or no response to treatment, or even occurrence of adverse effects, the clinician needs the genetic test tool in order to settle the correct therapy to each patient. The increase of this genetic testing need is reflected also by the United States Food and Drug Administration (FDA) that publishes on its web site the list containing those drugs with a genetic test, recommended or compulsory, in their drug label. Table 1 shows some examples of drugs with pharmacogenomic/genetic marker published in FDA website.

Pharmacogenetic Biomarkers in Drug Labels			
	Theraputic Area	**Biomarker**	**Label Sections**
Aripiprazole	Psychiatry	CYP2D6	Clinical Pharmacology
Azathioprine	Rheumatology	TPMT	Dosage and Administration, Warnings and Precautions, Drug Interactions, Adverse Reactions, Clinical Pharmacology
Carvedilol	Cardiovascular	CYP2D6	Drug Interactions, Clinical Pharmacology
Celecoxib	Analgesics	CYP2C9	Dosage and Administration, Drug Interactions, Use in Specific Populations, Clinical Pharmacology
Cetuximab	Oncology	EGFR	Indications and Usage, Warnings and Precautions, Description, Clinical Pharmacology, Clinical Studies
Cetuximab	Oncology	KRAS	Indications and Usage, Clinical Pharmacology, Clinical Studies
Maraviroc	Antivirals	CCR5	Indications and Usage, Warnings and Precautions, Clinical Pharmacology, Clinical Studies, Patient Counseling Information

Table 1. Examples of pharmacogenetic biomarkers in drug labels in FDA website (www.fda.gov, accession date: (24/06/2011).

On the other hand, Pharmacogenomics is responsible for discovering the relationships between genes and disease by means of the molecular etiology and pathways of each illness. The identification of these new associations opens a window to search for new drugs for novel therapeutic targets.

The aim of both disciplines is to obtain the highest therapeutic effect with the lowest risk, minimizing the adverse effects of the treatments. This should lead to a better control of the disease through personalized medicine.

In order to start explaining the main findings of Pharmacogenetics in the renal transplantation field, we need first to understand some basic concepts. The first one is Polymorphism, which is a monogenic mendelian character that is normally present in the population at least in 1% frequency. It is characterized by the presence of more than one allele in a same gene locus, and consequently, more than one phenotype. The polymorphisms that have a meaning in pharmacogenetics are those who represent different alleles in a gene related to the interaction of a drug with the organism. There are different types of polymorphisms: those were the change from one allele to the variant is only one nucleotide are called SNPs, Single Nucleotide Polymorphisms, and these will be the subject of most part of the research in the field, including our own work. But there are also other kind of polymorphisms as RFLPs, Restriction Fragment Lenght Polymorphisms, and VNTR, Variable Number Tandem Repeats. SNPs are the most common ones, representing 90% of the whole genetic variability. It is important not to mix this concept up with the term "mutation", although actually they are sometimes mixed. A mutation is usually less frequent than a polymorphism, being present in less than 1% of the population but also a mutation represents a very little part of the whole genetic variability and is mostly associated with the pathology concept: a mutation is most always the cause of a missfunction or disease, while a polymorphism will only show some biological effect under some concrete circumstances. For instance, if we are carriers of a variant in a polymorphic site, related to a better efficacy of a given drug, we will only notice this effect if we take that drug, but if we never take it, we will probably not find any biological effect in our body due to carrying that variant.

Another important concept to consider is the Haplotype. We refer to haplotype when we talk about alleles which tend to be inherited together because they are close to each other on the chromosomes. The haplotypes have been extensively studied by the HapMap project (www.hapmap.org). Currently, the investigations are more and more directed to the study of the effect of several combined SNPs, instead of aisled SNPs, especially those that form an haplotype. The reason for this is that most probably the biological effects that we could find are the result of the sum of the effect of several SNPs in different genes affecting several parts of the pathway of the drug. Moreover, the effect of a single SNP can be, in turn, enhanced, reduced or silenced by compensation by the effect of other SNPs. Related to the term haplotype we can also hear about Linkage Disequilibrium, LD, which is the occurrence of some combinations of alleles or genetic markers in a population more often or less often than would be expected from a random formation of haplotypes from alleles based on their frequencies. This aspect is also important in the study of SNPs, since in many cases, a SNP that apparently seems to have no clear biological meaning may be in disequilibrium with another SNP with a known effect and taking this into account, this property could help us infer the genotype of a patient in several SNPs, by only studying one or two of them if they are linked, and also it makes sense to study not only the SNPs with a clear direct effect, but those apparently non-functional but linked to the functional ones.

The application of these skills and expertise in the field of transplantation could be one of the great advances in current immunosupressive therapy. In the transplantation field, there are still many unanswered questions, its success depends on the fragile equilibrium between the risks and benefits of immunosuppression. Therapeutic drug monitoring helps to determine suitable immunosuppressant dose adjustments but usually the work is done by assay-error method so the challenge now is to combine pharmacokinetic with pharmacogenetic information to provide patients with the most suitable treatment. Many papers have been written about genetic variability based on SNPs influencing immunosuppressant blood levels but the results are still contradictory in many cases, probably due to the hidden effects of other SNPs not included in the study, the number of patients included, their ethnicity (SNP frequencies can be very different from one ethnicity to another) and so on.

Just focusing our review of the state of the art in tacrolimus and cyclosporine, two genes seem to be the most relevant on having pharmacogentic effects on these drugs: the ABCB1 gene, coding for the transporter P-glycoprotein, and the CYP3A5 gene, coding for an extensive drug-metabolizing enzyme of cytochrome P450 family.

Tacrolimus and cyclosporine are calcineurin inhibitors indicated for prophylaxis of renal, liver and heart transplant rejection. Cyclosporine has a broader use as immunosuppressive agent, as apart from preventing transplant rejection (kidney, liver, heart, lung and bone marrow) it is also employed in autoimmune diseases (uveitis endogenous, psoriasis, nephrotic syndrome, rheumatoid arthritis and atopic dermatitis). In the metabolism of both drugs, cytochrome P-450 plays an important role, specifically the CYP3A5 isoform, but also CYP3A4 in the case of cyclosporine. On the other hand, they are both transported out of cells by P-glycoprotein, encoded by the gene ABCB1. Changes in expression or function of these proteins will cause changes in the absorption, metabolism and distribution of both drugs and, therefore, can lead to changes in the response and toxicity of the treatment. The characterization of genetic variants, as for instance SNPs, that cause variations in expression or function can help in establishing effective doses and in minimizing adverse reactions (Astellas Pharma, S.A., 2010; Staatz et al., 2010).

The good correlation between these two drugs blood levels and their tissue concentration, makes them suitable for pharmacokinetic monitoring to prevent graft rejection or toxicity. If we add the inter- and intra-individual variability, a narrow therapeutic range and a clear correlation between high blood levels and appearance of toxicity, then we have two perfect candidates for the need of dose optimization. Other factors affecting tacrolimus and cyclosporine dosage/concentration after renal transplantation are consistent with the features of the patients (renal and hepatic function, age, race). Liver function, albumin, hematocrit, gastrointestinal disturbances and the effects of food are also important factors responsible for the variation of dosage/concentrations (Marqués et al., 2009).

The final goal of pharmacogenetics in transplantation is to find a clear link between genetic variations and pharmacokinetics/pharmacodynamics of the drugs employed, to allow us to find the optimal doses of both initial and maintenance periods, ensuring the success of the graft and reducing treatment toxicity. Amongst all the SNPs described in the literature included in genes related to these drugs, we need to validate those that really have an impact on actual clinical practice, those that really alter drug levels/efficacy/toxicity and we can only achieve that through research, in order to obtain individualized therapies as effective as possible. Contradictory results in the published studies seem to tarnish the utility of pharmacogenetics, but there are also many encouraging works, where clear correlations are found. Probably a good experimental design, without alteration of the real clinical setting could help to discriminate whether these studies will be useful or not in the therapeutic decisions, but certainly we need multiple approaches correlating genetics with kinetics and with safety/efficacy; good and accurate informatic tools to process such a great quantity of information; and finally, we do not have to forget other important factors involving the patient as concomitant drugs and donor genotype. In this chapter we are presenting a summary of some relevant published works and some of our own group's results in this area.

2. Tacrolimus

2.1 Absorption

Tacrolimus has a mean oral bioavailability ranging from 20 to 25%. After oral administration, peak concentrations (Cmax) are reached in an interval of 1 to 3 hours. Co-administration with food leads to a decrease in the speed and extent of absorption, being more accentuated in the case of fat rich food. Once in blood, it is highly found bound to erythrocytes and plasma proteins (> 98.8%), with preference for serum albumin and α-1 acid glycoprotein (Astellas Pharma, S.A., 2010).

2.2 Distribution

It is widely distributed throughout the body reaching a volume of distribution around 1,300 liters. It has a low clearance that, as with its half-life, differs depending on the type of transplantation performed and the age of the patients (total clearance in pediatric patients undergoing liver transplantation is twice that of adult patients with the same transplantation type). Generally, it has a long half-life that is affected by variations in clearance rates observed in transplantation patients (Astellas Pharma, S.A., 2010).

2.3 Metabolism

Tacrolimus is extensively metabolized in the liver but also has a minimal metabolism in the intestine. The primary responsible is the cytochrome P450. Several products of metabolism have been identified, but there is only one metabolite with immunosuppressive activity similar to that of tacrolimus, however, it does not contribute to the pharmacological activity, since it has not been detected in systemic circulation (Astellas Pharma, S.A., 2010).

2.4 Elimination

The main route of elimination of tacrolimus is the faeces. Only 2% is excreted in urine. Only 1% of the administered tacrolimus appears unchanged in feces and urine (Astellas Pharma, S.A., 2010).

3. Cyclosporine

3.1 Absorption

The new current formulation of cyclosporine microemulsion compared to conventional forms, has a faster absorption, leading to a reduction of 1 hour in the t max and Cmax increased by 59%, with an increase of 29% in AUC (Novartis Farmacéutica, S.A., 2010).

3.2 Distribution

Most of the cyclosporine is outside the blood compartment. In the blood it is preferently distributed in plasma (33 - 47%) and erythrocytes (41-58%). 90% is fixed to plasma proteins, primarily lipoproteins (Novartis Farmacéutica, S.A., 2010).

3.3 Metabolism

Biotransformation of cyclosporin is broad and leads to the formation of about 15 metabolites. There is not a main metabolic pathway and it suffers enterohepatic cycle (Novartis Farmacéutica, S.A., 2010).

3.4 Elimination

It is mainly performed via the bile. Only 6% of the oral dose is excreted in the urine (0.1% as unchanged drug) (Novartis Farmacéutica, S.A., 2010).

4. Genetic polymorphisms

A great number of genes are thought to be involved in different effects of immunosuppressive therapy (www.fda.gov; www. pharmgkb.org). Two genes in particular have demonstrated clear correlations in several studies: ABCB1 (or MDR1), which codes for the transporter P-glycoprotein and CYP3A5, which codes for an extensive drug metabolizing enzyme of the cytochrome P450 family.

4.1 ABCB1 genetic polymorphisms

P-glycoprotein is encoded by the multidrug resistance gene (MDR1), also known as the ABCB1 gene. The protein encoded by this gene is an ATP-dependent drug efflux pump for xenobiotic compounds with broad substrate specificity. It is responsible for decreased drug accumulation in multidrug-resistant cells and often mediates the development of resistance to anticancer drugs. This protein also functions as a transporter in the blood-brain barrier. ABCB1 is polymorphically expressed, with at least 50 SNPs identified to date (http://www.ncbi.nlm.nih.gov).

4.1.1 Influence on tacrolimus pharmacokinetics.

The results of the influence of ABCB1 on the pharmacokinetics of tacrolimus are controversial. Some studies talk about an increase in the ratio Co/dose and lower dose requirement in those individuals expressing variant ABCB1 3435 TT regarding the CC variant, related to a possible lower functional activity of P-glycoprotein in the carriers of TT variant (Staatz et al, 2010). This "3435 C>T" is the common nomenclature for the SNP cataloged as rs1045642 in the SNP database of NCBI website (http://www.ncbi.nlm. nih.gov), where C is the ancestral allele (also "wild type") and most frequent and T the less frequent one and they lead to three different genotypes: CC, CT and TT. In contrast, some other studies have failed to find an association between the ABCB1 3435C>T and changes in tacrolimus blood levels. In a prospective study with 96 renal transplant recipients, the effect of genetic polymorphisms of ABCB1 on tacrolimus whole blood levels was analyzed, concluding that ABCB1 1199G>A, 3435C>T and 2677G>T/A SNPs (rs2229109, 1045642, 2032582, respectively), appeared to reduce the activity of P-glycoprotein towards tacrolimus, increasing tacrolimus peripheral blood mononuclear cell concentrations. Nevertheless, the impact of ABCB1 genetic polymorphisms on tacrolimus blood concentrations was negligible (Capron et al., 2010). In another study on Chinese renal transplant recipients, MDR1 3435C>T polymorphism was not an important factor in tacrolimus pharmacokinetics (Rong et al., 2010). In a retrospective study of 81 renal transplant recipients the effect on tacrolimus dosages and concentration/dose ratio of four frequent MDR1 SNP possibly associated with P-gp function (T-129C in exon 1b, 1236C>T in exon 12, 2677G>T,A in exon 21, and 3435C>T in exon 26; corresponding to rs3213619, 1128503, 2032582 and 1045642, respectively). In the general caucasian population, the SNP in exons 12, 21, and 26 exhibited incomplete linkage disequilibrium, which means that the different variants of each SNP tend to be displayed together, but not in the 100% of the

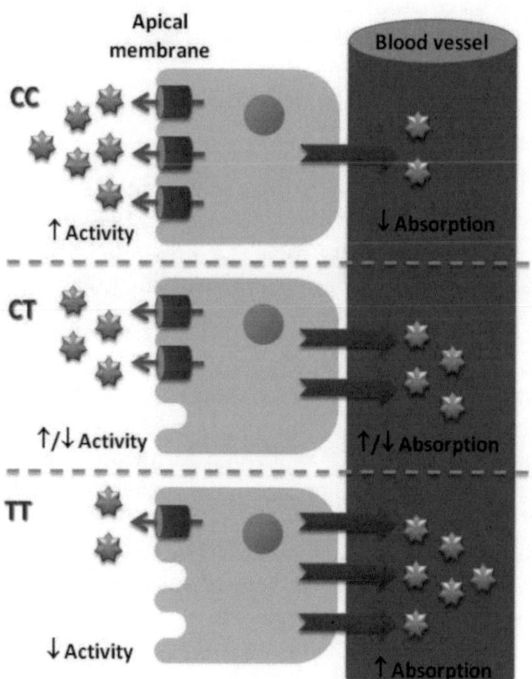

Fig. 1. Influence of the functional activity of glycoprotein-P (transporter in apical membrane) in the transport of tacrolimus (stars) in the intestine epithelium. The diagram shows the different degree of drug absorption due to variations in ABCB1/MDR1 polymorphic site rs1045642. Individuals with TT variant have a decreased transporter activity and hence greater absorption efficiency. CC variant causes more expulsion out of the cell, which decreases absorption.

individuals. One month after tacrolimus introduction, exon 21 SNP correlated significantly with the daily tacrolimus dose (P < or = 0.05) and the concentration/dose ratio (P < or = 0.02). Tacrolimus dose requirements were 40% higher in homozygous TT than in wild-type patients GG for this SNP. The concentration/dose ratio was 36% lower in the wild-type GG patients, suggesting that, for a given dose, their tacrolimus blood concentration is lower. Haplotype analysis substained these results and suggested that exons 26 and 21 SNPs may be associated with tacrolimus dose requirements (Anglicheau et al., 2003).

4.1.2 Influence on cyclosporine pharmacokinetics

Nowadays the data about ABCB1 influence on cyclosporine pharmacokinetics are not conclusive, either. Many studies have tried to find correlations with ABCB1 SNPs 3434C>T, 2677G>T/A and 1236C>T without significant findings. A recent meta-analysis that included 1036 renal transplantation recipients, concluded that there were no significant differences in the influence of ABCB1 3435C>T on cyclosporine pharmacokinetics (AUC_4/Dose, CL/F, Cmax/Dose or C_0/Dose). However, it was indicated in this meta-analysis that CC carriers had lower cyclosporine exposure presented as AUC 0–12 than those with at least one T allele (CT or TT). In a recent study that included 225 renal transplant recipients treated with cyclosporine, ABCB1 2677G>T SNP correlated significantly with dose-adjusted levels in patients, at 1, 3 and 6 months after renal transplantation. Recipients with the wild-type genotype of this SNP were associated with significantly lower dose-adjusted values and consequently required higher cyclosporine daily dose to attain the therapeutic level. ABCB1 1236C>T also had a minor influence on dose-adjusted C2/T0 levels (Singh et al, 2010).

4.2 CYP450 genetic polymorphisms

The cytochrome P450 proteins are monooxygenases which catalyze many reactions involved in drug metabolism and synthesis of cholesterol, steroids and other lipids. This proteins are localized in the endoplasmic reticulum and their expression is induced by glucocorticoids and some pharmacological agents (http://www.ncbi.nlm.nih.gov).

CYP3A5 is found in the liver, small intestine and kidney. One of the most relevants SNPs in this gene is rs776746, also know as 6986 A>G, being G the most frequent allele. Allele *3 is the wild type genotype, GG, while *1 is the variant homozygous AA and heterozygote A/G is known as *1/*3. There are clear ethnic differences in the prevalence of the CYP3A5*3 genotype. At the molecular level, the SNP is located in intron 3, and the change of base produces a splicing defect. The result is a nonfunctional protein (allele *3). The patients that show the allelic variant *3 in homozygosis G/G, also called non-expressors, are slow metabolizers of the immunosuppressant. In contrast, heterozygote A/G alleles *1/*3 are intermediate metabolizers, whereas those carriers of allele *1 in homozygosis A/A are normal metabolizers (Glowacki et al, 2011; Macphee et al, 2005; www.pharmgkb.org)

4.2.1 Influence on tacrolimus pharmacokinetics

CYP3A5 may play a more important role than CYP3A4 in the metabolism of tacrolimus in individuals who are CYP3A5 expressors, so we will focus on this enzyme. The intrinsic clearance of tacrolimus is approximately 2-fold higher for CYP3A5 than for CYP3A4 (Hesselink et al., 2008). This plasmatic clearance is higher in those individuals with genotype CYP3A5*1/*3 regarding those CYP3A5*3/*3 (Haufroid et al., 2006). In fact, CYP3A5*1 is responsible from about 60% of tacrolimus hepatic metabolism (Dai et al., 2006; Thervet et al., 2010), so it is of great interest studying it in order to establish optimal doses that reach quickly the efficient blood concentrations, avoiding toxicity but also assuring the necessary concentrations to avoid rejection. The studies performed so far indicate the need to administrate higher tacrolimus doses in patients CYP3A5*1/*1. In fact, in some of those studies there is even a recommendation of an initial double dose for those patients (Haufroid et al, 2006). In a study with forty kidney recipients, CYP3A5*1 variant was associated with significant lower tacrolimus dose adjusted concentration at 3, 6, 12 and 36 months after transplantation, concluding that CYP3A5*1 carriers need higher tacrolimus dose than CYP3A5*3 homozygotes to achieve the target blood concentration (Katsakiori et al., 2010). Similarly, in a study with 28 chinese renal transplant recipients, the patients with *1/*3 showed significantly lower tacrolimus blood levels than those with the *3/*3 in the first and second week after transplantation (Zhang et al., 2010). In another similar study, on Chinese renal transplant recipients, individuals who were CYP3A5*1 carriers required a higher dose of tacrolimus than CYP3A5*3/*3, indicating a significantly lower dose-adjusted AUC(0-12) of tacrolimus (Rong et al., 2010). The last reviewed work, with 200 patients objectifies that patients who were CYP3A5*3/*3 received significantly higher tacrolimus dose at 1 week, 6 months, and 1 year (Tavira et al., 2011). Some studies found that the weighted mean apparent oral clearance was 48% lower in CYP3A5 nonexpressors than CYP3A5 expressors (range, 26%-65%) (Barry & Levine, 2010). Recently, a study with 280 transplant recipients concludes that patients receiving a pharmacogenetic adaption of the daily dose of tacrolimus were associated with improved achievement of the target C_0 (Thervet et al, 2010).

4.2.2 Influence on cyclosporine pharmacokinetics

Unlike tacrolimus, CYP3A4 may play a more dominant role than CYP3A5 in the metabolism of cyclosporine. The intrinsic clearance of cyclosporine, calculated from total metabolite formation, is approximately 2.3-fold higher for CYP3A4 than for CYP3A5 (Dai et al., 2006). Still, the results of studies conducted so far do not indicate a clear relationship (Anglicheau et al., 2007) with 3A4 isoform. However, many papers continue studying the effect of both on the metabolism of cyclosporine. A recent meta-analysis with twelve studies includes the effects of CYP3A5 during cyclosporine dose adjustment. This meta-analysis showed that CYP3A5*3/*3 polymorphism is associated with cyclosporine dose-adjusted concentration (dose-adjusted trough and dose-adjusted peak concentrations) in renal transplant recipients and patients carrying the CYP3A5*3/*3 genotype will require a lower dose of cyclosporine to reach targets levels compared with the CYP3A5*1/*1 or 1*/*3 carriers (Zhu et al., 2011).

5. Our results

5.1 Objective

The aim of our studies was to evaluate the effect of the most relevant SNPs in ABCB1 and CYP3A5 genes, in renal transplant recipients and their donors, regarding blood concentrations of tacrolimus in the first two weeks post-transplantation.

5.2 Materials and methods

One blood sample, collected in anticoagulation tubes at routine extraction, was obtained in each of 97 renal transplant recipients and their donors (caucasians). The DNA was extracted from 200 μL of blood using a commercially available kit based on centrifugation in microcolumns (UltraClean BloodSpin DNA Isolation Kit; MoBioLaboratories, Inc, Carlsbad, California). After quantification using a spectrophotometer (NanoDrop Technologies Inc, Wilmington, Delaware) to determine the concentration and purity, DNA was stored at -20°C until use. A genetic analysis platform (MassARRAY; Sequenom, Inc, San Diego, California) was used to obtain the genotypes of each sample in the SNPs rs1045642 (3435C>T), rs2032582 (2677G>T/A), and rs1128503 (1236C>T) of the ABCB1 gene, and in the SNPs rs776746 (6986A>G, CYP3A5*3) and rs10264272 (267871G>A, CYP3A5*6) of the CYP3A5 gene. All the 97 patients received tacrolimus as the primary immunosuppression drug, at an initial dose of 0.2 to 0.3 mg/kg/24 h. Blood concentration of tacrolimus was measured routinely using a clinical chemistry system (Dimension; Siemens Healthcare, Deerfield, Illinois) to determine the trough level (C_0 , in nanograms per milliliter). Drug blood concentrations from the first and second weeks were determined, and all of the measured levels in the patients during that period were considered. The resulting values were plotted in the form of median and quartile range, 1 for each week in each group of recipients or recipient with their donors, according to genotypes. Normality tests of Kolmogorov-Smirnof and Shapiro-Wilk were performed and then differences between groups were evaluated using the Mann-Whitney test (nonparametric test that compares two groups)

5.3 Results

The SNP genotyping of the 167 samples showed similar frequencies to those expected for Caucasian population in public databases (SNP Database in NCBI site). Tables 2 to 4 show the relationship between the frequencies observed in recipients in our study regarding the expected ones according to the data from public data bases of the ABCB1 and CYP3A5 genes, in the most relevant genotyping assays in caucasian population. Tables 5 to 7 show the same information but regarding the donors of the transplanted kidneys. The data related to donors is a little bit outside the expected range, while there is a better fit in recipient's data. We associate these findings to the lower number of donors, thus we can appreciate that in recipients, having a larger number of samples, the frequencies fit better.

GENE	POLYMORFISMS	EXPECTED FREQUENCY (%)			FOUND FREQUENCY (%)		
		CC	CT	TT	CC	CT	TT
ABCB1	rs 1045642	12.5-15.5	50-60.3	37.5-24.1	22.68	52.28	24.74
	rs 1128503	32	41	27	34.02	46.39	24.05

Table 2. Recipients' genotypes frequency regarding the expected frequencies from public data bases.

GENE	POLYMORFISMS	EXPECTED FREQUENCY (%)					FOUND FREQUENCY (%)				
		AA	AG	GG	GT	TT	AA	AG	GG	GT	TT
ABCB1	rs 2032582	0	0	32.3-32.2	48.4-55.9	19.3-11.9	1.03	1.03	32.99	50.52	14.43

Table 3. Recipients' genotypes frequency regarding the expected frequencies from public data bases.

GENE	POLYMORFISMS	EXPECTED FREQUENCY (%)		FOUND FREQUENCY (%)	
		GG	GA	GG	GA
CYP3A5	rs 776746	88.3-95.5	11.7-4.5	81.44	18.55
	rs 1026427	100	0	97.94	2.06

Table 4. Recipients' genotypes frequency regarding the expected frequencies from public data bases.

GENE	POLYMORFISMS	EXPECTED FREQUENCY (%)			FOUND FREQUENCY (%)		
		CC	CT	TT	CC	CT	TT
ABCB1	rs 1045642	12.5-15.5	50-60.3	37.5-24.1	30.07	49.18	14.75
	rs 1128503	32	41	27	39.06	50	9.38

Table 5. Donors' genotypes frequency regarding the expected frequencies from public data bases.

GENE	POLYMORFISMS	EXPECTED FREQUENCY (%)					FOUND FREQUENCY (%)				
		AA	AG	GG	GT	TT	AA	AG	GG	GT	TT
ABCB1	rs 2032582	0	0	32.3-32.2	48.4-55.9	19.3-11.9	0	0	42.37	54.24	3.39

Table 6. Donors' genotypes frequency regarding the expected frequencies from public data bases.

GENE	POLYMORFISMS	EXPECTED FREQUENCY (%)		FOUND FREQUENCY (%)	
		GG	GA	GG	GA
CYP3A5	rs 776746	88.6-95.5	11.4-4.5	79.10	19.4
	rs 1026427	99	1	98.5	1.43

Table 7. Donors' genotypes frequency regarding the expected frequencies from public data bases.

5.3.1 ABCB1

According to the literature, rs1045642 seems to be the most relevant SNP in ABCB1 gene regarding its correlation with tacrolimus or cyclosporine blood levels.

Figure 2 shows tacrolimus levels as trough concentration, corrected by administered dose and weight of the patient ($C_0/Dc= C_0/(Dose/weight)$) during the first two weeks after renal transplantation, grouped in a way that we represent the data of those recipients whose donor has the same genotype as them (eg. CC/CC, means recipients CC whose donors were also CC). The data are represented as median inside the whole data range, remarking the interquartilic range which includes the 50% of the data. The statistical test applycated was Mann-Whitney two-tailed test. Statistically significant differences ($p<0,05$) were found between CC/CC vs TT/TT and also between CT/CT vs TT/TT in the second week after transplantation. With this kind of analysis we evaluate the global effect of the variant, C or T, without taking into account if the effect is greater in recipients or in donors.

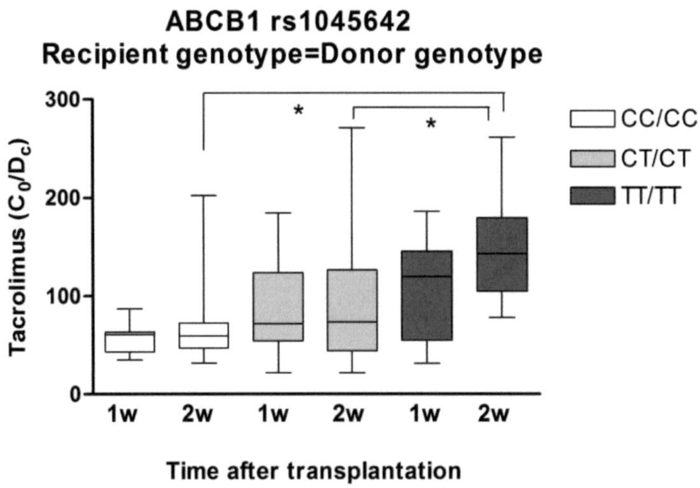

Fig. 2. Tacrolimus corrected trough concentration in renal recipients regarding single nucleotide polymorphism (SNP) rs1045642 genotype recipient/donor. Corrected trough concentration (C_0/(dose/weight)) (C_0: ng/mL; dose: mg/Kg/day; weight: Kg) regarding the patient and donor genotype, grouped so that both genotypes match, in SNP rs1045642 of ABCB1 gene, in the first (1w) and second week (2w) after transplantation. The horizontal line inside each bar is the median of the data, the bar is the interquartilic range, including 50% of the data, and the lines up and down the bars cover the whole data range for each set. A significant difference (*= p<0,05)was achieved in the second week between CC/CC and TT/TT, and also between CT/CT and TT/TT employing Mann-Whitney two-tailed test.

Figures 3, 4 and 5 show the same kind of analysis as in Figure 2 but with patients grouped by a single recipient variant comparing the three possible donors' genotype.

We could not find any statistically significant differences in Fig.3, applying Mann-Whitney non-parametric test, most probably because we only had one value for CC/TT in the first week, and two for the second. However, those three values show the expected trend of higher tacrolimus levels than the rest of the groups.

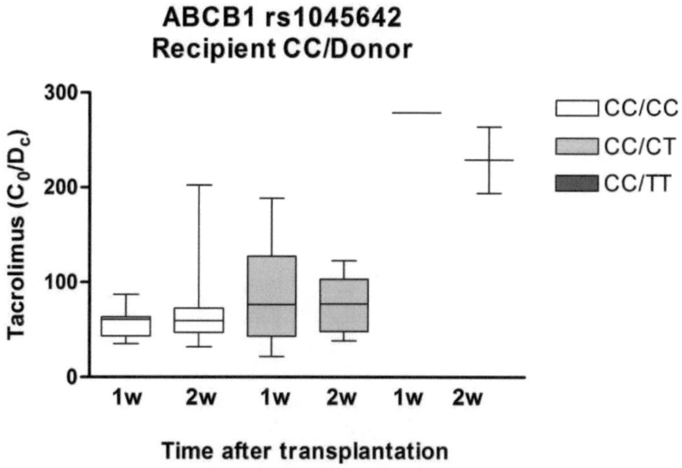

Fig. 3. Tacrolimus corrected trough concentration in renal recipients regarding single nucleotide polymorphism (SNP) rs1045642 in CC recipients. Corrected trough concentration (C_0/(dose/weight)) (C_0: ng/mL; dose: mg/Kg/day; weight: Kg) regarding the patient and donor genotype, showing the data from recipients CC divided in three different groups according to their donor genotype (recipient/donor), in the first (1w) and second week (2w) after transplantation. The horizontal line inside each bar is the median of the data, the bar is the interquartilic range, including 50% of the data, and the lines up and down the bars cover the whole data range for each set. No significant differences were found.

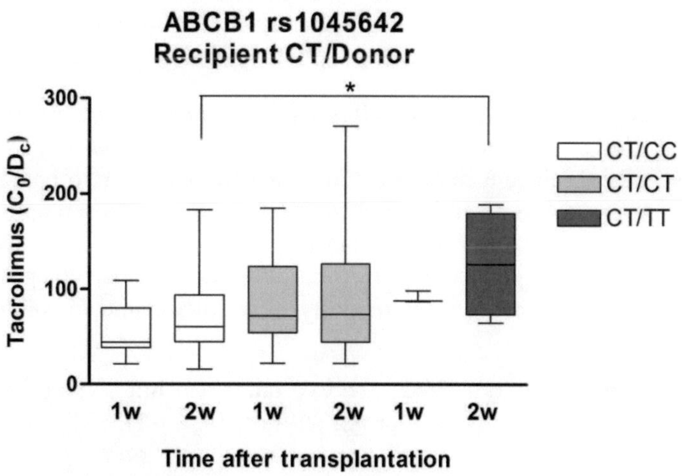

Fig. 4. Tacrolimus corrected trough concentration in renal recipients regarding single nucleotide polymorphism (SNP) rs1045642 in CT recipients. Corrected trough concentration (C_0/(dose/weight)) (C_0: ng/mL; dose: mg/Kg/day; weight: Kg) regarding the patient and donor genotype, showing the data from recipients CT divided in three different groups according to their donor genotype (recipient/donor), in the first (1w) and second week (2w) after transplantation. The horizontal line inside each bar is the median of the data, the bar is the interquartilic range, including 50% of the data, and the lines up and down the bars cover the whole data range for each set. Significant differences were found between CT/CC and CT/TT at week two ($p<0,05$) employing Mann-Whitney two-tailed test.

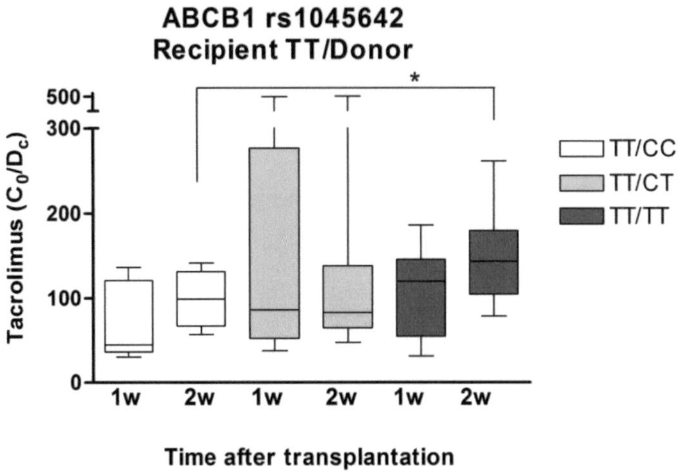

Fig. 5. Tacrolimus corrected trough concentration in renal recipients regarding single nucleotide polymorphism (SNP) rs1045642 in TT recipients. Corrected trough concentration (C_0/(dose/weight)) (C_0: ng/mL; dose: mg/Kg/day; weight: Kg) regarding the patient and donor genotype, showing the data from recipients TT divided in three different groups according to their donor genotype (recipient/donor), in the first (1w) and second week (2w) after transplantation. The horizontal line inside each bar is the median of the data, the bar is the interquartilic range, including 50% of the data, and the lines up and down the bars cover the whole data range for each set. Significant differences were found between TT/CC and TT/TT at week two ($p<0,05$) employing Mann-Whitney one-tailed test.

There is a clear trend of CC genotype in SNP rs1045642 to normalize tacrolimus levels, while there is always an increase related with T allele, especially in TT genotype, where most of the times, statistically significant differences are reached at week two post-transplantation. With these data, we can calculate an increase in the value of the median up to 286.53% when comparing the difference between the median in group CC/TT and the median in group CC/CC (fig. 2, second week) Table 8 shows the differences in percentage of the medians from figures 2, 3, 4 and 5, and also the quantity of recipients and tacrolimus level values included in each of the figures.

But we have not only studied rs1045642, also two other relevant SNPs in ABCB1 that have been described to be in linkage disequilibrium with the first: rs1128503 and rs2032582. With the genotype data for these three SNPs in our renal transplantation recipients, we constructed haplotype groups, being "Normal" those recipients carrying CC in rs1045642, CC in rs1128503 and GG in rs2032582, and "Variant" those carrying the rest of the possible combinations, containing at least one T allele in any of the three SNPs. The results correlating these genotypes with tacrolimus corrected trough level are shown in figures 6 and 7. In figure 6 the data are represented according to the donors' haplotype, with n=23 values for "normal"group in the first week and 29 in the second, and for "variant", 77 in the first week and 93 in the second. Figure 7 shows the data arranged according to the haplotype of the recipients, with 21, 19, 86 and 110 values, respectively. In both figures we find significant differences of $p<0,05$ between the two groups with Mann-Whitney two-tailed test.

GENOTYPE 1 (R/D)*	Nº PATIENTS	Nº SAMPLES	GENOTYPE 2 (R/D)*	Nº PATIENTS	Nº SAMPLES	Δ%
TT/TT	4	7	CC/CC	6	12	141.4
			CT/CT	15	33	94.6
			TT/CC	5	8	44.53
			TT/CT	9	20	71.88
CC/TT	1	2	CC/CC	6	12	286.53
			CC/CT	8	14	196.52
CT/TT	2	4	CT/CC	14	29	107.52
			CT/CT	15	33	71.29

Table 8. Percent increase (Δ%) of the median in the second week after transplantation, comparing different groups according to their genotype recipient/donor, as shown in figures 2-5. Columns 2 and 5 show the number of recipients in each group, and columns 3 and 6 show the number of tacrolimus levels included. *Recipient/Donor.

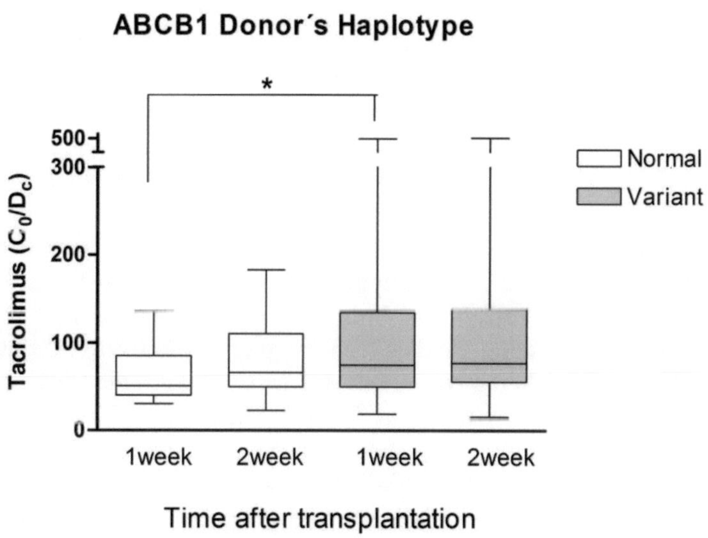

Fig. 6. Tacrolimus corrected trough concentration in renal recipients regarding SNPs rs1045642, rs1128503 and rs2032582 haplotype in their donors. Corrected trough concentration (C_0/(dose/weight)) (C_0: ng/mL; dose: mg/Kg/day; weight: Kg) regarding the patient's donor genotype, showing the data from recipients divided in two groups according to their donor's genotype being Normal those whose donors are CC/CC/GG in the three SNPs respectively, and Variant those with any of the other possible combinations. The results displayed correspond to the first (1w) and second week (2w) after transplantation. The horizontal line inside each bar is the median of the data, the bar is the interquartilic range, including 50% of the data, and the lines up and down the bars cover the whole data range for each set. Significant differences were found between the two groups at the first week ($p<0,05$) employing Mann-Whitney two-tailed test.

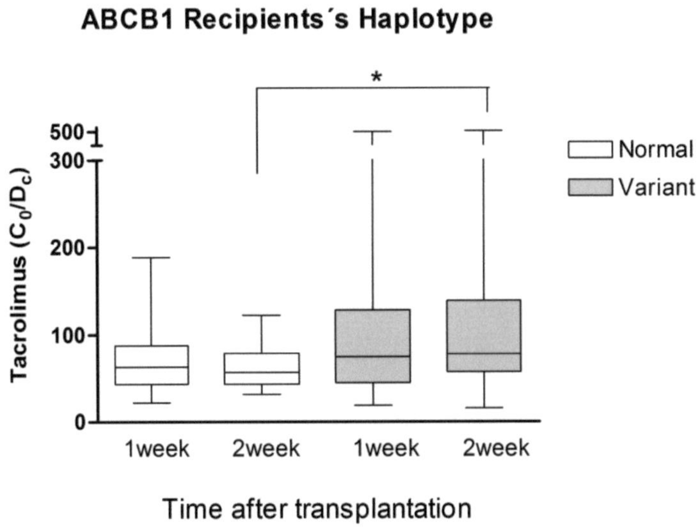

Fig. 7. Tacrolimus corrected trough concentration in renal recipients regarding SNPs rs1045642, rs1128503 and rs2032582 haplotype in the patients. Corrected trough concentration (C_0/(dose/weight)) (C_0: ng/mL; dose: mg/Kg/day; weight: Kg) regarding the recipients' genotype, showing the data from recipients divided in two groups according to their haplotype being Normal those CC/CC/GG in the three SNPs respectively, and Variant those with any of the other possible combinations. The results displayed correspond to the first (1w) and second week (2w) after transplantation. The horizontal line inside each bar is the median of the data, the bar is the interquartilic range, including 50% of the data, and the lines up and down the bars cover the whole data range for each set. Significant differences were found between the two groups at the second week ($p<0,05$) employing Mann-Whitney two-tailed test.

5.3.2 CYP3A5

The corresponding data for the analysis of SNPs rs776746 and rs10264272 of CYP3A5 showed the expected behavior, already described in the literature. In figure 8, we find a significant increase in tacrolimus concentration in patients GG, the non-expressors, regarding GA. We failed to have AA patients, which we would expect to have even lower concentrations than GA. Regarding SNP rs102642272, we only had one GA patient, so we could not perform any statistical analysis, however the only three values that we have from that recipient are consistent with the expected results of higher tacrolimus concentrations.

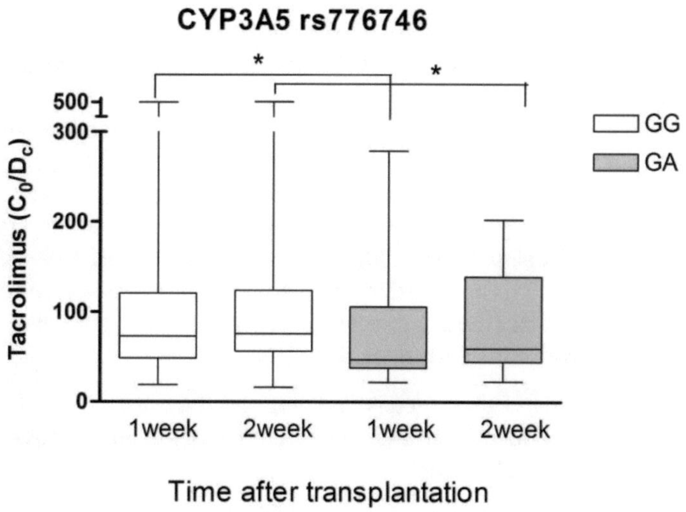

Fig. 8. Tacrolimus corrected trough concentration in renal recipients regarding SNP rs776746 genotype. Tacrolimus corrected trough concentration (C_0/Dc (dose/weight)) (C_0 ng/mL; dose mg/Kg/24 hours; weight Kg) is shown regarding recipient's genotype GG or GA, in the first (1w) and second (2w) week after transplantation. P<0,05 statistically significant difference was found between groups at both weeks by Mann-Whitney one-tailed test.

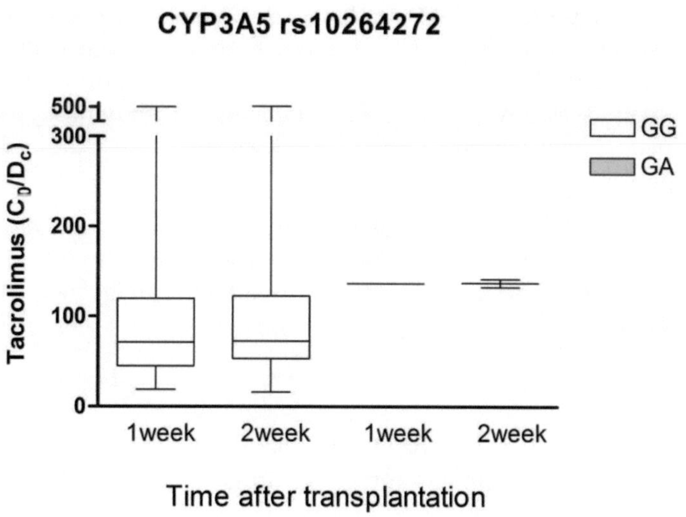

Fig 9. Tacrolimus corrected trough concentration in renal recipients regarding SNP rs10264272 genotype. Tacrolimus corrected trough concentration (C_0/Dc (dose/weight)) (C_0 ng/mL; dose mg/Kg/24 hours; weight Kg) is shown regarding recipient's genotype GG or GA, in the first (1w) and second (2w) week after transplantation. No statistical difference was found between groups.

6. Conclusions

The importance of obtaining the best results in terms of efficacy and safety, but also in terms of economic saving is out of discussion. With the personalized medicine we search for formulas that help us decide wich is the perfect treatment in drug and dose for each patient. This is actually possible nowadays with the help of tools as pharmacogenetics, but there is still a lot of work to do before this tool would really be useful in all the therapeutic areas in the daily work with the patient. There are a lot of published works about many genes and SNPs, but when we look deeply for the usefulness, not all of them pass the test. In this work we have confirmed with real patients' data, the expected effect of five different SNPs in ABCB1 and CYP3A5 genes. We have also demonstrated that there is an additional effect of the donor's genotype translated into the received organ, which is also playing a role in the transport (ABCB1) of tacrolimus (Herrero et al., 2010).

But there are still many other genes related to tacrolimus, and also to other immunosuppressants as cyclosporine and micophenolic acid, which have to be explored and validated in the real clinical setting.

Interdisciplinar groups are also necessary for a complete approach to the scenario, only summing the work of different professionals could we achieve the success. The results in other kinds of transplantation must also be taken in consideration (Jordán et al, 2011).

The effects of many other factors need also to be considered, as they may overlap or disguise a genotype effect.

With the data in our hands, we have found a clear effect of increased tacrolimus trough concentration associated with TT genotype in SNPs rs1045642, rs1128503 and rs2032582 in ABCB1 gene. And regarding CYP3A5, we have also found an increase of the mentioned levels in the non-expressor genotype GG. These data, in agreement with more published works by other groups (Haufroid et al. 2006, Thervet et al., 2010), makes us consider conducting an analysis to any patient before initiating an immunosuppressive therapy, before the transplantation is performed in order to know in advance the optimal dose based on the polymorphisms found.

Further studies with a higher number of patients, also in long term responses, relating several SNPs at the same time, building haplotypes and taking also into consideration the correlation with adverse effects are required to establish this "new" and promising Pharmacogenetic Tool.

7. References

Anglicheau, D., Legendre, C., Beaune, P., & Thervet, E. (2007). Cytochrome P450 3A polymorphisms and immunosuppressive drugs: an update. Pharmacogenomics, 8, 7, (July 2007), pp. (835-849)

Anglicheau, D., Verstuyft, C., Puig, Laurent-Puig, P., Becquemont, L., Schlageter, M., Cassinat, B., Beaune, P., Legendre, C., & Therver, E. (2003). Association of the Multidrug Resistance-1 gene single-nucleotide polymorphisms with the tacrolimus dose requirements in renal transplant recipients. *Journal of the American Society of Nephrology*, 14, 7, (July 2003), pp. (1889-1896)

Astellas Pharma, S.A. Prograf®. Technical. (August 2010) Available from: http://www.portalfarma.com

Barry, A., & Levine, M. (2010). A systematic review of the effect of CYP3A5 genotype on the apparent oral clearance of tacrolimus in renal transplant recipients. Therapeutic Drug Monitoring, 32, 6, (December 2010), pp. (708-714)

Capron, A., Mourad, M., De Meyer, M., De Pauw, L., Eddour, DC., Latinne, D., Elens, L., Haufroid, V., & Wallemacq, P. (2010). CYP3A5 and ABCB1 polymorphisms influence tacrolimus concentrations in peripheral blood mononuclear cells after renal transplantation. Pharmacogenomics, 11, 5, (May 2010), pp. (703-714)

Dai, Y., Hebert, MF., Isoherranen, N., Davis, CL., Marsh, C., Shen, DD., & Thummel, KE. (2006). Effect of cyp3a5 polymorphism on tacrolimus metabolic clearance in vitro. Drug metabolism and disposition, 34, 5, (May 2006), pp. (836-847)

FDA. June 2011. Avaiable from: www.fda.gov

Glowacki, F., Lionet, A., Buob, D., Labalette, M., Allorge, D., Provôt, F., Hazzan, M., Noël, C., Broly, F., & Cauffiez, C. (2011). CYP3A5 and ABCB1 polymorphisms in donor and recipient: impact on Tacrolimus dose requirements and clinical outcome after renal transplantation. Nephrology, dialysis, transplantaion, 0, (June 2011), pp. (1-5)

HapMap project, June 2011, available at www.hapmap.org

Haufroid, V., Wallemacq, P., VanKerckhove, V., Elens, L., De Meyer, M., Eddour, DC., Malaise, J., Lison, D., & Mourad, M. (2006). CYP3A5 and ABCB1 polymorphisms and tacrolimus pharmacokinetics in renal transplant candidates: Guidelines from an experimental study. *American Journal of Transplantation*, 6, 11, (November 2006), pp. (2706-2713)

Herrero, MJ., Sánchez-Plumed, J., Galiana, M., Bea, S., Marqués, MR., Aliño, SF. (2010). Influence of pharmacogenetic polymorphisms in routine immunosuppression therapy after renal transplantation. *Transplantation Proceedings*, 42, pp. (3134-3136)

Hesselink, DA., Van Schaik, RH., Van Agteren, M., De Fijter, JW., Hartmann, A., Zeier, M., Budde, K., Kuypers, DR., Pisarski, P., Le Meur, Y., Mamelok, RD., & Van Gelder, T. (2008). CYP3A5 genotype is not associated with a higher risk of acute rejection in tacrolimus-treated renal transplant recipients. *Pharmacogenetic and Genomics*, 18, 4, (april 2008), pp. (339-348)

Jordán, C., Herrero, MJ., Sánchez, I., Almenar, L., Poveda JL., Aliño, SF. (2011). Pharmacogenetic study of ABCB1 and CYP3A5 genes during the first year following heart transplantation regarding tacrolimus and cyclosporine levels. *Transplantation Proceedings, in press, 2011*

Katsakiori, PF., Papapetrou, EP., Sakellaropoulos, GC., Goumenos, DS., Nikiforidis, GC., & Flordellis, CS. (2010). Factors affecting the long-term response to tacrolimus in renal transplant patients: pharmacokinetic and pharmacogenetic approach. *International Journal of Medical Sciences*, 7, 2, (May 2010), pp. (94-100)

MacPhee, IA., Fredericks, S., & Holt, DW. (2005). Does pharmacogenetics have the potential to allow the individualization of immunosuppressive drug dosing in organ transplantation?. *Expert Opinion Pharmacotherapy*, 6, 11, (December 2005), pp. (914-919)

Macphee IA, Fredericks S, Mohamed M, Moreton M, Carter ND, Johnston A, Goldberg L, Holt DW. (2005). Tacrolimus pharmacogenetics: the CYP3A5*1 allele predicts low dose-normalized tacrolimus blood concentrations in whites and South Asians. Transplantation, 79, 4, (February 2005), pp. (499-502)

Marqués, MR., Gil, MI., & Fernández, MJ. (2009). Farmacocinética de los inmunosupresores, In: *Bases para la atención farmacéutica al paciente trasplantado*, Poveda, JL., Font, I., & Monte, E., pp. (93-104), Roche Farma, ISBN: 978-84-692-2583-7, Spain

NCBI. June 2011. Avaiable from: http://www.ncbi.nlm.nih.gov

Novartis Farmacéutica, S.A. Sandimmun Neoral®. Technical. (August 2010) Available from: http://www.portalfarma.com

Pharmgkb. June 2011. Avaiable from: www. pharmgkb.org

Rong, G., Jing, L., Deng-Qing, L., Hong-Shan, Z., Shai-Hong, Z., & Xin-Min, N. (2010). Influence of CYP3A5 and MDR1 (ABCB1) Polymorphisms on the Pharmacokinetics of Tacrolimus in Chinese Renal Transplant Recipients. *Transplantation Proceedings*, 42, 9, (November 2010), pp. (3455–3458)

Singh, R., Srivastava, A., Kapoor, R., & Mittal, RD. (2011). Do Drug Transporter (ABCB1) SNPs Influence Cyclosporine and Tacrolimus Dose Requirements and Renal Allograft Outcome in the Posttransplantation Period?. *The Journal of Clinical Pharmacology*, 51, 4, (June 2010), pp. (603-615)

Staatz, CE., Goodman LK., & Tett, SE. (2010). Effect of CYP3A and ABCB1 single nucleotide polymorphisms on the pharmacokinetics and pharmacodynamics of calcineurin inhibitors: Part I. *Clinical Pharmacokinetics*, 49, 3, (March 2010), pp. (141-175)

Tavira, B., Garciá, EC., Díaz-Corte, C., Ortega, F., Arias, M., Torres, A., Díaz, JM., Selgas, R., López-Larrea, C., Campistol, JM., & Alvarezca, V. (2010). Pharmacogenetics of tacrolimus after renal transplantation: analysis of polymorphisms in genes encoding 16 drug metabolizing enzymes. Clinical chemistry an laboratory medicine, 49, 5, (May 2011), pp. (825-833)

Thervet, E., Lariot, MA., Barbier, S., Buchler, M., Ficheux, M., Choukroun, G., Toupance, O., Youchard, G., Alberti, C., Pogamp, PL., Moulin, B., Meur, YL., Heg, AE., Subra, JF., Beaune, P., & Legendre, C. (2010). Optimization of initial tacrolimus dose using pharmacogenetic testing. *Clinical Pharmacology & Therapeutics*, 87, 6, (June 2010), pp. (721-726)

Zhang, J., Zhang, X., Liu, L., & Tong, W. (2010). Value of CYP3A5 genotyping on determining initial dosages of tacrolimus for Chinese renal transplant recipients. *Transplantation Proceedings*, 42, 9, (November 2010), pp. (3459-3464)

Zhu, HJ., Yuan, SH., Fang, Y., Sun, XZ., Kong, H., & ge, WH. (2011). The effect of CYP3A5 polymorphism on dose-adjusted cyclosporine concentration in renal transplant recipients: a meta-analysis. *The Pharmacogenomics Journal*, 11, 3, (June 2011), pp. (237-246)

11

Pharmacokinetics and Pharmacodynamics of Mycophenolate in Patients After Renal Transplantation

Thomas Rath[1] and Manfred Küpper[2]
[1]*Department of Nephrology and Transplantation Medicine, Westpfalz-Klinikum GmbH, Kaiserslautern*
[2]*HPLC-Laboratory, Institute for Immunology and Genetics, Kaiserslautern*
Germany

1. Introduction

Mycophenolic-acid (MPA) is a selective, non-competitive inhibitor of Inosine-Monophosphate-Dyhydrogenase (IMPDH) leading to the inhibition of the de-novo synthesis of guanosine-nucleotides. In human lymphocytes inhibition of IMPDH results in altered cellular proliferation with arrest in the S-phase of the cell cycle. Due to the absence of a salvage pathway, proliferating activated t-cells are severely affected by the inhibitory effects of MPA (1-3). For patients after renal transplantation MPA is used either as mycophenolate-mofetil (MMF, Cellcept) or as enteric-coated mycophenolate-Sodium (EC-MPS, Myfortic) in daily doses of 2000 mg respectively 1440 mg per day.

Since its introduction in immunosuppressive therapy more than ten years ago, Mycophenolate-Mofetil (MMF) is an established part of immunosuppressive therapy after renal transplantation. Still in the first publication of the landmark Tricontinental trial because of possibly dose related side effects of the drug (CMV-infection, gastrointestinal disturbances, and increased cancer risk) the need for individualization depending on clinical course or other factors was mentioned (4).

The usefulness of pharmacokinetic measurements of MMF was shown in early studies stating that the Area-under the curve (AUC) of MMF is predictive of the likelihood of allograft rejection after renal transplantation in patients receiving mycophenolate mofetil (5). To facilitate therapeutic drug monitoring different limited sampling strategies for adult and pediatric patients after renal transplantation were established (6-13).

The two available preparations of MPA (MMF, EC-MPS) showed equivalent drug exposure measured by MPA-AUC when applied to the patients in equimolar doses. Therefore, both preparations are seen as equipotent (14-16).

2. Pharmacokinetics of MPA

MPA trough levels show relevant inter- and intraindividual variability especially in patients with elevated serum creatinine and proteinuria (17-19). Clinically important, low trough levels are associated with an increased frequency of rejection (20), whereas elevated MPA trough levels are related to an increased risk for infections (21). Nevertheless, relevant correlations between MPA trough levels and MPA-AUC values could not be detected, therefore the usefulness of measuring trough levels in routine care of renal transplant recipients is doubted (22-24).

2.1 Effect of immunosuppressive therapy on MPA pharmacokinetics

Concomitant immunosuppressive therapy has major influence on MPA pharmacokinetics. For patients on Cyclosporine (CsA) therapy lower MPA trough levels are observed (25). In addition, MPA trough levels increased after discontinuation of CsA resulting in almost a doubling of MPA trough concentrations (26). In general, the variability of MPA-AUC in patients with concomitant cyclosporine and steroid therapy seems to be low (27). However, in 154 patients with an immunosuppressive therapy consisting of CsA, prednisone and MMF the mean MPA AUC increased after 21 days although mean MMF dose was reduced (28).

For patients treated with tacrolimus (TAC) increased MPA trough levels are reported (29). Additionally, a randomized trial with 150 participants, patients receiving TAC and MMF displayed significantly higher MPA trough levels and higher MPA exposure measured by MPA-AUC than those receiving CsA and the same dose of MMF. Equivalent MPA levels could only be attained in patients receiving CsA by increasing the MMF dose by 50% (30). Similar results were obtained for pediatric renal transplantation (31). Interestingly, at least in japanese renal transplant patients, a difference for MPA-AUC in patients with different tacrolimus-trough levels could not be detected (32). At least, for renal transplant recipients limited sample strategies for MPA-AUC with concomitant medication of tacrolimus are established (33).

In patients with Sirolimus (SRL) MPA exposure in the presence of SRL is higher than MPA exposure with CsA. Therefore it was recommended, that the MMF dose should be reduced to 0.75 g twice a day in patients receiving SRL to obtain MPA-AUC levels comparable to that in patients treated with CsA and MMF 1 g twice a day (8). These results were confirmed in a pharmacokinetic study in 31 renal transplant patients (34). It was also shown, that although MPA peak concentration and time to peak concentration was comparable, the MPA-AUC was higher in patients receiving SRL instead of CsA (35).

Steroids have been shown to induce the hepatic glucuronyltransferase (GT) expression enhancing the activity of uridine diphosphate-GT, the enzyme responsible for mycophenolic acid (MPA) metabolism. Therefore, also for steroids interactions with MPA are reported. During a steroid tapering and withdrawal phase in 26 patients MPA trough levels progressively increased and plasma MPA clearance declined (36).

2.2 Effect of concomitant therapy on MPA pharmacokinetics

For patients in the maintenance phase after transplantation it is known, that MPA-AUC increases with declining transplant function (37). This effect may be modulated by concomitant medication. Beside immunosuppression, patients after renal transplantation have to use antiviral prophylaxis. At least for Ganciclovir no effect on MPA clearance in kidney transplant recipients was reported (38).

With respect to the use of proton pump inhibitors the published results are unequivocally. In japanese patients, the peak MPA-concentrations were lower with 30 mg lansoprazole than with 10 mg rabeprazole or without PPI. For patients with cytochrome (CYP) 2C19, and multidrug resistance (MDR)1 C3435T polymorphisms this was also seen for the MPA-AUC (39).

Patients after heart transplantation with PPI co-medication show significantly lower MPA plasma concentrations resulting in lower drug exposure exposing the patients at a higher risk for acute rejection (40). Also in patients with autoimmune diseases the co-medication of pantoprazole with MMF significantly influences the drug exposure and immunosuppressive potency of MMF (41). In contrast, the recently published sub-analysis of the CLEAR-study reported no difference in MPA-AUC in patients with or without PPI-therapy when a 3g/d loading dose of MMF for 5 days used. However, MPA concentrations 2 h and 12 h after MMF intake were reduced (42).

At least for heart transplant recipients no influence of pantoprazole on EC-MPS pharmacokinetics could be disclosed (43).

Own results in 74 patients in the early and maintenance phase after renal transplantation showed a relevant reduction in normalized MPA-AUC (40,9 +/- 19,7 vs. 26,1 +/- 11,7 mg/l*h; p<0,01) in patients with PPI co-medication. A difference between patients using either omeprazole or pantoprazole in MPA-AUC could not be detected. (Rath et al., Congress of the German Transplantation Society, 2009)

3. Clinical relevance of MPA-AUC

3.1 MPA-AUC and acute rejection

In different clinical trials, MPA drug exposure was correlated with the occurrence of biopsy proven acute rejection (BPAR). In a double blind trial aiming for three predefined target MPA AUC values the incidence of BPAR was lower in patients with MPA AUC values between 30 and 60 µg x h/ml (28). Similar results were reported for a group of 46 stable patients after renal transplantation, with better graft function in patients with a MPA AUC > 40 µg/ml*h and for pediatric renal transplantation (20;44;45).

Three randomized trials, the OPTICEPT study, the APOMYGRE-trial (Adaption de Posologie du MMF en Greffe Renale) and the FDCC study (fixed-dose versus concentration controlled) investigated the benefit of therapeutic drug monitoring for MMF in renal transplant recipients.

The APOMYGRE Trial was a study in 137 allograft recipients treated with basiliximab, cyclosporine A, corticosteroids and MMF. Patients were randomized to receive either concentration-controlled doses or fixed-dose MMF. A novel Bayesian estimator of MPA AUC based on three-point sampling was used to individualize MMF doses. At month 12, the concentration-controlled group had fewer treatment failures and acute rejection episodes. Therefore, the authors conclude, that therapeutic MPA monitoring using a limited sampling strategy can reduce the risk of treatment failure and acute rejection in renal allograft recipients 12 months post-transplant with no increase in adverse events (46).

The FDCC study was a randomized trial in 901 patients after renal transplantation allocating patients to receive MMF either in a fix dose or in a concentration controlled manner aiming at a predefined MPA AUC of 45 mg*h/L. In general, there was no difference in the incidence of primary treatment failure or biopsy proved rejection. However, MPA-AUC levels at day 3 after transplantation predicts the incidence of BPAR in the first year (47).

The OPTICEPT study was a 2-year, open-label, randomized, multicenter trial comparing the efficacy and safety of concentration-controlled MMF dosing with a fixed-dose regimen in 720 kidney recipients. In patients with Tacrolimus, those with higher MMF exposure had less rejection episodes (48).

Similarly, a recently published substudy of the FDCC-trial in patients with delayed graft function disclosed significantly lower dose-corrected MPA AUC on Day 3 and Day 10 in this patient group (49).

3.2 MPA-pharmacokinetics and gastro-intestinal side effects

It is known, that side effects of MMF are causing dose reductions in approximately 60% of the patients leading to a cumulative and increasing risk for acute rejection (50). In addition, gastrointestinal (GIT) side effects affect medical adherence of the patients with consecutive risk for graft failure (51). In addition, dose reductions of MMF are related to increased costs, mainly due to frequent hospitalization of the patients (52).

USRDS data of 3589 patients with MMF prescription and GIT complaints revealed that dosage reduction or discontinuation of mycophenolate mofetil in the first 6 months after diagnosis of GI complications was associated with significantly increased risk of graft failure and increased healthcare costs in adult renal transplant recipients (53). Another report from USRDS data of 3675 patients with gastrointestinal complications under MMF and subsequent dose reduction also disclosed an increased risk for graft loss after dose reduction or discontinuation of MMF (54).

The enteric coated preparation of mycophenolate (EC-MPS) is attributed to a lower rate of gastrointestinal side effects, but in a prospective study based on patient questionnaires the rate of gastrointestinal side effects was nearly identical between the two formulations (55). In addition, a double-blind study comparing MMF and the newly developed enteric-coated formulation of MPA (EC-MPS) showed no advantage for either of the drugs (56). In contrast, a large, prospective study in more than 700 renal transplant recipients disclosed a significant improvement in gastrointestinal adverse events after conversion from MMF to EC-MPS (57). A study in patients with GIT complaints under MMF switching to EC-MPS indicates that converting patients with mild, moderate or severe GI complaints from MMF to EC-MPS significantly reduces GI-related symptom burden and improves patient functioning and well-being (58).

Also in liver transplant patients results are reported that converting patients with gastrointestinal complaints from MMF to equimolar doses of EC-MMF leads to a reduction of gastrointestinal-related symptom burden and frequency of stools (59).

There is some evidence from pharmacokinetic studies that elevated MPA exposure correlates with the occurrence of gastrointestinal side effects. Some authors suggest that gastrointestinal side effects are related to exposure of the active substance MPA (60). Others report, that the occurrence of possibly MMF-related side effects corresponds with MPA-AUC and MPA concentration 30 minutes after oral dose of 1000 mg (61). Also, a longitudinal study in 37 patients with 357 MPA measurements revealed higher trough levels in patients with MMF associated side effects(62). It is known that MPA trough levels >3 mg/l, peak levels >8.09 mg/l and MPA-AUC > 37.6 mg*h/l may lead to adverse effects (63). Also in 31 patients after renal transplantation higher MPA-AUC (>60 mg*h/l) was associated with side effects (64). Nevertheless, in a small pharmacokinetic study with 11 hispanic renal transplant patients treated with EC-MPS the MPA-AUC does not correlate with overall Gastrointestinal Symptom Rating Scale scores or subscale scores (65).

Also, a 5-year clinical follow-up study in 100 renal allograft recipients in whom MPA exposure was measured at 7 days, 6 weeks, 3 months, 1, 3, and 5 years post transplantation using abbreviated AUC measurements reported more episodes of leucopenia and anemia with MPA AUC(0-12h) ranges >60 mg/L x h(-1). However, no association between incident episodes of diarrhea or infection and target MPA AUC (0-12 h) ranges (66).

4. Pharmacodynamics of MPA

4.1 Inhibition of IMPDH-activity

Recently, pharmacodynamic measurement of MPA was introduced into clinical practice. Especially with the use of reversed-phase HPLC, it is possible to monitor the immunosuppressive effect of MPA in its target cell population by quantifying the activity of IMPDH. This nonradioactive method for specific measurement of IMPDH activity in isolated peripheral mononuclear cells was developed by direct chromatographic determination of produced xanthosine 5'-monophosphate (XMP). In the canine model MPA in therapeutic doses leads to an 50% inhibition of IMPDH-activity (67) . Application of a single dose of 1 g MMF in dialysis patients resulted in a significant inhibition of IMPDH activity in lysed mononuclear cells. IMPDH activity is inversely correlated to MPA blood concentrations and the IC (50) for in vitro inhibition of IMPDH activity was about 2 to 3 µg/l. (68). In addition, others report, that IMPDH-activity on peak concentration of MPA is approximately 40% and could be suppressed for 8 hours (69). In general, it is assumed, that IMPDH activity has a substantial interindividual, but low intraindividual variability (70). This was also shown in pediatric patients (71).

In addition, in renal allograft recipients an inverse relationship between plasma MPA and IMPDH activity within the dose interval was demonstrated and minimum IMPDH activity was a median 8 % of values pre-MMF dose, coinciding with the MPA peak. Six hours post-dose, IMPDH activity had returned to pre-dose values. Patients receiving MMF had a 4.5-fold higher pre-dose enzyme activity than transplanted patients without MMF (72). Long-term treatment with mycophenolate was associated with an induction of IMPDH activity (73). Also a study with 12 patients over two years showed an increase of type 1 IMPDH mRNA during the first 3 months following transplantation and reaching its maximal level during acute rejection episodes, whereas type2 IMPDH mRNA was stable (74). Interestingly, in 30 patients transplantation and the initiation of immunosuppressive therapy was associated with increased IMPDH1 and decreased IMPDH2 expression. In addition, patients with acute rejection during follow-up demonstrated higher IMPDH2 expression in pretransplant CD4+ cells than nonrejecting patients (75). Later, the same group described in detail the MMF concentration dependent modulation of IMPDH1 expression in renal allograft recipients (76).

4.2 IMPDH-activity and acute rejection

Measurement of IMPDH activity may be useful in estimating the degree of immunosuppression in individual patients in addition to applied MMF dose. When comparing three patients groups with MMF doses of 1.0, 1.5 and 2.0 g/d there was no correlation between MPA-AUC (0-12) values and MMF dose detectable. Also, the degree of inhibition of IMPDH activity was comparable in the three groups, indicating considerable interindividual pharmacodynamic variability (77). In a cross-sectional analysis patients experiencing acute rejection episodes had increased IMPDH activity during rejection episodes (78). Additional information was gained in a genotyping study in 191 kidney transplant patients. There, seventeen genetic variants were identified in the IMPDH1 gene with allele frequencies ranging from 0.2 to 42.7%. Two single-nucleotide polymorphisms, rs2278293 and rs2278294, were significantly associated with the incidence of biopsy-proven acute rejection in the first year post-transplantation (79). A similar study in 82 japanese transplant recipients found no difference in the incidence of subclinical acute rejection between IMPDH1 rs2278293 or rs2278294 polymorphisms ($p = 0.243$ and 0.735, respectively). However, the authors report that the risk of subclinical acute rejection for recipients who cannot adapt in therapeutic drug monitoring (TDM) of MPA seems to be influenced by IMPDH1 rs2278293 polymorphism (80). Also, in patients after renal transplantation high pre-transplant IMPDH-activity predisposes to subsequent MPA dose-reductions and increases the risk for acute rejection (81).

4.3 IMPDH activity and MMF or EC-MPS

There is some discussion about the degree of IMPDH suppression with either MMF or EC-MPS. In a single-center, crossover study in patients treated with MMF and EC-MPS IMPDH activity inversely followed MPA concentrations and was inhibited to a similar degree (approximately 85%) by both formulations. In addition, the calculated value for 50% IMPDH inhibition was identical for both drugs (16). However, when comparing the pharmacodynamic activity of MMF and EC-MPS a series of 260 measurements in 110 patients disclosed lower median IMPDH activity in the EC-MPS patients than in the MMF patients. This was especially pronounced in patients on 1440 mg/d EC-MPS compared with 2000 mg/d MMF (82).

Nevertheless, for EC-MPS a recently published pharmacokinetic study in 75 de-novo kidney transplant recipients randomly assigning the patients either to receive EC-MPS as standard dose or as intensified dose revealed in an exploratory analysis of IMPDH activity that the intensified regimen resulted in significantly lower IMPDH activity on day 3 after transplantation (83).

There is ongoing discussion about the effect of PPI therapy on pharmacokinetics of MMF and EC-MPS. In a cross-sectional analysis in 153 renal transplant recipients, we measured IMPDH-activity before the first daily dose of MMF or EC-MPS. We could not detect any statistical with respect to PPI intake, type or dosing of either MMF or EC-MPS (Congress of the German Transplant Society, 2009).

5. Measuring IMPDH-activity

5.1 Sample preparation

Peripheral blood is collected in 5ml tubes with Li-heparin as anti-coagulant and stored at room temperature. Heparin is superior to EDTA as anti-coagulant since it maintains cell viability for longer time. Within four hours after arrival of the sample to the lab, and within no more than two days of collection, the peripheral mononuclear cell fraction is isolated by density centrifugation according to a modified protocol from Glander et al. (2001). Li-heparinized blood (2.5ml) is mixed with an equal volume of phosphate-buffered saline (PBS), carefully layered on 4ml Lymphodex (InnoTrain, Germany) density gradient centrifugation medium in a 15ml screw-cap polypropylene tube, and centrifuged at 1200 x g for 15 min without brake at room temperature.

The mononuclear cell fraction is collected from the interphase and transferred into a fresh 15ml screw-cap tube with 5ml PBS for washing. The cells are washed only once with PBS since repeated washing steps might cause diffusion of mycophenolate from the cells, resulting in over-estimation of the residual IMPDH activity. After centrifugation at 1200 x g for 10 min at room temperature, the supernatant is removed quantitatively. This step is crucial with respect to the assay validity, since only a minute fraction of the total mycophenolate is contained within the cells, while the vast majority (estimated 99%) is present in the plasma. Any trace of the supernatant might therefore still contain considerable amounts of mycophenolate, hence leading to a vast underestimation of the residual IMPDH activity. The cell pellet is resuspended in 250µl ice-cold HPLC-grade water, and 125µl of the sample are transferred into each of two 2ml screw-cap vials, one designated as working sample, the second as back-up. The vials are deep frozen at -80°C until assayed. In the same way, control cells from healthy probands are prepared; these cells will be included in each assay as an incubation control.

5.2 IMPDH activity assay

The residual IMPDH activity is assayed in a cell-free system. The patient samples and control cells are thawed at room temperature and vigorously vortexed for 30 seconds to support cell lysis; insoluble cell fragments are removed by centrifugation at 4000 x g for 5 min at room temperature in a desktop centrifuge. Cell lysate (50µl) is added to 100µl incubation buffer containing 1 mmol/L inosine-monophosphate (IMP) as substrate, 0.5 mmol/L NAD as co-substrate, 72 mmol/L sodium dihydrogen-phosphate, and 180 mmol/L potassium chloride (pH = 7.5). After adjusting the volume to 180ml with distilled water, the samples are incubated at 37°C in a heating block. In presence of NAD, IMPDH converts inosine-monophosphate to xanthine 5′-mono-phosphate. In the subsequent high-performance liquid chromatography (HPLC) assay, the amount of synthesized xanthine 5′-monophosphate is determined together with the amount of AMP, which serves as an internal standard for normalization to the cell count.

After exactly 2.5 hours of incubation, the reaction is stopped by adding 20µl ice-cold 4mol/L perchloric acid. Precipitation of denatured protein is enhanced by incubating the samples at -20°C for 10 min. After centrifugation at 13000 rpm for 2 min in a desktop centrifuge, 170µl supernatant are transferred to a test tube containing 14µl 2.5 mol/L potassium carbonate solution for neutralization. The exact volume of potassium carbonate, required to achieve a final pH between pH 6 and pH 7, has to be determined for each lot of 4 mol/L perchloric acid and 2.5 mol/L potassium carbonate solution. Prior to HPLC analysis, the samples are deep-frozen at -20°C for at least 30 min, thawed, and centrifuged 5 min at 13000 rpm in a desktop centrifuge.

5.3 HPLC chromatography

Determination of the amounts of xanthine-monophosphate and adenosine-monophosphate is carried out by ion-pair reversed-phase high-performance liquid chromatography on a computerized isocratic HPLC system from Shimadzu (Kyoto, Japan) consisting of a system controller SCL-10A *VP*, an HPLC pump LC-10AT *VP*, an autoinjector SIL-10AF, a column oven CTO-10AS *VP*, and an UV-VIS detector SPD-10A *VP*, controlled by Shimadzu LC Solution data collection software.

For the assay 6µl of the samples are loaded onto a 250 mm x 3.1 mm Prontosil 120 to 5 ODS AQ column (Bischoff Chromatography, Leonberg, Germany). Column oven temperature is set to 40°C. Chromatographic separation is achieved using a mobile phase containing 50 mmol/L potassium-dihydrogen-phosphate, 7 mmol/L tetra-n-butyl-ammonium hydrogen sulfate, and 6% (v/v) methanol at a flow rate of 1 mL/min. The analytes are detected at 254-nm wavelength. Incubation efficacy is verified by including a sample from a healthy volunteer as incubation control in each incubation cycle. For calibration, two standards containing 500 and 2500 pmol xanthin-monophosphate and adenosin-monophosphate, respectively, in 0.4% BSA solution are processed in several independent experiments, and repeatedly measured, like the patient specimen: protein denaturation with perchloric acid followed by neutralization with potassium carbonate. This calibration curve allows to deduct the amount of XMP synthesized during incubation and the amount of AMP in the sample. The specific IMPDH activity is then expressed as pmol XMP synthesized per second, which is normalized to 1 pmol of AMP [pmol XMP/(pmol AMP s)].

6. Summary and conclusion

Mycophenolic-acid (MPA) is a selective, non-competitive inhibitor of Inosine-Monophosphate-Dyhydrogenase (IMPDH) leading to the inhibition of the de-novo synthesis of guanosine-nucleotides. In human lymphocytes inhibition of IMPDH results in altered cellular proliferation with arrest in the S-phase of the cell cycle. Due to the absence of a salvage pathway, proliferating activated t-cells are severely affected by the inhibitory effects of MPA.

In patients after renal transplantation, MPA is a well-established part of immunosuppressive therapy, applied either as mycophenolate-mofetil (MMF, Cellcept) or as mycophenolate-sodium (MPS, Myfortic). MMF is used in prophylaxis of kidney rejection for nearly 15 years in daily doses of 2 - 3 g/d. The enteric-coated MPS is available since a few years; the recommended daily dose is 1440 mg/d. Both preparations are equipotent, when given in equimolar doses.

In recent years drug monitoring of MPA gained more and more attention proving its usefulness in clinical setting. Relevant information could be collected by measuring MPA drug exposure by calculating the MPA-Area under the curve (MPA-AUC) with pharmacokinetic modeling allowing estimating the degree of immunosuppression.

In different clinical studies MPA-AUC target concentrations of 30 - 60 µg*h/ml were correlated to a low rate of rejections and less occurrence of drug induced side effects. Clinically important, MPA metabolism is influenced not only by the choice of immunosuppressive medication, but also by renal function and concomitant medication.

Recently pharmacodynamic measurement of MPA was introduced into clinical practice. Especially with the use of reversed-phase HPLC, it becomes possible to monitor the immunosuppressive effect of MPA in its target cell population by quantifying the activity of IMPDH. IMPDH activity is inversely correlated to MPA blood concentrations. Maximum inhibition of IMPDH activity ranges between 60% and 80% and the reported IC (50) of IMPDH activity corresponds to MPA blood levels of 2-3 μ/l. In renal transplant recipients, IMPDH shows relevant inter-individual variability. However, pre-transplant IMPDH activity was predictive for increased risk of rejection when additional dose reductions of MMF were necessary. In a cross-sectional studies better transplant function was associated with lower IMPDH-activity and probably the usage of EC-MPS. Pharmacokinetic and pharmacodynamic parameters of MPA are influenced by additional immunosuppression. In addition, concomitant therapy especially the use of proton-pump inhibitors affects MPA-levels, whereas an effect of IMPDH-activity, at least in renal transplant recipients could not be disclosed. Therefore, it can be concluded, that pharmacokinetic and pharmacodynamic measurements of MPA adds relevant information to improve clinical care of renal transplant recipients.

7. References

[1] Allison AC, Eugui EM. Purine metabolism and immunosuppressive effects of mycophenolate mofetil (MMF). Clin Transplant 1996 Feb;10(1 Pt 2):77-84.

[2] Cohn RG, Mirkovich A, Dunlap B, Burton P, Chiu SH, Eugui E, et al. Mycophenolic acid increases apoptosis, lysosomes and lipid droplets in human lymphoid and monocytic cell lines. Transplantation 1999 Aug 15;68(3):411-8.

[3] Dayton JS, Lindsten T, Thompson CB, Mitchell BS. Effects of human T lymphocyte activation on inosine monophosphate dehydrogenase expression. J Immunol 1994 Feb 1;152(3):984-91.

[4] A blinded, randomized clinical trial of mycophenolate mofetil for the prevention of acute rejection in cadaveric renal transplantation. The Tricontinental Mycophenolate Mofetil Renal Transplantation Study Group. Transplantation 1996 Apr 15;61(7):1029-37.

[5] Hale MD, Nicholls AJ, Bullingham RE, Hene R, Hoitsma A, Squifflet JP, et al. The pharmacokinetic-pharmacodynamic relationship for mycophenolate mofetil in renal transplantation. Clin Pharmacol Ther 1998 Dec;64(6):672-83.

[6] Johnson AG, Rigby RJ, Taylor PJ, Jones CE, Allen J, Franzen K, et al. The kinetics of mycophenolic acid and its glucuronide metabolite in adult kidney transplant recipients. Clin Pharmacol Ther 1999 Nov;66(5):492-500.

[7] Willis C, Taylor PJ, Salm P, Tett SE, Pillans PI. Evaluation of limited sampling strategies for estimation of 12-hour mycophenolic acid area under the plasma concentration-time curve in adult renal transplant patients. Ther Drug Monit 2000 Oct;22(5):549-54.

[8] El HW, Ficheux M, Debruyne D, Rognant N, Lobbedez T, Allard C, et al. Pharmacokinetics of mycophenolic acid in kidney transplant patients receiving sirolimus versus cyclosporine. Transplant Proc 2005 Mar;37(2):864-6.

[9] Miura M, Satoh S, Niioka T, Kagaya H, Saito M, Hayakari M, et al. Limited sampling strategy for simultaneous estimation of the area under the concentration-time curve of tacrolimus and mycophenolic acid in adult renal transplant recipients. Ther Drug Monit 2008 Feb;30(1):52-9.

[10] Mohammadpour AH, Nazemian F, Abtahi B, Naghibi M, Gholami K, Rezaee S, et al. Estimation of abbreviated mycophenolic acid area under the concentration-time curve during early posttransplant period by limited sampling strategy. Transplant Proc 2008 Dec;40(10):3668-72.

[11] Filler G. Abbreviated mycophenolic acid AUC from C0, C1, C2, and C4 is preferable in children after renal transplantation on mycophenolate mofetil and tacrolimus therapy. Transpl Int 2004 Mar;17(3):120-5.

[12] Schutz E, Armstrong VW, Shipkova M, Weber L, Niedmann PD, Lammersdorf T, et al. Limited sampling strategy for the determination of mycophenolic acid area under the curve in pediatric kidney recipients. German Study Group on MMF Therapy in Pediatric Renal Transplant Recipients. Transplant Proc 1998 Jun;30(4):1182-4.

[13] Weber LT, Schutz E, Lamersdorf T, Shipkova M, Niedmann PD, Oellerich M, et al. Therapeutic drug monitoring of total and free mycophenolic acid (MPA) and limited sampling strategy for determination of MPA-AUC in paediatric renal transplant recipients. The German Study Group on Mycophenolate Mofetil (MMF) Therapy. Nephrol Dial Transplant 1999;14 Suppl 4:34-5.

[14] Arns W, Breuer S, Choudhury S, Taccard G, Lee J, Binder V, et al. Enteric-coated mycophenolate sodium delivers bioequivalent MPA exposure compared with mycophenolate mofetil. Clin Transplant 2005 Apr;19(2):199-206.

[15] Arns W, Breuer S, Choudhury S, Taccard G, Lee J, Binder V, et al. Enteric-coated mycophenolate sodium delivers bioequivalent MPA exposure compared with mycophenolate mofetil. Clin Transplant 2005 Apr;19(2):199-206.

[16] Budde K, Bauer S, Hambach P, Hahn U, Roblitz H, Mai I, et al. Pharmacokinetic and pharmacodynamic comparison of enteric-coated mycophenolate sodium and mycophenolate mofetil in maintenance renal transplant patients. Am J Transplant 2007 Apr;7(4):888-98.

[17] Merkel U, Lindner S, Vollandt R, Sperschneider H, Balogh A. Trough levels of mycophenolic acid and its glucuronidated metabolite in renal transplant recipients. Int J Clin Pharmacol Ther 2005 Aug;43(8):379-88.

[18] Fernandez A, Marcen R, Pascual J, Martins J, Villafruela JJ, Cano T, et al. Mycophenolate mofetil levels in stable kidney transplant recipients. Transplant Proc 2007 Sep;39(7):2182-4.

[19] Fernandez A, Martins J, Villlafruela JJ, Marcen R, Pascual J, Cano T, et al. Variability of mycophenolate mofetil trough levels in stable kidney transplant patients. Transplant Proc 2007 Sep;39(7):2185-6.

[20] Oellerich M, Shipkova M, Schutz E, Wieland E, Weber L, Tonshoff B, et al. Pharmacokinetic and metabolic investigations of mycophenolic acid in pediatric patients after renal transplantation: implications for therapeutic drug monitoring. German Study Group on Mycophenolate Mofetil Therapy in Pediatric Renal Transplant Recipients. Ther Drug Monit 2000 Feb;22(1):20-6.

[21] Smak Gregoor PJ, van Gelder T, van Riemsdijk-van Overbeeke IC, Vossen AC, Ijzermans JN, Weimar W. Unusual presentation of herpes virus infections in renal transplant recipients exposed to high mycophenolic acid plasma concentrations. Transpl Infect Dis 2003 Jun;5(2):79-83.

[22] Mardigyan V, Giannetti N, Cecere R, Besner JG, Cantarovich M. Best single time points to predict the area-under-the-curve in long-term heart transplant patients taking mycophenolate mofetil in combination with cyclosporine or tacrolimus. J Heart Lung Transplant 2005 Oct;24(10):1614-8.

[23] Jirasiritham S, Sumethkul V, Mavichak V, Na-Bangchang K. The pharmacokinetics of mycophenolate mofetil in Thai kidney transplant recipients. Transplant Proc 2004 Sep;36(7):2076-8.

[24] Pape L, Ehrich JH, Offner G. Long-term follow-up of pediatric transplant recipients: mycophenolic acid trough levels are not a good indicator for long-term graft function. Clin Transplant 2004 Oct;18(5):576-9.

[25] Smak Gregoor PJ, van Gelder T, Hesse CJ, van der Mast BJ, van Besouw NM, Weimar W. Mycophenolic acid plasma concentrations in kidney allograft recipients with or without cyclosporin: a cross-sectional study. Nephrol Dial Transplant 1999 Mar;14(3):706-8.

[26] Gregoor PJ, de Sevaux RG, Hene RJ, Hesse CJ, Hilbrands LB, Vos P, et al. Effect of cyclosporine on mycophenolic acid trough levels in kidney transplant recipients. Transplantation 1999 Nov 27;68(10):1603-6.

[27] Sumethkul V, Na-Bangchang K, Kantachuvesiri S, Jirasiritham S. Standard dose enteric-coated mycophenolate sodium (myfortic) delivers rapid therapeutic mycophenolic acid exposure in kidney transplant recipients. Transplant Proc 2005 Mar;37(2):861-3.

[28] van Gelder T, Hilbrands LB, Vanrenterghem Y, Weimar W, de Fijter JW, Squifflet JP, et al. A randomized double-blind, multicenter plasma concentration controlled study of the safety and efficacy of oral mycophenolate mofetil for the prevention of acute rejection after kidney transplantation. Transplantation 1999 Jul 27;68(2):261-6.

[29] Hubner GI, Eismann R, Sziegoleit W. Drug interaction between mycophenolate mofetil and tacrolimus detectable within therapeutic mycophenolic acid monitoring in renal transplant patients. Ther Drug Monit 1999 Oct;21(5):536-9.

[30] Zucker K, Rosen A, Tsaroucha A, de Faria L, Roth D, Ciancio G, et al. Unexpected augmentation of mycophenolic acid pharmacokinetics in renal transplant patients receiving tacrolimus and mycophenolate mofetil in combination therapy, and analogous in vitro findings. Transpl Immunol 1997 Sep;5(3):225-32.

[31] Filler G, Zimmering M, Mai I. Pharmacokinetics of mycophenolate mofetil are influenced by concomitant immunosuppression. Pediatr Nephrol 2000 Feb;14(2):100-4.

[32] Kagaya H, Miura M, Satoh S, Inoue K, Saito M, Inoue T, et al. No pharmacokinetic interactions between mycophenolic acid and tacrolimus in renal transplant recipients. J Clin Pharm Ther 2008 Apr;33(2):193-201.

[33] Pawinski T, Hale M, Korecka M, Fitzsimmons WE, Shaw LM. Limited sampling strategy for the estimation of mycophenolic acid area under the curve in adult renal

transplant patients treated with concomitant tacrolimus. Clin Chem 2002 Sep;48(9):1497-504.

[34] Picard N, Premaud A, Rousseau A, Le MY, Marquet P. A comparison of the effect of ciclosporin and sirolimus on the pharmokinetics of mycophenolate in renal transplant patients. Br J Clin Pharmacol 2006 Oct;62(4):477-84.

[35] Cattaneo D, Merlini S, Zenoni S, Baldelli S, Gotti E, Remuzzi G, et al. Influence of co-medication with sirolimus or cyclosporine on mycophenolic acid pharmacokinetics in kidney transplantation. Am J Transplant 2005 Dec;5(12):2937-44.

[36] Cattaneo D, Perico N, Gaspari F, Gotti E, Remuzzi G. Glucocorticoids interfere with mycophenolate mofetil bioavailability in kidney transplantation. Kidney Int 2002 Sep;62(3):1060-7.

[37] Gonzalez-Roncero FM, Gentil MA, Brunet M, Algarra G, Pereira P, Cabello V, et al. Pharmacokinetics of mycophenolate mofetil in kidney transplant patients with renal insufficiency. Transplant Proc 2005 Nov;37(9):3749-51.

[38] Wolfe EJ, Mathur V, Tomlanovich S, Jung D, Wong R, Griffy K, et al. Pharmacokinetics of mycophenolate mofetil and intravenous ganciclovir alone and in combination in renal transplant recipients. Pharmacotherapy 1997 May;17(3):591-8.

[39] Miura M, Satoh S, Inoue K, Kagaya H, Saito M, Suzuki T, et al. Influence of lansoprazole and rabeprazole on mycophenolic acid pharmacokinetics one year after renal transplantation. Ther Drug Monit 2008 Feb;30(1):46-51.

[40] Kofler S, Deutsch MA, Bigdeli AK, Shvets N, Vogeser M, Mueller TH, et al. Proton pump inhibitor co-medication reduces mycophenolate acid drug exposure in heart transplant recipients. J Heart Lung Transplant 2009 Jun;28(6):605-11.

[41] Schaier M, Scholl C, Scharpf D, Hug F, Bonisch-Schmidt S, Dikow R, et al. Proton pump inhibitors interfere with the immunosuppressive potency of mycophenolate mofetil. Rheumatology (Oxford) 2010 Nov;49(11):2061-7.

[42] Kiberd BA, Wrobel M, Dandavino R, Keown P, Gourishankar S. The role of proton pump inhibitors on early mycophenolic acid exposure in kidney transplantation: evidence from the CLEAR study. Ther Drug Monit 2011 Feb;33(1):120-3.

[43] Kofler S, Wolf C, Shvets N, Sisic Z, Muller T, Behr J, et al. The proton pump inhibitor pantoprazole and its interaction with enteric-coated mycophenolate sodium in transplant recipients. J Heart Lung Transplant 2011 May;30(5):565-71.

[44] Cattaneo D, Gaspari F, Ferrari S, Stucchi N, Del PL, Perico N, et al. Pharmacokinetics help optimizing mycophenolate mofetil dosing in kidney transplant patients. Clin Transplant 2001 Dec;15(6):402-9.

[45] Weber LT, Shipkova M, Armstrong VW, Wagner N, Schutz E, Mehls O, et al. The pharmacokinetic-pharmacodynamic relationship for total and free mycophenolic Acid in pediatric renal transplant recipients: a report of the german study group on mycophenolate mofetil therapy. J Am Soc Nephrol 2002 Mar;13(3):759-68.

[46] Le Meur Y, Buchler M, Thierry A, Caillard S, Villemain F, Lavaud S, et al. Individualized mycophenolate mofetil dosing based on drug exposure significantly improves patient outcomes after renal transplantation. Am J Transplant 2007 Nov;7(11):2496-503.

[47] van GT, Silva HT, de Fijter JW, Budde K, Kuypers D, Tyden G, et al. Comparing mycophenolate mofetil regimens for de novo renal transplant recipients: the fixed-dose concentration-controlled trial. Transplantation 2008 Oct 27;86(8):1043-51.

[48] Gaston RS, Kaplan B, Shah T, Cibrik D, Shaw LM, Angelis M, et al. Fixed- or controlled-dose mycophenolate mofetil with standard- or reduced-dose calcineurin inhibitors: the Opticept trial. Am J Transplant 2009 Jul;9(7):1607-19.

[49] van GT, Silva HT, de FH, Budde K, Kuypers D, Mamelok RD, et al. How delayed graft function impacts exposure to mycophenolic acid in patients after renal transplantation. Ther Drug Monit 2011 Apr;33(2):155-64.

[50] Knoll GA, MacDonald I, Khan A, Van Walraven C. Mycophenolate mofetil dose reduction and the risk of acute rejection after renal transplantation. J Am Soc Nephrol 2003 Sep;14(9):2381-6.

[51] Takemoto SK, Pinsky BW, Schnitzler MA, Lentine KL, Willoughby LM, Burroughs TE, et al. A retrospective analysis of immunosuppression compliance, dose reduction and discontinuation in kidney transplant recipients. Am J Transplant 2007 Dec;7(12):2704-11.

[52] Tierce JC, Porterfield-Baxa J, Petrilla AA, Kilburg A, Ferguson RM. Impact of mycophenolate mofetil (MMF)-related gastrointestinal complications and MMF dose alterations on transplant outcomes and healthcare costs in renal transplant recipients. Clin Transplant 2005 Dec;19(6):779-84.

[53] Machnicki G, Ricci JF, Brennan DC, Schnitzler MA. Economic impact and long-term graft outcomes of mycophenolate mofetil dosage modifications following gastrointestinal complications in renal transplant recipients. Pharmacoeconomics 2008;26(11):951-67.

[54] Bunnapradist S, Lentine KL, Burroughs TE, Pinsky BW, Hardinger KL, Brennan DC, et al. Mycophenolate mofetil dose reductions and discontinuations after gastrointestinal complications are associated with renal transplant graft failure. Transplantation 2006 Jul 15;82(1):102-7.

[55] Kamar N, Oufroukhi L, Faure P, Ribes D, Cointault O, Lavayssiere L, et al. Questionnaire-based evaluation of gastrointestinal disorders in de novo renal-transplant patients receiving either mycophenolate mofetil or enteric-coated mycophenolate sodium. Nephrol Dial Transplant 2005 Oct;20(10):2231-6.

[56] Budde K, Glander P, Diekmann F, Dragun D, Waiser J, Fritsche L, et al. Enteric-coated mycophenolate sodium: safe conversion from mycophenolate mofetil in maintenance renal transplant recipients. Transplant Proc 2004 Mar;36(2 Suppl):524S-7S.

[57] Sanchez-Fructuoso A, Ruiz JC, Rengel M, Andres A, Morales JM, Beneyto I, et al. Use of mycophenolate sodium in stable renal transplant recipients in Spain: preliminary results of the MIDATA study. Transplant Proc 2009 Jul;41(6):2309-12.

[58] Chan L, Mulgaonkar S, Walker R, Arns W, Ambuhl P, Schiavelli R. Patient-reported gastrointestinal symptom burden and health-related quality of life following conversion from mycophenolate mofetil to enteric-coated mycophenolate sodium. Transplantation 2006 May 15;81(9):1290-7.

[59] Robaeys G, Cassiman D, Verslype C, Monbaliu D, Aerts R, Pirenne J, et al. Successful conversion from mycophenolate mofetil to enteric-coated mycophenolate sodium (myfortic) in liver transplant patients with gastrointestinal side effects. Transplant Proc 2009 Mar;41(2):610-3.

[60] Arns W. Noninfectious gastrointestinal (GI) complications of mycophenolic acid therapy: a consequence of local GI toxicity? Transplant Proc 2007 Jan;39(1):88-93.

[61] Mourad M, Malaise J, Chaib ED, De MM, Konig J, Schepers R, et al. Correlation of mycophenolic acid pharmacokinetic parameters with side effects in kidney transplant patients treated with mycophenolate mofetil. Clin Chem 2001 Jan;47(1):88-94.

[62] Lu YP, Zhu YC, Liang MZ, Nan F, Yu Q, Wang L, et al. Therapeutic drug monitoring of mycophenolic acid can be used as predictor of clinical events for kidney transplant recipients treated with mycophenolate mofetil. Transplant Proc 2006 Sep;38(7):2048-50.

[63] Mourad M, Malaise J, Chaib ED, De Meyer M, Konig J, Schepers R, et al. Pharmacokinetic basis for the efficient and safe use of low-dose mycophenolate mofetil in combination with tacrolimus in kidney transplantation. Clin Chem 2001;47(7):1241-8.

[64] Mourad M, Malaise J, Chaib ED, De Meyer M, Konig J, Schepers R, et al. Correlation of mycophenolic acid pharmacokinetic parameters with side effects in kidney transplant patients treated with mycophenolate mofetil. Clin Chem 2001 Jan;47(1):88-94.

[65] Shah T, Tellez-Corrales E, Yang JW, Qazi Y, Wang J, Wilson J, et al. The pharmacokinetics of enteric-coated mycophenolate sodium and its gastrointestinal side effects in de novo renal transplant recipients of Hispanic ethnicity. Ther Drug Monit 2011 Feb;33(1):45-9.

[66] Kuypers DR, de JH, Naesens M, de LH, Halewijck E, Dekens M, et al. Current target ranges of mycophenolic acid exposure and drug-related adverse events: a 5-year, open-label, prospective, clinical follow-up study in renal allograft recipients. Clin Ther 2008 Apr;30(4):673-83.

[67] Langman LJ, Shapiro AM, Lakey JR, LeGatt DF, Kneteman NM, Yatscoff RW. Pharmacodynamic assessment of mycophenolic acid-induced immunosuppression by measurement of inosine monophosphate dehydrogenase activity in a canine model. Transplantation 1996 Jan 15;61(1):87-92.

[68] Glander P, Braun KP, Hambach P, Bauer S, Mai I, Roots I, et al. Non-radioactive determination of inosine 5'-monophosphate dehydro-genase (IMPDH) in peripheral mononuclear cells. Clin Biochem 2001 Oct;34(7):543-9.

[69] Langman LJ, LeGatt DF, Halloran PF, Yatscoff RW. Pharmacodynamic assessment of mycophenolic acid-induced immunosuppression in renal transplant recipients. Transplantation 1996 Sep 15;62(5):666-72.

[70] Glander P, Hambach P, Braun KP, Fritsche L, Waiser J, Mai I, et al. Effect of mycophenolate mofetil on IMP dehydrogenase after the first dose and after long-

term treatment in renal transplant recipients. Int J Clin Pharmacol Ther 2003 Oct;41(10):470-6.

[71] Fukuda T, Goebel J, Thogersen H, Maseck D, Cox S, Logan B, et al. Inosine Monophosphate Dehydrogenase (IMPDH) Activity as a Pharmacodynamic Biomarker of Mycophenolic Acid Effects in Pediatric Kidney Transplant Recipients. J Clin Pharmacol 2010 Apr 23.

[72] Vethe NT, Mandla R, Line PD, Midtvedt K, Hartmann A, Bergan S. Inosine monophosphate dehydrogenase activity in renal allograft recipients during mycophenolate treatment. Scand J Clin Lab Invest 2006;66(1):31-44.

[73] Sanquer S, Breil M, Baron C, Dhamane D, Astier A, Lang P. Induction of inosine monophosphate dehydrogenase activity after long-term treatment with mycophenolate mofetil. Clin Pharmacol Ther 1999 Jun;65(6):640-8.

[74] Sanquer S, Maison P, Tomkiewicz C, Macquin-Mavier I, Legendre C, Barouki R, et al. Expression of inosine monophosphate dehydrogenase type I and type II after mycophenolate mofetil treatment: a 2-year follow-up in kidney transplantation. Clin Pharmacol Ther 2008 Feb;83(2):328-35.

[75] Bremer S, Mandla R, Vethe NT, Rasmussen I, Rootwelt H, Line PD, et al. Expression of IMPDH1 and IMPDH2 after transplantation and initiation of immunosuppression. Transplantation 2008 Jan 15;85(1):55-61.

[76] Bremer S, Vethe NT, Rootwelt H, Bergan S. Expression of IMPDH1 is regulated in response to mycophenolate concentration. Int Immunopharmacol 2009 Feb;9(2):173-80.

[77] Brunet M, Martorell J, Oppenheimer F, Vilardell J, Millan O, Carrillo M, et al. Pharmacokinetics and pharmacodynamics of mycophenolic acid in stable renal transplant recipients treated with low doses of mycophenolate mofetil. Transpl Int 2000;13 Suppl 1:S301-S305.

[78] Chiarelli LR, Molinaro M, Libetta C, Tinelli C, Cosmai L, Valentini G, et al. Inosine monophosphate dehydrogenase variability in renal transplant patients on long-term mycophenolate mofetil therapy. Br J Clin Pharmacol 2010 Jan;69(1): 38-50.

[79] Wang J, Yang JW, Zeevi A, Webber SA, Girnita DM, Selby R, et al. IMPDH1 gene polymorphisms and association with acute rejection in renal transplant patients. Clin Pharmacol Ther 2008 May;83(5):711-7.

[80] Kagaya H, Miura M, Saito M, Habuchi T, Satoh S. Correlation of IMPDH1 gene polymorphisms with subclinical acute rejection and mycophenolic acid exposure parameters on day 28 after renal transplantation. Basic Clin Pharmacol Toxicol 2010 Aug;107(2):631-6.

[81] Glander P, Hambach P, Braun KP, Fritsche L, Giessing M, Mai I, et al. Pre-transplant inosine monophosphate dehydrogenase activity is associated with clinical outcome after renal transplantation. Am J Transplant 2004 Dec;4(12):2045-51.

[82] Rath T, Kupper M. Comparison of inosine-monophosphate-dehydrogenase activity in patients with enteric-coated mycophenolate sodium or mycophenolate mofetil after renal transplantation. Transplant Proc 2009 Jul;41(6):2524-8.

[83] Glander P, Sommerer C, Arns W, Ariatabar T, Kramer S, Vogel EM, et al. Pharmacokinetics and pharmacodynamics of intensified versus standard dosing of mycophenolate sodium in renal transplant patients. Clin J Am Soc Nephrol 2010 Mar;5(3):503-11.

12

Malignant Neoplasms in Kidney Transplantation

S. S. Sheikh[1], J. A. Amir and A. A. Amir[2]
[1]*Chief, Pathology and Laboratory Services*
[2]*Consultant Nephrologist*
Dhahran Health Center, Saudi Aramco, Dhahran
Saudi Arabia

1. Introduction

Renal transplantation is the preferred renal replacement therapy for patients with end stage renal disease (ESRD) as this modality provides better quality of life, improved overall survival, and lower treatment cost than dialysis. Malignancy is a known complication among transplant recipients, and is likely to become even more common in these patients as donation criteria are extended to allow older donors, the age of patients on waiting list is increased, and transplant recipients live longer (Gallagher et al, 2010). However still there is a continuous struggle to keep the delicate balance between reducing the immunosuppression and maintaining the graft survival. Majority of post-transplant morbidity and mortality is related to immunosuppression. Post-transplant patients are subjected to high rate of infections, medication nephrotoxicity, cardiovascular disorders, and development of malignancies. The life expectancy in kidney transplant patients is only half of that in general population. Although cardiovascular diseases are the most common cause of death in patients with functioning graft, malignancy is a significant cause of mortality. Malignancy is the third most common cause of death in renal transplant recipients after cardiovascular events and infections. There is a substantial three to five fold increase in the incidence of malignancy after solid organ transplantation as compared to the general population. Moreover the cancer incidence is also higher in transplant recipients than that seen in dialysis patients (Rama & Grinyó, 2010). As the risk of acute rejection and subsequent organ loss diminished due to the introduction of better immunosuppressive agents, infection and malignancy incidence has increased. Recently the life-threatening infections have also been declining due to the more judicious use of immunosuppressive agents and improved treatment regimen for infections. As cardiovascular diseases poses the greatest risk to the long-term graft and patient survival, efforts are being undertaken to reduce these risks by the use of less atherogenic immunosuppressive regimens, aggressive treatment of hyperlipidemia and better blood pressure control. Based on these observations it is estimated that malignancy will surpass cardiovascular complications as the leading cause of death post-transplant within the next 2 decades (Buell et al, 2005).

2. Epidemiology

There are several factors that lead to development of malignancy among transplant recipients. These include impaired immunosurveillance of tumor cells, DNA damage and impaired DNA repair mechanism, exposure to oncogenic viruses, and upregulation of cytokines that may promote tumor growth such as vascular endothelial growth factor, transforming growth factor β1 (TGF-β1), and interleukin-10. Certain neoplasms have a much higher incidence in post-transplant patients such as skin cancers including squamous cell carcinoma, basal cell carcinoma, merkel cell cancer, and melanoma, kaposi's sarcoma, lymphoma, carcinoma of oropharynx, anogenital cancer, liver cancer, in-situ carcinoma of cervix , renal cell carcinoma, and several sarcomas. In contrast, solid tumors that are most commonly seen in general population such as breast, colorectal, prostate, and invasive cervical cancer have only a modest increase in post-transplant patients. The largest study on the rate and types of malignancies was on 35,000 first time renal transplant recipients of deceased and living donor kidney transplants. As compared to the general population, the incidence of tumors was found to be as follows (kasiske et al, 2004):

- 2 fold increase: most common solid tumors in general population such as breast, colon, prostate, lung, ovary, stomach, pancreas, and esophagus.
- 3 fold increase: testicular and bladder carcinoma.
- 5 fold increase: melanoma, leukemia, hepatobiliary, cervical, and vulvovaginal tumors.
- 15 fold increase: renal cell carcinoma.
- 20 fold increase: nonmelanoma skin cancer, non-Hodgkins lymphoma(NHL), and kaposi's sarcoma (KS).

Certain malignancies tend to occur at a higher rate in transplant recipients as compared to patients on transplant waiting list (Morath et al, 2004). These include non-melanoma skin cancer (2.6 fold), melanoma (2.2 fold), KS (9 fold) NHL (3.3 fold), oral cancer (2.2 fold), and renal cell carcinoma (39% higher) (Kasiske et al, 2004). Malignancy development is 2-4 fold more common in heart transplant than renal transplant patients as a result of increased immunosuppression required in heart transplantation. In general, the post-transplant carcinomas tend to behave more aggressively and have a worse outcome. The incidence of second primary cancer is similar to that of the first malignancy with an exception of non-melanoma skin cancer with recurrent Squamous cell carcinoma. Malignancies develop in 15-20% of transplant recipients after 10 years. After 20 years of immunosuppressive therapy, approximately 40% of recipients develop cancer. However the real incidence still could be underestimated as follow-up is usually short in many patients (Pita-Fernandez et al, 2009).

The average latency of malignancy development after transplant is approximately 3-5 years. Different tumors have a distinct time interval between transplant and tumor presentation (Brennan et al, 2011):

- Kaposi's sarcoma : 13-21 months
- Lymphomas: 32 months. The risk is highest during the first year when the immunosuppression is intense and the risk of viral infection is highest.
- Epithelial carcinomas (including skin): 69 months
- Anogenital region carcinomas: 84-112 months. The latency is longer in children transplant recipients who may develop tumors during adulthood.

3. Common malignancies in transplant recipients

3.1 Skin carcinomas

Non-melanoma skin cancers such as squamous cell and basal cell carcinomas are common after transplant. They account for approximately 37% of all cancers, and can result in significant morbidity and mortality rate of 5-8%. As compared to general population, the transplant recipients develop these tumors 15-20 years earlier with an average time of development of 4-9 years post- transplant. The incidence of these tumors can vary between different geographic locations. Risk factors include increase age, male gender, fair skin, HLA A11, B27, and DR7, presence of HPV, use of cyclosporine, or Azathioprin, sun exposure, and the geographic location. Rapamycin has been reported to potentially decrease the risk of developing these tumors after transplant (Comeau et al, 2008). The overall incidence of skin cancer rises progressively as transplanted graft longevity increases with a cumulative risk increase from 7.5% to 28.6% after 5 years and 15 years respectively. The anatomic distribution of these tumors in transplant recipients is similar to the general population. The development of skin cancer is also strongly related to the patient's age and sex at the time of the transplantation (Naldi et al, 2000).

3.1.1 Squamous cell carcinoma (SCC) and basal cell carcinoma (BCC)

Non-melanoma skin cancers are the commonest tumors following solid organ transplant. They are reported to occur approximately 8 years after renal transplant in recipients aged 40 years or younger, and 3 years post-transplant in recipients 60 years and older. SCC and BCC account for more than 90% of these tumors. The risk of SCC is 60-250 times greater than the general population whereas the risk of BCC is 10 times higher. Interestingly, SCC is more common than BCC in transplant patients which is in contrast to the general population where the ratio of BCC:SCC is 4:1. Both tumors generally occur at a younger age, involve multiple sites, behave more aggressively, and tend to recur after treatment. The most important risk factors are prior exposure to ultraviolet radiation, and for SCC, development of premalignant lesions such as Bowen's disease, premalignant keratosis and warts, and keratoacanthoma.

3.1.2 Melanoma

The risk of developing melanoma is 3.6 times greater than in the general population. The risk is positively associated with increasing age at transplant, and use of depleting anti-lymphocyte antibodies. On the other hand, increasing time since transplant, female sex, and non-Caucasian race are associated with a reduced risk of melanoma development.

3.1.3 Merkel cell carcinoma (MCC)

MCC is an aggressive neuroendocrine carcinoma of skin which has an even more aggressive outcome in transplant patients.it is more common in transplant recipients with an average of 7 years post-transplant and mean survival of 18 months after diagnosis. Merkel cell polyomavirus (MCV) is believed to be a contributing factor.

3.1.4 Carcinomas of anogenital region

The incidence of these tumors is 100 fold higher in renal transplant recipients. These tumors often present as pigmented maculopapular lesions or warts. They tend to involve multiple sites including anus, and or perianal skin, and external genitalia of both sexes. They are usually extensive, in particular in women, one third of whom have concurrent cervical cancer.

3.2 SCC of the eye

The incidence of SCC of the eye is 20 fold higher in transplant recipients than in the general population. The incidence is also higher in HIV patients.

3.3 Urinary tract malignacy

There is an increased risk of developing tumors of the native urinary tract in patients with an exposure to cyclophosphamide, analgesic nephropathy, and nephropathy-induced by Chinese herbs (Morath et al, 2004).

3.3.1 Renal cell carcinoma (RCC)

The incidence of RCC after renal transplant is increased by more than 15 fold. Primary RCC occurs in approximately 3% of the general population, and 4.6% of renal transplant patients. The risk is increased in African-Americans, men, older donor age of more than 50 years, recipient age at least 65 years, patients with microscopic hematuria, acquired cystic kidney disease, analgesic nephropathy, and longer pre-transplant dialysis interval. More than 70 % of these tumors arise in native kidneys with only few cases reported in allografts. Once a RCC is diagnosed in an allograft, it is crucial to know the origin of the tumor cells whether they are of donor or recipient origin. RCC originating from renal allograft can be distinguished from RCC of the native kidney. Most RCCs of native kidney present as incidental tumors (90%) that are of low-grade, low-stage, and have a good prognosis. Post-transplant RCCs, on the other hand, are multifocal in 40% of cases, and bilateral in 20%. Clear cell carcinoma is the most common subtype, although papillary subtype is seen more frequently than in non-transplanted patients. If the RCC develops 6 months after transplant, it is assumed to be de novo. Although multiple risk factors have been identified, the exact risk factor dependent screening protocol is yet to be determined (Klatte & Marberger, 2011, & Boix, et al, 2009, & Tydén et al, 2000).

3.3.2 Bladder carcinoma

Among the urologic malignancies that develop after transplant, bladder cancers are associated with worse prognosis, aggressive behavior, and high risk of recurrence than the general population. Most bladder carcinomas reported among solid organ transplant recipients are seen after kidney transplant. Yearly screening for non-glomerular hematuria is indicated in patients exposed to prolonged cyclophosphamide therapy due to the increased risk of bladder cancer. These patients should undergo cystoscopy as cytology may miss low grade lesions.

3.4 Lung carcinoma

In comparison to renal and liver transplant recipients, the incidence of lung tumors tends to be much higher in heart and lung transplant patients.

3.5 Kaposi's sarcoma (KS)

The incidence of KS is much higher in renal transplant recipients with a male predilection (male:female ratio of 3.3:1). It is caused by Human Herpes virus 8 (HHV-8) and is commonly seen in patients of Mediterranean, Arabic, Jewish, Caribbean, or African descent, mostly corresponding to the geographic distribution of HHV-8. The choice of immunosuppressive agent also plays a role in development of this entity as calcineurin inhibitors are associated with a higher risk of developing KS than other immunosuppressive agents. Clinical presentation is similar to the classic KS with angiomatous lesions involving the lower extremities. Approximately 90% of patients have cutaneous involvement with 10% showing visceral involvement which is associated with a worse prognosis. The incidence of visceral involvement is lower in renal transplant than in heart or lung transplant recipients.

3.6 Gastrointestinal (GI) carcinomas

Approximately 50% of GI malignancies affect the large intestine. Other organs at increased risk are liver, esophagus, and stomach (Lutz & Heemann, 2003). Colorectal carcinomas occur almost 3 times more frequently in renal transplant than age- and gender- matched general population. Significant risk factors include male gender, > 50 years of age, and the duration of immunosuppression (Nafar et al, 2009). GI malignancies have poor prognosis. Cancer survival by stage is also much worse in transplant recipients. The 5 year survival for localized cancer is 74% in transplant patients as compared to 90% in the general population.

3.6.1 Hepatocellular carcinoma

Infection with oncogenic hepatitis B and C viruses increases the risk of hepatocellular cancer. Transplant recipients with known hepatitis B and C cirrhotic liver disease should have serum alpha-fetoprotein (AFP) and hepatic ultrasound screen every 12 months (Kasiske et al, 2010). AFP has high specificity (>90%) but low sensitivity (20-60%) for detection of small hepatocellular carcinomas. The abdominal ultrasound, on the other hand, is more sensitive than serum AFP (80-85%) for detection of small hepatocellular carcinoma (1-5 cms in size). Patients with suspicious lesions should undergo contrast-enhanced CT (Brennan et al, 2011).

3.7 Post-transplant lymphoproliferative disorder (PTLD)

PTLD is characterized by abnormal proliferation of lymphoid cells with majority representing malignant lymphoproliferative lesions. The most recent 2008 WHO classification of PTLD stratifies the subgroups into monoclonal or polyclonal. These are further subdivided according to their morphologic features and characteristics to monomorphic, if cells are homogenous, or polymorphic if cells are heterogenous. (Table 1) (Mucha et al, 2010). PTLD varies from polyclonal B cell proliferation with normal cytogenetics and no evidence of immunoglobulin gene rearrangement to polyclonal B cell proliferation with early malignant transformation associated with clonal cytogenetic abnormalities and or immunoglobulin gene rearrangements to monoclonal B cell proliferation with malignant cytogenetic abnormalities and immunoglobulin gene rearrangements, the latter accounting for about 15% of cases (Nalesnik et al, 1988). 80-90% of these PTLDs representing B-cell malignancies are associated with EBV infection. Most PTLDs are of recipient origin with only few that are of donor cell origin. The recipient-origin

Early Leions	• **Plasmacytic Hyperplasia** • **Infectious-mononucleosis like lesions**
Polymorphic PTLD	
Monomorphic PTLD	• **B Cell Neoplasms** o **Diffuse large B-cell lymphoma** o **Burkitt lymphoma** o **Plasma cell myeloma** o **Plasmacytoma-like lesions** • **T Cell Neoplasms** o **Peripheral T-cell lymphoma, not otherwise specified** o **Hepatosplenic T-cell lymphoma**
Classical Hodgkins Lymphoma-type PTLD	

Table 1. Pathologic Classification of PTLD (Morgans et al, 2009).

PTLDs clinically present with a multisystem disease that occurs after an average of 76 months post-transplant. On the other hand, the donor-origin PTLDs are usually limited to the allograft, develop after an average of 5 months, and regress with reduction of immunosuppression. Although, most of these disorders are of B-cell origin, however T-cell derived lesions are rarely reported. Data obtained from United States Renal Data System related to 66,159 renal transplant recipients, reported the development of malignant lymphoid proliferation in 1.8% of patients over 10 year follow-up, with 70% representing NHL, 14% multiple myeloma, 11% lymphoid leukemias, and 5% Hodgkins lymphoma (HL) (Caillard et al, 2006). The incidence was higher in the first year. NHLs in these patients have a more aggressive clinical course with more extranodal involvement occurring in 30-70% of cases, and worse prognosis. The lymphoproliferative disorders occurring in post-transplant behave differently than those in general population. NHL accounts for 65% of lymphomas in the general population whereas it accounts for 93% in post-transplant patients. Most of these NHLs are large cell lymphomas, majority of B-cell origin. For early detection of these disorders, a high level of suspicion is required, and when diagnosed the management should be handled by an experienced team to overcome this life-threatening complication (Morgans et al, 2009). Although the prognosis varies with clonality and extent of disease, the overall survival rate ranges from 25-35%. Mortality with monoclonal malignancies has been reported to be as high as 80%. T cell lymphomas in general have an extremely poor prognosis. Additional prognostic factors associated with worse outcome are identified for PTLD that include the performance status of > 2 as per the Eastern Cooperative Oncology Group criteria and more than one site involvement. The International Prognostic Index useful in determining prognosis in immunocompetent patients with NHL, is less beneficial in this setting. Adverse prognostic indicators include the presence of hypoalbuminemia, and involvement of central nervous system (CNS) and bone marrow. Increase mortality rates have been associated with a diagnosis within 6 months versus after 6 months from surgery (64% versus 54%), increasing age, no surgical intervention (100% versus 55%), allograft plus other organ involvement versus allograft involvement alone (64% versus 31%), and multiple versus single sites (73% versus 53%) and the risks are additive (Friedberg et al, 2011).

4. Pathogenesis

Malignancy can develop in transplant recipients in three different ways (Morath et al, 2004):

- **De novo malignancy occurrence.** The risk is approximately 0.2%.
- **Recurrent malignancy in the recipient.**
- **Transmission of malignancy from the donor.** Despite all efforts to secure a safe organ for transplantation, transmission of diseases such as malignancies, and infections may occur. Donor transmission of solid cancers is an unlikely event (Pedotti et al, 2004). These tumors may represent metastasis from malignancies diagnosed in the donor at the time of transplant (Donor-transmitted malignancy) or tumors develop de novo in transplanted donor tissue (Donor-derived malignancy). The risk of cancer developing in recipients receiving kidney from a donor with known or incidentally discovered cancer is 45%. In a population based study by the United Network for Organ Sharing analysed 257 donors who donated 650 organs over a period of 33 months (Birkeland & Storm, 2002), both cadaveric and living-related donors were seen to have a concealed malignancy. In general, diagnosis of a malignant tumor in a donor is a contraindication for organ donation, except from those with in-situ carcinoma of cervix, low-grade cancers of skin, and primary tumors of CNS. CNS tumors may metastasize in less than 2.3% of cases with only few reports of transmission to recipients (Detry et al, 1997 & 2000 & Wallace et al, 1996).

4.1 Risk factors

Multiple factors are associated with development of de novo malignancy in transplant recipients. The risk of oncogenesis after transplantation is related to the types and duration of exposure to immunosuppressive therapy. Disruption of both antitumor immune surveillance and antiviral activity likely play a role. Chronic antigen stimulation from transplanted organs, repeated infections, or transfusion of blood products may overly stimulate a partially depressed immune system, resulting in the development of post-transplant lymphoproliferative disorder (Buell et al, 2005, Chapman and Campistol, 2007).

4.1.1 Immunosuppression

There is strong evidence that the intensity of immunosuppression after transplant affects the risk of post-transplant malignancy development. This observation is supported by the fact that the incidence of malignancy is higher in heart and lung transplant patients who routinely require more intense immunosuppression than renal transplant recipients. In addition, the risk of development of PTLD is highest in the first year post-transplant when the degree of immunosuppression is at its maximum. Episodes of graft rejection in the first year post-transplant increase the likelihood of developing a second malignancy most likely due to the increased level of immunosuppression required.

4.1.1.1 Calcineurin inhibitors (CNI)

Both cyclosporine and tacrolimus have been associated with increased levels of TGF-β that might lead to tumor growth since both agents have long been linked to the development of post-transplant malignancies including PTLD and solid organ cancers. Some authors suggest that tacrolimus is safer than cyclosporine in this regards. In addition, cyclosporine also induces production of VEGF, thus promoting carcinogenesis, and enhances the apoptotic effect of taxol and INF-gamma on human gastric and bladder carcinomas (Buell et al, 2005). Patients receiving low dose cyclosporine have a lower incidence of malignancy development (19.8% versus 32%) in particular skin carcinomas. In animal model, cyclosporine and tacrolimus have a direct effect on the tumor cells, promote invasiveness, and facilitate metastases. Data suggest that the CNI promote metastatic spread of the pre-existing tumor cells rather than convert a non-malignant cell into a cancer cell (Suthanthiran, 2009).

4.1.1.2 Azathioprin

Azathioprine is an antimetabolite that has long been recognized as an etiologic agent in the development of neoplasia. It is in particular associated with increased incidence of non-melanoma skin cancer especially SCC. It also may lead to the development of myelodysplastic syndrome. Azathioprin has been reported to increase photosensitivity and also allows ultraviolet A to directly damage the DNA by intercalating DNA level, inhibiting repair splicing, eliciting codon misreads, and development of microsatellite DNA instability (Buell et al, 2005 & O'Donovan et al, 2005).

4.1.1.3 Antilymphocyte therapy

The use of anti-T-cell therapy (antilymphocyte serum or muromonab-CD3), but not IL-2 receptor antibodies, has been shown to predispose solid organ transplant recipients to EBV-associated PTLD. Transplant patients on monoclonal antilymphocyte antibody (anti-CD3) as the sole induction agent, show a 72% increase in in the risk of PTLD, however despite this relation anti-CD3 has not been found to show any association in the development of other solid organ malignancies. Anti-CD52 appears safer with no increased risk of de novo malignancy development (Buell et al, 2005).

4.1.1.4 Sirolimus

Sirolimus, an inhibitor of the mammalian target of rapamycin (m-TOR), suppresses the growth and proliferation of tumors. It has antineoplastic effect mainly due to inhibition of p70 S6K, IL-10, cyclins, and vascular endothelial growth factors A and C, with direct inhibition of cell replication, induction of apoptosis, and inhibition of tumor angiogenesis. Some studies show a decreased incidence of malignancy in patients receiving Sirolimus than other immunosuppressive therapies. Post-transplant patients treated with Sirolimus appear to have a lower incidence of de novo malignancy when compared with a triple immunosuppressive regimen treated group (CNI, antimetabolite, and corticosteroids). In addition the use of Sirolimus in place of cyclosporine has been associated with complete regression of KS in the vast majority of renal transplant recipients (Buell et al, 2005). Newer sirolimus analogues, such as temsirolimus, have become a focus in pure oncological research for their antineoplastic effects on a variety of malignancies (Kapoor, 2008, & Campistol, 2007).

4.1.1.5 Mycophenolate Mofetil (MMF)

MMF impairs lymphocyte function by inhibiting enzyme inosine monophosphate dehydrogenase leading to purine biosynthesis block. Several cancers including leukemias and some solid tumors produce dramatic elevation of this enzyme. Some studies suggest that the risk of malignancy is not increased and even may be even decreased with MMF (Rama & Grinyó, 2010 & Brennan et al, 2011). Recent studies show a distinctive antineoplastic effect of MMF against colorectal and prostatic carcinomas, and its inhibiting effect on the adhesion of colonic adenocarcinomatous cells to endothelial cells (Eng, 2005, & Leckel, 2003). The use of MMF is clearly associated with a distinctive decrease in the incidence of post-transplant PTLD (Buell et al, 2005).

4.1.2 Conventional risk factors

Exposure to ultraviolet radiation is associated with increased risk of skin cancer. Other common risk factors are also associated with development of post-transplant malignancy such as advanced age, smoking, and analgesic abuse. History of phenacetin abuse is associated with striking increase in urothelial carcinoma. Renal transplant recipients also have higher incidence of development of carcinomas in the native kidneys in particular if they have been on long term dialysis. The incidence is almost 100 times greater than expected and is in part related to ESRD, tubular hyperplasia, cyst formation, and in some cases malignant transformation.

4.1.3 Genetic factors

Transplant recipients who had history of invasive carcinoma before transplant have a higher risk (relative risk 2.38) of developing a second invasive carcinoma post-transplant. Some primary renal disorders such as von Hippel-Lindau disease are associated with higher risk of developing renal cell carcinoma that behave more aggressively. In addition, patients with Wiskott-Aldrich syndrome and Drash syndrome are also associated with an increased risk of carcinoma development in particular lymphoma and Wilms tumor.

4.1.4 Coexisting oncogenic viral infection

Certain viral infections are associated with increased predisposition of transplant patients to development of specific tumors. At least 4 viruses may be cocarcinogenic in transplant patients.

4.1.4.1 EBV

Most PTLDs are associated with EBV infection. EBV is a gamma herpes virus. It is present worldwide and EBV antibodies are seen in almost 90-95% of the population. In immunosuppressed patients, EBV infection can lead to cell transformation. Latent membrane protein-1 (LMP-1) of EBV has the major role in EBV-associated PTLD development as it engages the signaling proteins from tumor-necrosis-factor-receptor-associated factors (TRAFs) that lead to cell growth and transformation. There is increased risk of PTLD among EBV-seronegative recipients of EBV positive donors. The incidence of PTLD for EBV seronegative recipients is reported to be 24 times higher than EBV seropositive recipients. EBV negative PTLDs present much later (2324 days versus 546 days post-transplant), and have a much more virulent behavior (Friedberg et al, 2011).

4.1.4.2 HHV-8

All types of KS including classic, endemic, AIDS-related, and post-transplant KS are all associated with HHV-8 presence in tumor tissue. There is convincing evidence of transmission of HHV-8 from the donor to transplant recipients, with one study showing evidence of donor-derived tumor cells transmitted to transplant recipients. HHV-8 is necessary but not sufficient for KS development, with transplant related immune dysfunction being an important contributing cofactor. Pretransplant antibody screening of recipients as well as donors in high seroprevalent areas may be useful. However seropositivity for HHV-8 is not always associated with increased risk of development of KS. Studies from Saudi Arabia show the proportion of patients with antibodies against HHV-8 is higher among patients who developed KS post-transplant than those who did not. In addition the incidence of KS is higher in patients with HHV-8 infection at the time of transplant than among those who did not have infection (15-28% versus <1%) (Diociauiti et al, 2000, & Cattani et al, 2001, & Regamey et al, 1998). A study from Saudi Arabia revealed 10 fold higher incidence of KS in Saudi transplant recipients than in Western countries. In addition, there was a markedly higher incidence of specific anti-HHV-8 antibodies in patients with KS as compared to those without it (92% versus 28%) (Qunibi et al, 1998).

4.1.4.3 Human papilloma virus (HPV)

There is an extremely diverse group of HPV subtypes that can be found in various benign, premalignant, and malignant skin lesions in transplant recipients. Multiple subtypes can be seen in a single lesion. HPV DNA is detected in 65-90% of skin tumors in transplant recipients. However a causative role of HPV in development of secondary skin cancers is not proven. Interestingly, HPV has been detected in normal hair follicles of transplant patients (Boxman et al, 1997, & Berkhout et al, 2000).

4.1.4.4 Merkel cell virus (MCV)

MCV is believed to be a contributing factor to MCC.

4.1.5 Geographic differences

Literature review shows widely variable relative frequency of the different types of post-transplant malignancies in different geographic areas. In Saudi Arabia the most common tumors in transplant recipients are KS, skin cancers (melanoma being more common in children than in adults), anogenital cancers, and lymphomas particularly in children (al-Sulaiman & al-Khader, 1994). In Japan the most common post-transplant tumors are those of digestive tract including stomach, liver, colon, and rectum. On the contrary, the incidence of lymphoma and skin tumors in Japan is low. In Australia the risk of skin cancer development is the highest, most likely due to the excessive sun exposure of the fair-skinned population. In South East Asia the frequency of liver cancer is high where hepatitis B and C infections are endemic. In United Kingdom lymphomas, renal cell carcinomas, bronchial cancer, and tumors of digestive tract are the most commonly encountered tumors in post-transplant recipients (Morath et al, 2004). In South Africa, the incidence of post-transplantation malignancy development is reported to be 5.6%, the commonest tumors being PTLD, followed by non-melanoma skin cancer, KS, gastrointestinal carcinoma, cervical cancer, and vulval cancer (Maharaj & Assounga, 2010). The Northern Italy Transplant program studied 3,521 patients over a 10 years period in 10 local Transplant centers. The average cancer incidence was 4.9%. The commonest tumors were KS, PTLD, renal and skin cancers followed by colorectal, breast, gastric, lung, and bladder carcinomas, and mesothelioma (Pedotti et al, 2003). In India, the incidence of malignancy after transplant is lower than the Western countries. PTLD is the commonest malignancy there especially in the first year followed by oropharyngeal cancer. Skin cancer incidence of both melanoma as well as non-melanoma cancer is much lower mostly attributed to the high cutaneous melanin content (Joshi and Jha, 2009).

4.1.6 Renal transplant tourism

Despite the international abandonment of commercial organ trafficking, many patients continue to travel to different countries to receive commercial transplants. Commercial cadaveric renal transplant was compared to domestic cadaveric renal transplant in China. The 10 year cumulative cancer incidence of the touring group, primarily of Taiwan origin, (21.5%) was significantly higher than the domestic group (6.8%). This might be related to older age at transplantation, more depleting antibody induction therapy, and omitted pre-transplant cancer screening. The graft and patient survival in transplant tourism group is inferior as compared to the domestic group. Hepatocellular and urothelial carcinoma were the most prevalent malignancies in renal transplant tourism patients from Taiwan when compared to Western patients. This can be explained by the high incidence of viral hepatitis in Taiwan and the use of Chinese herbal medications. The use of Chines herbal medications containing anistolochic acid, which is associated with urothelial carcinoma development, facilitates diuresis and is a common practice in ESRD patients who do not accept dialysis. It is interesting that transplant tourism is considered to be an independent risk factor for post-transplant malignancy development (Tsai et al, 2011).

4.1.7 Blood groups

Types of blood groups does not seem to be related to increased incidence of cancer development (Pedotti et al, 2003).

4.1.8 Transplant center selection

Selection of a particular transplant centers does not appear to be related to an increase in incidence of cancer development (Pedotti et al, 2003).

4.1.9 HLA match

There is a strong influence of HLA matching on graft outcome (Opelz, 2001). However the association is indirect and related to the aggressive immunosuppression required for low degree HLA matching.

5. Incidence of post-transplantation malignancy in children

The pattern of malignancies that occur in pediatrics post-transplant population is different from the adult post-transplant patients and the general pediatric population. In a study of 219 children who underwent renal transplant, 7.3% developed malignancy. The cumulative incidence of cancer development was found to be 1.9% at 1 year, 4.0% at 5 year, 6.9% at 10 years, and 10.2% at 15 years. The 10 years incidence of PTLD was 4.5% when the mortality rate was 25%. Other commonly encountered tumors in post-transplant children recipients are HL, Burkitt lymphoma, renal papillary carcinoma, thyroid papillary carcinoma, recurrent ovarian seminoma, and skin cancer. The occurrence of skin cancer is rare in children and usually occurs during early adulthood. Screening and early detection of these tumors in children is of great importance. In addition regular screening for EBV viral load is recommended for patients at risk for developing PTLD (Koukourgianni et al, 2010).

6. Transplantation in patients with pre-existing malignancy

The recurrence rate of malignancy is 22% in patients treated before transplantation and 27% in those treated after transplantation. There is however variability in recurrence rate according to the type of tumor (Barrett et al, 1993, & Trofe et al, 2004, & Kasiske et al, 2001):

- 0-10%: Localized renal cell carcinoma, cervical, testicular, and thyroid carcinoma, and Hodgkins as well as non-Hodgkins lymphoma.
- 11-25%: Wilm's tumor, and cancer of colon, uterus, prostate, and breast.
- Over 25%: Advanced renal cell carcinoma, bladder cancer, myeloma, sarcoma, and skin cancer including melanoma and non-melanoma skin tumors.

Patients with low risk tumors such as in-situ carcinoma, low grade bladder carcinoma, and basal cell carcinoma should have no waiting period for transplantation. Patients with tumors that have a high risk of recurrence such as melanoma, colorectal and breast cancer should wait for at least 5 years before translantation. For most other tumors a delay of 2 years is often considered sufficient (Table 2) (Morath et al, 2004).

Type of Cancer	Recommendation (years)
Breast cancer	> 5 (> 2 for early disease)
Colorectal cancer	> 5 (> 2 for Dukes Stage A or B1)
Melanoma	> 5 (> 2 melanoma in situ)
Uterine cervical cancer	> 2 (> 5 for more advanced cervical cancer)
Renal cell carcinoma/Wilms tumor	> 2 (> 5 for large cancers; no wait for incidental tumor < 5 cm)
Bladder cancer	> 2
Kaposi sarcoma	> 2
Leukemia	> 2 (limited data to make recommendation)
Lung cancer	> 2
Lymphoma	> 2 (possibly > 5)
Prostate cancer	> 2 (possibly less for localized disease)
Testicular cancer	> 2
Thyroid cancer	> 2
Skin (nonmelanoma) cancer	0-2 (no wait for basal cell carcinoma)
Liver cancer	Unable to give recommendation
Myeloma	Unable to give recommendation

Table 2. Recommended Wait Time (Years) Based on Type of Cancer Before Listing for Transplantation (Kasiske et al, 2001).

7. Multiple independent primary cancers or second tumor in transplant recipients

Excluding the non-melanoma skin cancers, the risk of developing a second primary cancer is almost the same as the incidence of first cancer. The risk of developing a second primary in this group could be related to persistence of environmental risk factors associated with the first cancer such as tobacco, genetic factors responsible for development of second primary cancer, and individual susceptibility to carcinogens. A study of a network of cohort of transplanted patients shows the incidence of second primary cancer development to be 0.3%. The incidence of developing second primary cancer is 1-5%. Excluding skin cancers, transplant patients with first cancer diagnoses should follow regular screening procedures and do not appear to require a special program (Taioli et al, 2006).

Skin cancer is the commonest second malignancy among transplant recipients (Morath et al, 2004). The North Italy Transplant program reported the prevalence of second primary cancer to be 1.7% and development of multiple independent primary cancers arising in the same patient to have a prevalence of 3.6% (Pedotti et al, 2003). The risk of developing a second non-melanoma skin cancer is high in renal transplant recipients who developed a first non-melanoma skin cancer. The risk is, in particular, high of SCC but is also substantially increased for BCC. The risk is much lower for SCC in renal transplant recipients who present with BCC, however after the diagnosis of first SCC the subsequent risk for SCC appears to be the same. The 3 year cumulative risk is approximately 59% of non-melanoma skin cancers and 62% of subsequent SCC. The 3 year risk of BCC is 37% and the 5 year risk of subsequent BCC is 51%. Renal transplant recipients who develop SCC mostly develop SCC as subsequent skin cancer and recipients who have BCC as first malignancy mostly develop subsequent BCC. This difference could be related to the difference in the lifestyle as the risk of SCC is associated with chronic cumulative sun exposure whereas BCC is more associated with intermittent intense sun exposure. Longer time between transplantation and development of first SCC is also associated with an increased risk of subsequent SCC. The type of maintenance immunosuppression is the most important risk factor of subsequent development of SCC. Patients on Azathioprin have an approximately 3 times higher risk of subsequent SCC as compared to cyclosporine-based regimen. The duration of immunosuppression also influences the development of subsequent SCC after the first SCC. Sun exposure is an important risk factor for multiple lesions development. Fair skin of patients and light color of the hair and the eyes are predictive of multiple SCC development (Euvrard et al, 2006). Male sex is also a risk factor for multiple skin cancer development, especially the BCC. In addition, BCC is more commonly seen in living-related kidney transplant than the cadaveric kidney transplant recipients (Wisgerhof et al, 2010).

8. Prevention and screening for early detection

Regular cancer screening is recommended when a patient is considered for renal transplant. Screening and early detection of cancers should be incorporated into the pre-transplant evaluation of ESRD patients. Screening may also detect premalignant lesions quite early allowing for a timely intervention (Kiberd, 2005). The rising age and the prolonged duration on transplant waiting list increases patients' risk of being transplanted with an undetected malignancy (Morath et al, 2004). Careful screening should be performed for the recipient as

Target Organ or Cancer	Test*	Frequency	Age of Screening
Breast	Mammography	Every 1-2 years	> 40 years
Colon/rectum	Occult blood and Sigmoidoscopy or Colonoscopy	Annually Every 5 years Every 10 years	> 50 years > 50 years > 50 years
Prostate gland	Digital rectal exam PSA	Annually	> 50 years
Kidney	Imaging study†	Once	All patients
Bladder	Cystoscopy	Not routine	> 50 years and all high-risk patients
Uterine cervix	Pap smear Pelvic exam	Every 1-3 years	> 20 years or any sexually active patient
Testicle	History and physical exam	Once	All male patients
Kaposi sarcoma	History and physical exam HHV-8 assay	Once	All patients All high-risk patients
Skin	History and physical exam	Once	All patients
Melanoma	History and physical exam	Once	All patients
Liver	Imaging study†	Once, high risk annually	All patients
Lung	CXR	Once	All patients
Lymphoma	History and physical exam EBV assay	Annually	All patients
Leukemia	CBC	Annually	All patients
Myeloma	Immunoelectropheresis	Once	> 50 years

PSA = prostate specific antigen; HHV-8 = human herpes virus 8; CXR = chest x-ray;
EBV = Epstein-Barr virus; CBC = complete blood count
*Abnormalities on screening tests may indicate the need for additional tests. For example, suspicious lung lesions on the chest x-ray should be followed up with a computed tomography scan.
†Ultrasound, CT scan, or magnetic resonance imaging scan.

Table 3. Possible Pretransplant Screening Strategies for the Potential Kidney Transplant Recipient (Kasiske et al, 2001).

well as the donor. The 2009 Kidney Disease: Improving Global Outcomes (KDIGO) clinical practice guidelines on monitoring and treatment of kidney transplant recipients were developed to help practitioners caring for these patients. These guidelines were based on evidence and systemic review of treatment trials. A set of recommendations were developed for screening and risk assessment of renal transplant recipients (Kasiske et al, 2010). Patients with failed transplant returning to dialysis have a higher mortality than those on transplant waiting list (Cattran & Fenton, 1993).

The Clinical Practice Guidelines Committee of the American Society of Transplantation (AST) has published guidelines for outpatient evaluation of pediatric and adult kidney transplant candidates that include recommendations for screening and early detection of malignancies. Some of these recommendations are represented in Tables 3 and 4 (Kasiske et al, 2001 & Kiberd, 2005, & Kalble et al, 2009, & AST Kidney-Pancreas committee, 2009).

Target Organ or Cancer	Who	Test*	Frequency	Age of Screening
Breast	Selected*	Mammography	Every 1-2 years	> 40 years
Colon/ rectum	Selected*	Occult blood and Sigmoidoscopy or colonoscopy	Annually Every 5 years Every 10 years	> 50 years > 50 years > 50 years
Prostate gland	Selected†	Digital rectal exam PSA	Annually	> 50 years
Uterine cervix	Female	Pap smear Pelvic exam	Every 1-3 years	> 20 years or any sexually active patients
Kaposi sarcoma	All	History and physical	Annually	All high-risk patients
Nonmelanoma skin	All	History and physical	Annually	All patients
Melanoma	All	History and physical	Annually	All patients
Liver	Selected‡	Imaging study	High risk annually	All patients
Lymphoma	All	History and physical	As clinically indicated	All patients

PSA = prostate specific antigen
*Patients with good life expectancy and good allograft function
†Male patients at high risk, including black patients
‡Patients with cirrhosis

Table 4. Posttransplant Screening Strategies for the Kidney Transplant Recipient (Kiberd, 2005).

8.1 Skin and lip cancer

Introduction of patient education programs is recommended in particular in countries with high incidence of non-melanoma skin carcinoma secondary to high sun exposure. Patients should also be educated about their increased risk of such cancers especially if they are fair skinned, have high sun exposure level, or have prior history of skin cancer. Patients should reduce their sun exposure, perform self-examination, and have an annual skin and lip examination by qualified Health care provider. Oral acitretin should be given to patients with prior history of skin cancer to prevent development of new malignancy.

8.2 Non-skin cancer

The recommendations for transplant patients with moderately increased risk of developing non-skin cancer are non-specific. However they reinforce the same recommended screening strategies as for the general population. These include pap smear, self-breast examination, mammography, and colonoscopy. In addition annual liver ultrasound and α-fetoprotein monitoring is also recommended in patients with cirrhosis ((Rama & Grinyó, 2010).

8.3 PTLD

Since development of PTLD is related to the degree of immunosuppression, and infection with EBV and CMV, prevention largely relies on limiting patient exposure to aggressive immunosuppression, and anti-viral prophylaxis. There is a relatively high incidence of PTLD reported with introduction of tacrolimus and therefore rapid tapering of tacrolimus may limit the development of PTLD (Friedberg et al, 2011). In one review of PTLD in children, the incidence of PTLD development was 17% in children who received renal allograft with tacrolimus as compared to 4% in children who underwent aggressive tapering of tacrolimus (Shapiro et al, 1995). There is higher incidence reported of PTLD among EBV-seronegative recipients of EBV-seropositive donors that suggests that treatment of early EBV infection may decrease subsequent development of PTLD (Holmes et al, 2002 & Funch et al, 2005). In addition prophylactic antiviral therapy is also associated with a reduced risk of PTLD development. The use of prophylactic anti-CMV during the first 3-6 months after renal transplant significantly reduces the incidence of PTLD in the first year post-transplant but not in the subsequent 5 years (Kasiske et al, 2010, & Opelz et al, 2007).

8.4 Colorectal carcinoma

Community-level screening for colorectal carcinomas using fecal occult blood is now a standard practice in most developed countries. Studies in the general population have shown that the benefits of starting screening at a younger age were little and costly as compared to starting at age of 50. However renal transplant patients have an age-shifted increase in the risk of colorectal carcinoma and screening at a younger age in this population seems therefore justifiable (Wong et al, 2008).

9. Treatment

Reduction or cessation of immunosuppression is particulary useful in renal transplant recipients as loss of graft secondary to rejection is not a fatal event in this group as compared to the heart, lung, or liver transplant recipients. Immunosuppression reduction may lead to spontaneous regression of some tumors such as some cases of PTLD, some skin cancers, KS, and donor-derived malignancies. In KS reduction of CNI may be particularly important. Despite the association of CNI and cancer development, some authors recommend discontinuation of antimetabolite and use of CNI and Prednisone as first line approach in transplant recipients with malignancy. This is because rejection is less likely to occur with double therapy (CNI and prednisone) than combination of antimetabolite and prednisone. An exception to this is the very well matched HLA transplant recipients with 0 HLA, B, or DR mismatch, in which the risk of rejection is low with the use of antimetabolite in combination with prednisone (Brennan et al, 2011, & Bosman and Verpooten, 2007).

9.1 Skin, non-melanoma carcinomas

Once a skin lesion is detected there is no evidence of benefits from stopping azathioprin . Treatment of these patients requires several strategies including preventive strategy, specific treatment, and medical adjunct therapy because these tumors may present with multiple lesions, and large areas of skin involvement. Despite this, dedicated surveillance programs are lacking for most patients. Surgery remains the mainstay of managing these tumors and it may be destructive in large or multiple skin tumors. Studies in immunocompetent patients show recurrence in almost 100% of cases with incomplete surgical excision and therefore tumors that are not completely excised should be treated by additional methods (Jemec & Holm, 2003).

9.1.1 SCC

Premalignant lesions can be treated with topical retinoids or in combination with low dose systemic retinoids. Although systemic retinoids reduce actinic keratosis and prevent development of new dysplastic lesions in transplant patients, the treatment is frequently discontinued due to drug adverse events such as mucocutaneous xerosis, pruritis, arthralgia, and hyperlipidemia. Once treatment is discontinued, the lesions tend to recur rapidly. Superficial cancers can be treated with cryotherapy or electrocautery and curettage. More aggressive local therapy is required for invasive SCC as they may have metastasis at presentation and are more likely to develop recurrence. These invasive tumors need surgical excision with negative margins. Although there are no clear established guidelines about margins of SCC excision, Mohs micrographic surgery is typically recommended for these high risk tumors especially those seen in cephalic location, a diameter of > 2 cms, or rapid growth. Metastasis in a single lymph node is considered potentially curable. Adjuvant radiation, systemic chemotherapy, and or immunotherapy are not of benefit. Several reports show beneficial effect to immune response modifier Imiquimod, however, the safety and efficacy of this agent has not been adequately assessed (Brennan et al, 2011).

9.1.2 BCC

Development of frequent BCCs should prompt reduction in immunosuppression. The management otherwise is similar to that in non-immunocompromised patients.

9.1.3 MCC

Although management of MCC is similar to that in non-immunocompromised patients, the overall prognosis is poorer in transplant patients as compared to the general population with 2 year survival of 44% versus 65-75%. Distant metastasis may regress temporarily with cyclosporine discontinuation (Brennan et al, 2011).

9.2 Skin, melanoma

Multiple strategies are required to treat melanoma including wide local excision with or without sentinel lymphadenectomy, and reduction of immunosuppression.

9.3 KS

Discontinuation of immunosuppression should be the first line of treatment as majority of patients with KS may show complete regression of the lesions. The disappearance of KS by reducing immunosuppression is about 17% with mucocutaneous disease and 16% with visceral involvement. Substitution of Sirolimus for cyclosporine has also been associated with complete regression (Stallone et al, 2005). Patients who do not regress spontaneously should be treated the same way as non-immunosuppressed patients are treated. In the CONVERT study, a randomized prospective study to evaluate the effect of conversion to sirolimus from CNI, displayed a significantly lower malignancy rate (3.8%) at 24 months compared with those who continued CNI based therapy (11%). An mTOR-inhibitor CNI-free regimen should be considered for transplant recipients at high risk for cancer development and for those who develop malignancies over the post-transplant course (Alberú, 2010, & Schena, 2009).

9.4 Anogenital carcinomas

Anogenital Intra-epithelial neoplasia / in-situ carcinomas are treated with laser therapy, topical fluorouracil, or electrocautery. Reduction of immunosuppression is beneficial and may lead to regression of the in-situ lesions. Invasive carcinomas, on the other hand, require wide local excision with inguinal lymphadenectomy for tumors that are >1 mm thick. Adjuvant therapy is given to only selected patients.

9.5 Bladder carcinomas

9.5.1 Non-muscle invasive bladder carcinoma

Bacillus Calmette-Guerin is still the only intravesical therapy that has shown a significant reduction in recurrence-free and possibly progression-free survival.

9.5.2 Muscle-invasive bladder tumor

The mean time between organ transplant and bladder tumor development is 2.8 and 4 years. Most patients presenting with muscle-invasive bladder carcinoma have extravesical disease or lymphadenopathy at the time of surgery. In general, there has been little to no improvement in the survival after radical cystectomy. A reasonable cancer-specific survival and renal allograft preservation is achieved after aggressive surgical therapy in only a few patients. (Wallerand et al, 2010).

9.6 Other solid organ tumors

The course of these malignancies is more aggressive than the general population and the outcome is mostly determined by the stage of tumor at the time of presentation. Visceral malignancies are treated with surgical intervention, chemotherapy, and radiation therapy. If chemotherapy is needed, azathioprine should be discontinued to avoid myelosuppression. Early invasive and in-situ carcinomas can be cured by surgery. The outcome is poor in advanced disease with majority of the patients dying within 1-2 months (Brennan et al, 2011).

9.7 Donor-derived tumors

If the cancer is shown to be of donor origin, reduction of immunosuppression should theoretically lead to rejection of the tumor. This has been shown to be effective in PTLD but the data is not very supportive in other solid organ tumors. In RCC with no metastatic disease, total transplant nephrectomy is curative, however the patient has to go back to dialysis. Some authors suggest nephron sparing surgery in non-metastatic RCC that are located peripherally and are < 4 cms in size. Recipients with metastatic RCC should be treated with transplant nephrectomy, reduction in immunosuppression, and immune therapy (Muruve & Shoskes, 2005).

9.8 PTLD

9.8.1 Reduction of immunosuppression

The most important treatment modality for PTLD is reduction of immunosuppression which allows restoration of the natural T-cell mediated immune response against EBV-infected B cells. The goal by reducing the immunosuppression is to find the correct dose that will allow restoration of the patient's immune response against the PTLD without causing rejection of the transplanted organ. Transplant rejection occurs in approximately 39% of transplant recipients regardless of whether they respond to treatment or not. The risk of rejection also varies with the type of transplanted organ, with highest risk among heart and lung transplant recipients. The reduction of immunosuppression has no standard approach and it has to be individualized for each patient depending on various characteristics such as transplant type, relative risk of transplant rejection, extent and severity of PTLD, and selection of immunosuppressive agents. In general, MMF and azathioprine are discontinued first and the doses of CNI and steroids are reduced. There are several predictive factors to response to reduction of immunosuppression. Interestingly, EBV serostatus does not predict response and therefore this modality of treatment should be used for both EBV seronegative as well as EBV seropositive patients. Multiple factors are associated with poor response that include lactate dehydrogenase level of > 2.5 times the upper limit of normal, bulky disease, multiple visceral sites being involved, and organ dysfunction. Patients lacking these features show a response rate to reduction of immunosuppression as good as 89% (Morgans et al, 2009). The vast majority of polyclonal lymphoproliferative lesions and EBV-related plasmacytomas show significant improvement or complete resolution by immunosuppression reduction. The response is best in patients with early onset disease in whom the level if immunosuppression is a major risk factor as compared to patients with late onset or extensive disease who are much less likely to benefit. One potential regimen for patients who are severely ill and have extensive disease is to reduce prednisone and stopping all other immunosuppressive agents. For patients who are less severely ill and have only limited disease, one regimen is to reduce cyclosporine or tacrolimus and prednisone by at least 50% and the discontinuation of azathioprine or MMF. If necessary another 50% reduction of immunosuppression can be considered. Immunosuppressive regimens with the fewest possible toxic effects are desirable for transplant recipients. The ELITE-Symphony Study which is the largest prospective study in kidney transplantation evaluated the effects of standard dose versus low dose immunosuppression. The primary end point of the study was the estimated glomerular filtration rate and the secondary end points included acute rejection events and allograft survival. Over 3 years, daclizumab induction, MMF, steroids and low-dose tacrolimus proved highly efficacious, without the negative effects on renal function commonly reported for standard CNI regimens. (Ekberg et al, 2007, 2009).

9.8.2 Antiviral prophylaxis

Initially antiviral prophylaxis was used to eradicate EBV from the patient's system thereby preventing reactivation of any latent infection and abnormal cellular proliferation that may lead to PTLD. Currently there is no supportive evidence of antiviral therapy efficacy for treatment of PTLD. The nucleoside analogues acyclovir and gancyclovir inhibit the replication of multiple members of herpes virus family including CMV and herpes simplex virus. Although theoretically these medications should be effective against EBV, in vivo they are not effective against EBV. These agents need intracellular phosphorylation by a viral-encoded thymidine kinase which is not expressed in infected latent B cells. One approach to overcome this limitation is to use these agents in combination with arginine butyrate which induces the lytic phase of EBV gene expression and thus can induce expression of thymidine kinase. This may enable gancyclovir to be phosphorylated into its active form. Several studies are investigating the efficacy of these 2 agents used in combination in both solid organ as well as bone marrow transplant patients with PTLD and have shown moderate success (Morgans et al, 2009 & Friedberg et al, 2011).

9.8.3 Local therapy

Localized PTLD involving skin or a single GI lesion can be managed by surgery or radiation without the use of systemic therapy. This will spare the patient side effects of systemic therapy and withdrawal of immunosuppression. Local treatment in conjunction with immunosuppression reduction has resulted in very low PTLD-related mortality. Rituximab in combination with surgery or radiation has shown some success. Patients requiring palliative and emergent therapy for advanced disease can benefit from local field radiation therapy (Morgans, 2009).

9.8.4 Anti-B-cell antibody

Since most PTLDs are of B-cell origin, the use of medications that target B-cell antigens is proven beneficial with a reasonable response rate of 50-80%. In earlier studies the use of antiCD21 and antiCD24 has achieved complete response rates of 63% and long-term survival of 46%. However, in the past 10 years, more and more emphasis is on the use of antiCD20, the rituximab in the treatment of CD20 positive PTLDs. AntiCD20 binds to B cells, induces clearance of cells and destruction by antibody-dependant complement-mediated apoptosis. It may activate patient's immune system against EBV-infected B cells helping destruction of tumor and preventing its recurrence. These proposed mechanisms of action would explain the better efficacy of rituximab in patients with PTLD than the usual NHLs. Risk factors for poor response to anti B-cell therapy include late onset PTLD (onset > 1 years after transplantation), and involvement of CNS and multiple viscera. Rituximab has been reported to induce complete remission of PTLD in some patients with solid organ and bone marrow transplant. Early treatment with rituximab along with reduction of immunosuppression appears to be the evolving standard of care for CD20 positive PTLDs (Friedberg et al, 2011). Other anti-B-cell antibodies have not been fully evaluated systemically in PTLD. There are newer anti-CD20 antibodies such as tositumomab (anti-CD20 coupled with radioactive iodine-131), ibitumomab (anti-CD20 with yttrium-90), epratuzumab (anti-CD22), and galiximab (antiCD 80) that are currently being investigated (Morgans et al, 2009).

9.8.5 Cytotoxic chemotherapy

For patients in whom reduction of immunosuppression is ineffective and who have rapidly progressive or life-threatening disease, chemotherapy can be used as an alternative or additional treatment. Several chemotherapy regimens similar to those used in NHLs are offered for treating patients with monoclonal PTLD such as cyclophosphamide with prednisone, CHOP (cyclophosphamide, doxorubicin, vincristine, prednisone), dose-adjusted ACVBP (doxorubicin, cyclophosphamide, vindesine, bleomycin, prednisone), and other new regimens. Unfortunately although these chemotherapy agents are highly effective, they are associated with serious side-effects that significantly affect patient morbidity and mortality. Studies show that using CHOP after reduction of immunosuppression is associated with a complete remission rate of 63% and median disease-free survival of 10.5 years. The overall response rate of patients to rituximab is 68%. Patient with EBV-positive disease are more likely to respond to rituximab and achieve a complete response rate than those with EBV-negative disease. Patients who received chemotherapy show an overall response rate of 74%. Several factors limit the use of chemotherapy in PTLD. These include suboptimal performance status, drug-to-drug interaction, high likelihood of infectious complications, and dose-limiting organ-dysfunction. Although the overall response rate is somewhat higher for chemotherapy, the associated toxic effects are significant. Approximately 50% of these patients get hospitalized for infections and about 6% eventually die of complications. The debate regarding when to use rituximab as opposed to chemotherapy and how to use them in combination is still ongoing with no consensus recommendations (Morgans et al, 2009 & Friedberg et al, 2011).

9.8.6 Cellular immunotherapy

Cellular immunotherapy of PTLD involves reinfusion of T-cells into a recipient targeting the EBV-related lymphoma. T-cell targeting is HLA specific and EBV-specific and therefore cytotoxic T lymphocytes (CTL) must be HLA-matched to the recipient. Autologous pre-transplant-harvested CTLs are shown to be effective in reducing the EBV viral loads. More recently several tissue banks have been storing EBV-specific CTLs for various HLA types.

The overall response rate after these infusions is close to 52% and the results are thought to have a better response at 6 months in patients receiving closest HLA-matched CTLs (Morgans et al, 2009).

9.8.7 Retransplant

Kidney transplant recipients can be treated with complete withdrawal of immunosuppression and even removal of transplanted organ as it is not a life-sustaining organ unlike heart and lung transplant. Successful treatment of PTLD can result in years of continous transplant function. Patients with transplant failure due to PTLD may safely go through re-transplantation after 1-2 years. In addition, relapse of PTLD after re-transplantation only rarely occurs (Morgans et al, 2009).

10. Conclusion

Malignancy is a common cause of death after renal transplantation. Early detection and treatment of post-transplant malignancies is an important challenge. An even greater challenge is to prevent the development of these malignancies. Screening these patients for malignancies while they are on the waiting list for transplant and post-transplantation is crucial. It is also recommended to use the lowest planned doses of maintenance immunosuppressive medications by 2-4 months after transplantation, if there has been no acute rejection (Kasiske et al, 2010). The approach in these patients should start with preventive measures including minimizing immunosuppression, avoidance of carcinogenic factors such as ultraviolet radiation, avoidance of repeated exposure to depleting anti-lymphocyte antibodies, and screening of donors and recipients for cancer. There is also growing interest in the potential antioncogenic characteristics of the immunosuppressive agent - mTOR inhibitor. Once malignancy is detected, it should be managed with specific therapy. Reducing CNI dose is a good first approach in patients who develop lymphoma, skin cancer, or KS. Substitution of CNI for mTOR can lead to complete regression of early, small, or low grade KS in renal transplant recipients. Regression of PTLD has also been reported with conversion of CNI by mTOR. Long term studies are needed confirm the beneficial effects of mTOR in regression of cancer in transplant recipients.

11. References

Alberu, J. (November 2010). Clinical insights for cancer outcomes in renal transplant patients. *Transplant Proc.*, Vol. 42, pp. S36-S40

Al-Sulaiman, M. & Al-Khader, A. (1994). Kaposi Sarcoma in Renal Transplant Recipients. *Transplant Sci*, Vol. 4, pp. 46-60

American Society of Transplantation (AST) Kidney-Pancreas Committee. (May 29, 2009). Guidelines of Post-Kidney Transplant Management in the Community Setting. In: AST, July 5, 2011, http://www.a-s-t.org/public-policy/guidleines-post-kidney-transplant-management-community

Barrett, W.; First, M.; Aron B. & Penn I. (1993). Clinical Course of Malignancies in Renal Transplant Recipients. *Cancer*, Vol. 72, pp. 2186-2189

Berkhout, R.; Bouwes-Bavinck, J. & Ter Schegget, J. (2000). Persistence of Human Papilloma Virus DNA in Benign and (Pre)Malignant Skin Lesions from Renal Transplant Recipients. *J Clin Microbiol*, Vol. 38, No. 6, pp. 2087-2096

Birkeland, S. & Storm, H. (November 27, 2002). Risk for tumor and other disease transmission by translplantation: a population-based study of unrecognized malignancies and other diseases in organ donors. *Transplantation*, Vol. 74, No. 10, pp. 1409-1413, ISSN 0041-1337/02/7410-1409/0

Boix, R.; Sanz, C.; Mora, M.; Quer, A.; Beyer, K.; Musulen, E.; Gonzalez, C.; Bayona, S.; Saladie, J. & Ariza, A. (April 15, 2009). Primary Renal Cell Carcinoma in a Transplanted Kidney: Genetic Evidence of Recipient Origin. *Transplantation,* Vol. 87, No. 7, pp. 1057-1061, ISSN 0041-1337/09/8707-1057

Bosmans, J. & Verpooten, G. (2007). Malignancy after kidney transplantation: still a change. *Kidney international,* Vol. 71, pp. 1197-1199

Boxman, I.; Berkhout, R.; Mulder, L.; Wolkers, M.; Bouwes-Bavinck, J.; Vermeer, B. & Ter Schegget, J. (1997). Detection of Human Papilloma Virus DNA Plucked Hairs from Renal Transplant Recipients and Healthy Volunteers. *J Invest Dermatol,* Vol. 108, No. 5, pp. 712-715

Brennan, D.; Rodeheffer, R. & Ambinder, R. (February 15, 2011). Development of Malignancy Following Solid Organ Transplantation. In: UpToDate, June 22, 2011, http://www.uptodate.com/contents/development-of-malignancy-following-solid-organ-transplantation

Buell, J.; Gross, T. & Woodle, E. (October 15, 2005). Malignancy after transplantation. *Transplantation,* Vol. 80, No. 2S, pp. S254-S264, ISSN 0041-1337/05/8002S-254

Caillard, S.; Agodoa, L.; Bohen, E. & Abbott, K. (2006). Myeloma, Hodgkin Disease, and Lymphoid Leukemia after Renal Transplantation: Characteristics, Risk Factors and Prognosis. *Transplantation*, Vol. 81, No. 6, pp. 888-895

Campistol, J. et al. (2007). Use of proliferation signal inhibitors in the management of post-transplant malignancies-clinical guidance. Neprol Dial Transplant, Vol. 22, pp. i36-i41

Cattani, P. et al. (2001). Kaposi's Sarcoma Associated With Previous Human Herpes virus 8 Infection in Kidney Transplant Recipients. *J. Clin. Microbiol.,* Vol. 39, pp. 506-508

Cattran, D. & Fenton, S. (1993). Contemporary management of renal failure: outcome of the failed allograft recipient . Kidney Intl Suppl, Vol. 41, pp. S36-S39

Chapman, J. & Campistol, J. (2007). Malignancy in Renal Transplantation: Opportunities with Proliferation Signal Inhibitors. *Nephrol Dial Transplant,* Vol. 22, pp. i1-i3

Comeau, S.; Jensen, L.; Cockfield, S.; Sapijaszko, M. & Gourishankar, S. (August 27, 2008). Non-Melanoma Skin Cancer Incidence and Risk Factors after Kidney Transplantation: A Canadian Experience. *Transplantation,* Vol. 86, No. 4, pp. 535-541, ISSN 0041-1337/08/8604-535

Detry, O.; Bonnet, P.; Honore, P. et al. (1997). What is the risk of transferral of an undetected neoplasm during organ transplantation? *Transplant Proc,* Vol. 29, pp. 2410-2415

Detry, O.; Honore, P.; Hans, M. et al. (2000). Organ donors with primary central nervous system tumor. *Transplantation,* Vol. 70, pp. 244-248

Diociaiuti, A. et al. (2000). HHV8 in Renal Transplant Recipients. *Transpl. Int.,* Vol. 13, pp. S410-S412

Ekberg, H. et al. (August 9, 2009). Calcineurin minimization in the symphony study: observational results 3 years after transplantation. *Am J Transplant,* Vol. 8, pp. 1876-1885

Ekberg, H. et al. (December 20, 2007). Reduced exposure to calcineurin inhibitors in renal transplantation. *N Engl J Med*, Vol. 357, No. 25, pp. 2562-2575

Euvrard, S.; Kanitakis, J.; Decullier, E. et al. (2006). Subsequent skin cancer In kidney and heart transplant recipients after the first squamous cell carcinoma. *Transplantation*, Vol. 81, pp. 1093-1100

Engl, T. et al. (2005). Mycophenolate mofetil modulates adhesion receptors of the beta 1 integrin family on tumor cells: impact on tumor recurrence and malignancy. *BMC Cancer*, Vol. 5, pp.4

Friedberg, J.; Jessup, M. & Brennan, D. (March 30, 2010). Lymphoproliferative Disorders Following Solid Organ Transplantation. In: Uptodate, June 22, 2011, http://www.uptodate.com/contents/lymphoproliferative-disorders-following-solid-organ-transplant

Funch, D. et al. (2005). Ganciclovir and acyclovir reduce the risk of post-transplant lymphoproliferative disorder in renal transplant recipients. *Am J Transplant*, Vol. 5, pp. 2894-2900

Gallagher, M. et al. (2010). Long-term cancer risk of immunosuppressive regimens after kidney transplantation. *J Am Soc Nephrol*, Vol. 21, pp. 852-858

Holmes, R. & Sokol, R. (2002). Epstein-Barr virus and post transplant lymphoproliferative disease. *Pediatr Transplant*, Vol. 6, pp. 456-464

Joshi, K & Jha, V. (2009). Malignancies following kidney transplantation. *Journal of nephrology and renal transplantation (JNRT)*, Vol. 2, No. 1, pp. 94-105

Jemec, G. & Holm, E. (February 15, 2003). Nonmelanoma Skin Cancer in Organ Transplant Patients. *Transplantation*, Vol. 75, No. 3, pp. 253-257, ISSN 0041-1337/03/7503-253/0

Kalble, T.; Alcaraz, A.; Budde, K.; Humke, U.; Karam, G.; Lucan, M.; Nicita, G. & Susal, C. (March 2009). Guidelines on Renal Transplantation. *European Association of Urology*, pp. 72-77

Kapoor, A. (2008). Malignancy in kidney transplant recipients. *Source Drugs*, Vol. 68, pp. 11-19

Kasiske, B.; Snyder, J.; Gilbertson, D. & Wang, C. (2004) Cancer after Kidney Transplantation in the United States. *Am J Transplant*, Vol. 4, No. 6, pp. 905-913

Kasiske, B.; Cangro, C.; Hariharan, S. et al. (2001). The Evaluation of Renal Transplant Candidates: Clinical Practice Guidelines. Recommendations of Outpatient Surveillance of Renal Transplantation, *Am J Transplant*, Vol. 2, pp. 5-95

Kasiske, B., Zeier, M. et al. (2010). KDIGO clinical practice guideline for the care of kidney transplantatnt recipients: a summary. *Kidney International*, Vol. 77, pp. 299-311

Kiberd, B. (2005). Screening and Early Detection: Cancer in the Kidney Transplant Recipient. In: Medscape, May 5, 2011, http:// Medscape.com

Klatte, T. & Marberger, M. (2011). Renal Cell Carcinoma of Native Kidneys in Renal Transplant Patients. *Current Opinion in Urology*, Vol. 21, pp. 1-4, ISSN 0963-0643

Koukourgianni, F.; Harambat, J.; Ranchin, B.; Euvrard, S.; Bouvier, R.; Liutkus, A. & Cochat, P. (2010). Malignancy Incidence after Renal Transplantation in Children: A 20-year Single Center Experience. *Nephrol Dial Transplant*, Vol. 25, No. 2, pp. 611-616,

Leckel, K. et al. (2003). The immunosuppressive drug mycophenolate mofetil impairs the adhesion capacity of gastrointestinal tumour cells. *Clin Exp Immunol*, Vol. 134, pp. 238-245

Lutz, J. & Heeman, U. (2003). Tumours after kidney transplantation. *Current opinion in urology*, Vol. 13, pp. 105-109

Maharaj, S. & Assounga, A. (July 27, 2010). Post transplant cancer in kidney allograft recipients in Durbam South Africa: a single center experience. *Supplement to transplantation*, Vol. 90. Pp. 3022

Morath, C.; Mueller, M.; Goldschmidt H.; Schwenger V.; Opelz G. & Zeier, M. (2004). Malignancy in Renal Transplantation. *J Am Soc Nephrol*, Vol. 15, pp. 1582-1588, ISSN 1046-6673/1506-1582

Morgans, A.; Reshef, R. & Tsai, D. (January 2010). Post transplant Lymphoproliferative Disorder Following Kidney Transplant. *American Journal of Kidney Diseases*, Vol. 55, No. 1, pp. 168-180, ISSN 0272-6386/09/5501-0023

Mucha, K.; Foroncewicz, B.; Ziarkiewicz-Wrovlewska, B.; Krawczyk, M.; Lerut, J. & Paczek, L. (2010). Post-transplant lymphoproliferative disorder in view of the new WHO classification: a more rational approach to a protean disease. *Nephrol. Dial. Transplant*, Vol. 25, No. 7, pp. 2089-2098

Muruve, N. & Shoskes, D. (2005). Genitourinary malignancies in solid organ transplant recipients. *Transplantation*, Vol. 80, pp. 709-716

Nafar, M. et al. (2009). Gastrointestinal and Liver Malignancies after Renal Transplantation: A Multicenter Study. *Int J Nephrol Urol*, Vol. 1, No. 1, pp. 33-38,

Naldi, L. et al. (November 27, 2000). Risk of Nonmelanoma Skin Cancer in Italian Organ Transplant Recipients. A Registry-Based Study. *Transplantation*, Vol. 70, No. 10, pp. 1479-1484, ISSN 0041-1337/00/7010-1489/0

Nalesnik, M.; Jaffe, R.; Starzl, T.; Demetris, A.; Porter, K.; Burnham, J.; Makowka, L.; Ho, M. & Locker, J. (1988). The Pathology of Post Transplant Lymphoproliferative Disorders Occurring in the Setting of Cyclosporine A-Prednisone Immunosuppression. *Am J Pathol*, Vol. 133, No. 1, pp. 173-192

O'Donovan, P. et al. (2005). Azathioprine and UVA light generate mutagenic oxidative DNA damage. *Science*, Vol. 309, pp. 1871-1874

Opelz, G. (2001). New Immunosuppressants and HLA matching. *Transplant Proc*, Vol. 3, pp. 467-478

Opelz, G. et al. (2007). Effect of cytomegalovirus prophylaxis with immunoglobulin or with antiviral drugs on post-transplant non-Hogkin lymphoma: a multicenter retrospective analysis. *Lancet Oncol*, Vol. 8, pp. 212-218

Pedotti, P et al. (February 15, 2004). Epidemiologic study on the origin of cancer after kidney transplantation. *Transplantation*, Vol. 77, No. 3, pp. 426-428, ISSN 0041-1337/04/7703-426/0

Pedotti, P. et al. (November 27, 2003). Incidence of cancer after kidney transplant: results from the north Italy transplant program. *Transplantation*, Vol. 76, No. 10, pp. 1448-1451, ISSN 0041-1337/03/7610-1448/0

Pita-Fernandez, S.; Valdes-Canedo, Francisco.; Pertega-Diaz, S.; Pillado, M. & Seijo-Bestilleiro, Rocio. (August 22, 2009). Cancer Incidence in Kidney Transplant Recipients: A Study Protocol. *BMC Cancer*, Vol. 9, pp. 294-299

Qunibi, W, Al-Furayh, O; Almeshari, K. et al. (1998). Serologic Association of Human Herpes Virus Eight with Post transplant Kaposi's Sarcoma in Saudi Arabia. *Transplantation*, Vol. 65, pp. 583-585

Rama, I. & Grinyo, J. (September 2010). Malignancy after Renal Transplantation: The Role of Immunosupression. *Nature Reviews Nephrology*, Vol. 6, pp. 511-519, ISSN 1759-5061

Regamey, N. et al. (1998). Transmission of Human Herpes Virus 8 Infection from Renal-Transplant Donors to Recipients. *N. Engl. J. Med.*, Vol. 339, pp. 1358-1363

Shapiro, R. et al. (1995). FK506 in pediatric kidney transplantation primary and rescue experience. *Pediatr Nephrol,* Vol. 9

Schenna, F. et al. (January 2009). Conversion from calcineurin inhibitors to sirolimus maintenance therapy in allograft recipients: 24-month efficacy and safety results from the convert trial. *Transplantation,* Vol. 87, No. 2, pp. 233-242

Stallone, G. et al. Sirolimus for Kaposi's Sarcoma in Renal-Transplant Recipients. (2005). *N Eng J Med,* Vol. 352, pp. 1317-1323

Suthanthiran, M.; Hojo, M.; Maluccio, M.; Boffa, D. & Luan, F. (2009). Post-transplantation malignancy: a cell autonomous mechanism with implications for therapy. *Transactions of the American clinical and climatological association*, Vol. 120, pp. 369-388

Taioli, E. et al. (April 15, 2006). Incidence of second primary cancer in transplanted patients. *Transplantation,* Vol. 81, No. 7, pp. 982-985, ISSN 0041-1337/06/8107-982

Trofe, J.; Buell, J.; Woodle, E. et al. (2004). Recurrence Risk after Organ Transplantation in Patients with A History of Hodgkin Disease or Non-Hodgkin Lymphoma. *Transplantation*, Vol. 78, pp. 972-977

Tsai, MK.; Yang, CY.; Lee, CY.; Yeh, CC.; Hu, RH. & Lee, PH. (2011). De Novo Malignancy is Associated with Renal Transplant Tourism. *Kidney International*, Vol. 79, pp. 908-913,

Tyden, G.; Wernersson, A.; Sandberg, J. & Berg, U. (December 15, 2000). Development of Renal Cell Carcinoma in Living Donor Kidney Grafts. *Transplantation,* Vol. 70, No. 11, pp. 1650-1656, ISSN 0041-1337/00/7011-1650/0

Wallace, C.; Forsyth, P.; Edwards, D. (1996). Lymph node metastases from glioblastoma multiforme. *AJNR Am J Neuroradiol*, Vol. 17, pp. 1929-1931

Wallerand, H.; Ravaud, A. & Ferriere JM. (2010). Bladder Cancer in Patients after Organ Transplantation. *Current Opinion in Urology,* Vol. 20, pp. 432-436, ISSN 0963-0643

Wisgerhof, H. et al. (May 27, 2010). Subsequent squamous and basal cell carcinoma in kidney transplant recipients after the first skin cancer: cumulative incidence and risk factors. *Transplantation,* Vol. 89, No. 10, pp. 1231-1238, ISSN 0041-1337/10/8910-1231

Wong, G. et al. (February 27, 2008). Cost-effectiveness of colorectal cancer screening in renal transplant recipients. *Transplantation,* Vol. 85, No. 4, pp. 532-541, ISSN 0041-1337/08/8504-532

13

Osteonecrosis of Femoral Head (ONFH) After Renal Transplantation

Yan Jie Guo and Chang Qing Zhang
Department of Orthopedicsm,
The Sixth Poeple's Hospital Affiliated Shanghai Jiao Tong University, Shanghai,
P. R. China

1. Introduction

Approximately 25,000 patients undergo renal transplantation every year worldwide due to end-stage renal disease(ESRD). Renal transplantation is expected to lead to a progressive correction of the established renal bone disease, and osteonecrosis of the femoral head(ONFH) is a common and severe complication in these patients. It induces deformity of the hip joint and reduces the quality of life, especially in the young population ranging from 20 to 50 years old. Total hip replacement is not reasonable in this population due to the finite lifespan of implants. Clinical results suggest that free vascularized fibular grafting(FVFG) can slow or potentially halt the progression of osteonecrosis, it offers an alternative method for preserving the femoral head in younger renal transplant recipients.

2. Clinical backgroud

Chronic renal failure(CRF) and end-stage renal disease(ESRD) are associated with many disturbances of bone structure and metabolism due to deficiency of calcitriol, hypocalcemia, retention of phosphate, metabolic acidosis, secondary hyperparathyroidism. Renal transplantation can improve the metabolism disturbances of ESRD, but osseous complications like osteoporosis, consequent fracture, bone pain and osteonecrosis are not rare. It is reported that up to 40% of renal graft recipients have spontaneous osteoporotic pain. A major obstacle to the investigation of renal osteodystrophy in transplant recipients has been its unpredictable evolution under the multiple biochemical and hormonal influences that regulate mineral metabolism and bone turnover independently. Its course after transplantation depends on persisting abnormalities such as hypercalcaemia, hypophosphataemia and hypomagnesaemia as well as on the type, dose and duration of immunosuppressive medications that are needed to minimize allograft rejection.

2.1 Morbidity of ONFH in the recipients

Osteonecrosis of the femoral head (ONFH), an aseptic and ischemic disease, is especially common in the transplant recipients. Kubo documented femoral head MRI abnormalities of osteonecrosis in 25% of 51 renal allograft recipients; Marston reported 20% of 52 patients and 11% of 103 hips developed ONFH within 1 year after transplantation; Lopez-Ben reported 4%

of 48 patients and three of 96 hips had ONFH within 6 months after renal transplantation; In the study of Lee, ONFH developed in 6.3% of the 237 patients and 4.9% of the 473 femoral heads from 8 months to 16 months after renal transplantation. In the report of Children by Nishiyama *et al*, 141 renal transplants were performed in 129 children(72 boys and 57 girls), aged from 2 to 17 years. Osteonecrosis occurred in seven patients, in the following sites: the femoral head in four children including two bilateral cases: and the femoral condyle in Three children, with two bilateral cases. The mean period from transplantation to the diagnosis of OHFH was 18 months, 75% appeared more than 9 months after transplantation.

2.2 Etipathogenesis

2.2.1 Use of corticosteroids

High doses of corticosteroids are used after renal transplantation to reduce rejection and improve graft survival. They have also been implicated as the major predisposing factor for post-transplant bone loss and osteonecrosis, and It takes a few years to develop osteonecrosis after the start of corticosteroids therapy. Although corticosteroids therapy represents a pathogenetic key factor other immunosuppressive drugs such as cyclosporine, tacrolimus, azathioprine and rapamycin clearly contribute to its prevalence and expression through their pleiotropic pharmacological effects. These drugs have been shown to increase overall bone turnover and/or to stimulate loss of bone mass independently. Long-term glucocorticoid administration and possibly cyclosporine treatment may chronically activate osteoclasts in spongy and/or cortical bone while osteoblast activity is inhibited, and the highest tertiles of cumulative glucocorticoid were significantly associated with BMD loss and osteonecrosis. A prospective study using MRI in renal transplant patients showed the occurrence of ONFH within several months after the initiation of steroid treatment, and a time discrepancy between the occurrence of ONFH and onset of symptom.

2.2.2 Dose-related risk of osteonecrosis

Furthermore, an appreciable dose-related risk of osteonecrosis was also found in patients receiving long-term steroid therapy. Hirota *et al* reported the relationship between ONFH and the daily dosage of steroid (#16.6 mg in terms of prednisolone) or the highest daily dose (#80mg in terms of prednisolone) and concluded that higher steroid dosage per day contributed to increasing the frequency of ONFH in renal transplant patients. In a retrospective study of the medical records of 750 patients who had received a renal transplant during the period of 1968-1995, Lausten showed an 11.2% incidence of symptomatic osteonecrosis with high-dose glucocorticoids(cumulative mean dose of prednisolone 12.5g at 1 year post-transplant) and 5.1% with low-dose(cumulative mean dose of prednisolone average dose 6.5g). This difference in numbers of femoral head necroses was highly significant ($p < 0.005$); The cohort of Kopecky *et al* showed an osteonecrosis incidence of 22%, had a prednisolone equivalent dose of 7±3.25g prednisolone during the first 90 days after transplantation; The cohort of Lopez-Ben *et al* showed an osteonecrosis incidence of 4%, had a slightly lower cumulative steroid dosage (2.1g prednisolone at 3 months after transplantation) compared to previously reported cohorts; Lee *et al* also found a low incidence of ONFH in renal transplantation patients at the time of 1 year post-transplantation, which seems to be related with low cumulative steroid dosage. There is no known threshold dose. In clinical practice, some patients fail to benefit from daily doses as low as 2.5–7.5 mg of prednisone, whereas daily doses >7.5 mg will definitively induce osteoporosis and osteonecrosis in the majority of patients.

2.2.3 Main mechanism

The mechanism of ONFH after renal transplantation includes: 1. Thrombus due to the steroid-induced hypercoagulable state(Hypercoagulability of plasma was found after 3 months of steroid treatment in previous studies). 2. Reduction of blood flow in bone(Femoral head blood flow was 2-3 fold lower after 2 week high dose steroid treatment, decreased arterial inflow or increased venous outflow resistance can reduce intraosseous blood flow) 3. Osteoporosis of femoral(Steroid can decrease the absorption of calcium from intestine and increase its elimination via the kidneys. Direct and indirect effects on PTH secretion, changes in bone protein matrix, increased osteoclastic activity, and decreased protein synthesis all lead to a reduction in bone mass after renal transplantation, inhaled corticosteroids in doses above 1.5 mg/d may be associated with a significant reduction in bone density). 4. Metabolism disorder. 5. Fat embolism of femoral head. 6. Rise of intraosseous pressure(In the rigid intraosseous compartment, growth of fat cells may cause a rise in intraosseous pressure, and thereby compress the thin-walled sinusoids, with a subsequent decrease in bone blood flow). 7. Degenerative changes of the hip capsule(Degenerative changes in the arteries and arterioles of the capsule of the hip and the femoral head have been found in cadavers of renal transplant patients without clinical hip symptoms. There was thickening of the intima, gross diminution in the number and calibre of the vessels in the arteries of the femoral head and infarcts of subchondral bone).

2.2.4 Other risk factors

The type of donor, dialysis duration, acute rejection rate, and postoperative weight gain. The age of the graft recipients also matters. An age of less than forty years is a risk factor for osteonecrosis of the femoral head.

2.3 Contradiction during the treatment

ONFH continues to be a difficult problem to manage, especially in renal transplant recipients. Both the patients and surgeons were concerned about changes of renal function and survival of the graft. They paid little attention to the hip joint, although early signs of osteonecrosis were present. High doses of steroids were used in a continuous manner, neglecting the abnormal joint function, which hastened the deterioration of the femoral head. ONFH was diagnosed at a mean of 3.5 years after transplantation, it can progress to severe osteoarthritis and seriously impair the life quality of transplant recipients. Early hip joint symptoms, including progressing hip pain and joint dysfunction, always appear 9 to 19 months after transplantation, But in most of the clinical cases, severe joint pain and irreversible collapse of the femoral head had already developed when the diagnosis was established. Furthermore, steroid-induced ONFH following transplantation tends to have larger necrotic areas, and bilateral involvement is more common than unilateral involvement. the natural history of femoral head osteonecrosis has shown evidence that a large majority of clinically diagnosed cases will progress to femoral head collapse. The treatment of ONFH depends on the staging and severity of the clinical symptoms.

3. Therapy methods

3.1 Core decompression and THA

Joint-preserving operations like core decompression cannot arrest the progression of the disease effectively. Total hip replacemen(THA)t is also unsuitable for younger patients because of their higher activity level and longer remainder of life. So Osteonecrosis of the femoral head continues to be a difficult problem to manage, especial in the patient with various kinds of renal diseases(such like IgA nephropathy, focal segmental glomerular sclerosis, membranous nephropathy, mesangial proliferative glomerulonephritis, crescent glomerulonephritis, lupus nephritis, minimal change nephropathy and renal transplantation after end-stage renal diseases). Many patients with renal diseases inevitably lose the ability to live independently due to advanced stages of osteoarthritis.

3.2 FVFG

FVFG showed favorable outcomes. Compared with core decompression of femoral head, FVFG had a significantly lower conversion rate to total hip arthroplasty(stage II and III hips), because it can enhance the revascularization of bone tissue and arrest the progression of the necrosis. It is also an alternative method for younger patients without severe osteoarthritis of the hip joint.

3.2.1 Advantages of FVFG

The advantage of FVFG lies in the combination of femoral head decompression(Extensive decompression of the femoral head along with removal of necrotic bone theoretically interrupts the cycle of increased intraosseous pressure and ischemia and allows for revascularization of the femoral head), removal of necrotic bone, introduction of osteoinductive cancellous bone(Filling the defect with fresh cancellous bone provides both osteoinductive and osteoconductive stimulation of healing), and vascularized cortical bone support of the subchondral surface(The vascularized fibula provides a viable cortical bone strut to support the subchondral bone from collapse and further enhances the revascularization process). This procedure may benefit young patients with more advanced osteonecrosis of the femoral head by halting progression of collapse, prolonging reduction of symptoms, and postponing total hip replacement.

3.2.2 Clinical application of FVFG

With the emergence of microsurgical techniques, Judet *et al* first treated ONFH with FVFG in the late 1970s. The long-term results cover 68 hips in 60 patients with 18 of these classified as early failures requiring conversion to THA. The remaining 50 hips were followed on average for 18 years. Thirty-five hips scored good or very good, which corresponds to a 52% success rate, the data clearly show an increase in good results for patients younger than 40 years, and an increase in the rate of failures for patients older than 40 years. Specifically, of the patients younger than 40 years, 80% had good and very good results, whereas of the patients between 40 and 50 years, only 57% had good and very good results. After systemic research and long-term clinical study, Urbaniak *et al* improved the surgical technique. The results for 103 consecutive hips(eighty-nine patients) that had been treated with FVFG because of symptomatic osteonecrosis of the femoral head were reviewed in a prospective study. total arthroplasty had been performed in thirty-one hips: five (23 per cent) of the twenty-two that were in stage III; seventeen (43 per cent) of the forty that were in stage IV; and seven (32 per cent) of the twenty-two that were in stage V. Harris hip scores had improved at the latest follow-up evaluation, compared with the preoperative values ($p < 0.001$). For the stage-II hips, the average score improved from 56 to 80 points; for the stage-III hips, from 52 to 85 points; for the stage-IV hips, from 41 to 76 points; and for the stage-V hips, from 36 to 75 points. 59 percent of the hips did not limit or only slightly limited the patient's ability to carry out daily activities, and 62 percent did not limit or only slightly limited the patient's ability to work. FVFG had decreased the need for pain medication for 86 percent of the hips that had not been subsequently treated with an arthroplasty. Regardless of whether or not a subsequent arthroplasty was done, 81 per cent of the patients (81 per cent of the hips) were satisfied with their decision to have fibular grafting.

FVFG became widely performed in their clinical activities. Some other clinical research also showed good results. Zhang *et al* treated 56 hips in 48 patients with FVFG and followed patients for a mean duration of 16 months. Roughly 69.6% of femoral heads showed improvement on radiographs, and the Harris hip scores showed improvement ranging from 11-13 points. Most patients had full weight-bearing ability and took part in their daily activities. Aldridge *et al* reported an 88% success rate associated with FVFG in the femoral heads without collapse and a success rate of 78% with subchondral collapse. The results showed that FVFG is the most promising technique because it had satisfactory mid-term and long-term outcomes. Fibular grafts have also been proven to be alternative for the post-collapse stage of ONFH, It is also a worthwhile procedure in patients with postcollapse osteonecrosis. 188 patients (224 hips) who had undergone free vascularized fibular grafting, between 1989 and 1999, for the treatment of osteonecrosis of the hip that had led to collapse of the femoral head but not to arthrosis. The mean preoperative Harris hip score was 51.5 points, and it increased to 81 points for the patients in whom the surgery succeeded; 63% of the patients in that group had a good or excellent result, Patients with postcollapse, predegenerative osteonecrosis of the femoral head appear to benefit from FVFG, with good overall survival of the joint and significant improvement in the Harris hip score. FVFG is a well accepted treatment option for all symptomatic stages of the disease ,with proper patient selection, middle and long-term outcomes appear promising. FVFG continues to be a primary treatment option to provide relief of symptoms and preserve bone stock, especially in the younger patient population.

3.2.3 Attampts on the renal transplant recipients

FVFG has been rarely systematically reported in renal transplant recipients, although ONFH after renal transplantation is not rare in the clinical work. Recipients with renal insufficiency and unstable general conditions cannot withstand the excessive blood loss and traumatic stress of a hip operation. Postoperative renal graft dysfunction, severe anemia, electrolyte disorder, and infection are life-threatening complications. Therefore, laboratory indices, including the HB, WBC, ESR, BUN, SCr, UA, electrolyte, 24 hours urine volume, and urine protein quantity, are indispensable. In addition, the CRP and ESR should also be included as a nonspecific marker of the activation of the immune system in order to provide early signs of postoperative graft dysfunction and infection. Furthermore, the surgery should be rapid and less invasive. The use of toxic renal medicine should be avoided as well. Guo report three renal transplant recipients with ONFH who underwent FVFG in the orthopedics department of Shanghai Sixth Poeple's Hospital. Of the three cases, two cases showed radiographic improvement, one case showed radiographic unchanged. All the three cases have been living in good health and are satisfied with their joint function. The hip joint pain was significantly relieved and joint motion was also improved, The Harris hip score elevated 22 points in average, and the Visual Analogue Scale (VAS) was decreased by 37.3 points. Their quality of life has been greatly improved and the gait can return to normal after positive rehabilitation training. The patients were able to walk without aid, even engaged in sports. After operation, the patients returned to full activities with a better quality of life due to normal joint and kidney function. The follow-up results demonstrated that FVFG is safe, effective, and feasible for transplant recipients without serious renal graft dysfunction, anemia, or other systemic diseases. However, the safety of the operation should also be attributed to proficient surgical technique, meticulous laboratory monitoring, and deliberate postoperative supportive treatment.

3.2.4 Indication discussion

According to our previous experience, indications for using FVFG to treat ONFH in patients after the renal transplantation include: 1) A patient younger than 50 years who is not suitable for total hip replacement; 2) Severe hip pain that greatly impairs daily activity; 3) Necrosis of the femoral head less than Steinberg stage V (osteoarthritis stage); 4) The recipient's general physical condition is stable without renal graft dysfunction, serious anemia, metabolic disorder, or any other systemic diseases; 5) The recipient is active and in need of a high quality of life; 6) To take the safety of operation into account, FVFG ought to be performed at least one year after transplantation.

4. Clinical example

A 39-year-old man who was diagnosed with IgA nephropathy by renal biopsy and histopathological examination in January 1998. The disease developed to chronic renal failure six years later. The patient was maintained on hemodialysis for 10 months until unilateral renal transplantation in May 2005. He received steroid therapy for 18 months after the operation. The accumulative dose of corticosteroids was 7.5g (converted to prednisone dose). Tacrolimus (FK-506) 15mg per day and MMF 2.0g was also taken each day at the same time. He visited our hospital in November 2006 because of severe hip joint pain on the left side. The symptom became aggravated quickly, and the patient had to take 0.6mg Ibuprofen per day to maintain his daily activities. He was diagnosed with left side ONFH upon hip X-ray and MRI (classified as Steinberg stage III, Fig 1 a, b). A physical exam revealed a gait abnormality, deep inguinal region pain, positive Thomas sign, and Trendelenburg sign on the affected side. A decreased range of motion occurred in abduction and flexion. The Harris hip score was 72 points, and the VAS pain score was 80 points. All routine laboratory examination results were normal upon admission (shown in Table 1). FVFG on the left side was performed uneventfully one week later. The laboratory exam showed no significant change, except for a slight elevation of the WBC to $11.2\times10^9/L$ on postoperative day 1. The body temperature rose to 37.9°C. The WBC returned to $8.6\times10^9/L$ on day 3 and $7.4\times10^9/L$ on day 7 after antibiotic treatment (intravenous Cefuroxime 3.0g drip bid for 3 days), and the patient's temperature also returned to normal. The patient was discharged within 2 weeks in good health. No signs of infection or renal graft dysfunction were discovered during the 1 year and 8 months of follow-up. The latest radiograph results showed improvement (Fig 1 c). The left joint pain and stiffness were significantly relieved. A daily pain-killer was no longer needed. The patient's gait also returned to normal after positive rehabilitation training. He returned to his full activities with a better quality of life due to normal joint and kidney function. The Harris hip score rose to 89 points, and the VAS pain score decreased to 28 points.

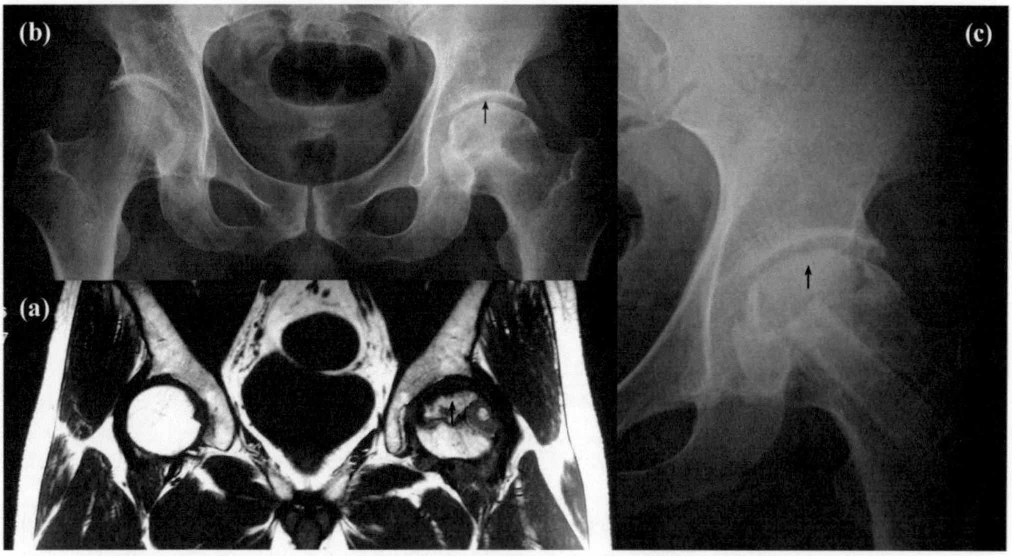

Fig. 1. (a) Preoperative radiograph (b) T1-weighted MRI (c) Radiograph 1 year and 8 months after FVFG showed revascularization of the necrosis area. The femoral head did not collapse.

5. References

[1] A.Y. Plafseychuk, S.Y. Kim and B.C. Park *et al.*, Vascularized compared with nonvascularized fibula grafting for the treatment of osteonecrosis of the femoral head, *J Bone Joint Surg Am* 85 (2003), p. 589.

[2] H. Hedri, M. Cherif and K. Zouaghi *et al.*, Avascular osteonecrosis after renal transplantation, *Transplant Proc* 39 (2007), p. 1036.

[3] J.M. Aldridge and J.R. Urbaniak, Free vascularized fibular grafting for the treatment of osteonecrosis of the femoral head, *Tech orthop* 23 (2008), p. 44.

[4] M.E. Steinberg, G.D. Hayken and D.R. Steinberg. A quantitative system for staging avascular necrosis, *J Bone Joint Surg Br* 77 (1995), p. 34.

[5] H.L Hoeksma, C.H.M. Van den Ende, H.K. Ronday *et al.*, Comparison of the responsiveness of the Harris Hip Score with generic measures for hip function in osteoarthritis of the hip, *Ann Rheum Dis* 62 (2003), p. 935.

[6] Holdgate, S. Asha, J. Craig *et al.*, Comparison of a verbal numeric rating scale with the visual analogue scale for the measurement of acute pain, *Emerg Med* 15 (2003), p. 441

[7] J.G. Heaf, Bone disease after renal transplantation, *Transplantation* 75 (2003), p. 315.

[8] T.R. Mikuls, B.A. Julian and A. Bartolucci *et al.*, Bone mineral density changes within six months of renal transplantation, *Transplantation* 75 (2003), p. 49.

[9] S. Tang, T.M. Chan and S.L. Lui *et al.*, Risk factors for avascular bone necrosis after renal transplantation, *Transplant Proc* 32 (2000), p. 1873.

[10] W. Drescher, T. Schneider and C. Becker *et al.*, Selective reduction of bone blood flow by short-term treatment with high-dose methylprednisolone, An experimental study in pigs. *J Bone Joint Surg Br* 83 (2000), p. 274.

[11] G.S. Dean, R.C. Kime and R.D. Fitch *et al.*, Treatment of osteonecrosis in the hip of pediatric patients by free vascularized fibular graft, *Clin Orthop Relat Res* 386 (2001), p. 106.

[12] H. Judet and A. Gilbert, Long-term results of free vascularized fibular grafting for femoral head necrosis, *Clin Orthop Relat Res* 386 (2001), p. 114.

[13] J.R. Urbaniak, P.G. Coogan and E.B. Gunneson *et al.*, Treatment of osteonecrosis of the femoral head with free vascularized fibular grafting: A long-term follow-up study of one hundred and three hips, *J Bone Joint Surg* Am 77 (1995), p. 681.

[14] C.Q. Zhang, B.F. Zeng and Z.Y. Xu, *et al.*, Treatment of femoral head necrosis with free vascularized fibular grafting: a preliminary report, *J Microsurg* 25 (2005), p. 305.

[15] K.R. Berend, E.B. Gunneson and J.R. Urbaniak, Free vascularized fibular grafting for the treatment of postcollapse osteonecrosis of the femoral head, *J Bone Joint Surg Am* 85 (2003), p. 987.

[16] A.M. Cueto-Manzano, L.E. Morales-Buenrostro and L. Gonzalez-Espinoza *et al.*, Markers of inflammation before and after renal transplantation, *Transplantation* 80 (2005), p. 47.

[17] C. Reek, S. Conrad and H. Huland, The role of C-reactive protein in graft dysfunction after renal transplantation, *J Urol* 161 (1999), p. 1463.

[18] Y. J. Guo, D. X. Jin, C.Q. Zhang, *et al.*, Curative Effect and Safety of Vascularized Fibula Grafting in Renal Transplant Recipients With Osteonecrosis of the Femoral Head: Three Case Reports, *J Transplant Proc* 41(2009), P. 3731.

[19] H. Sperschneider, G. Stein, Bone disease after renal transplantation, *J Nephrol Dial Transplant* 18(2003), P.874

[20] E. Lee, K. Lee, W. Huh, *et al.*, Incidence and radio-uptake patterns of femoral head avascular osteonecrosis at 1 year after renal transplantation: a prospective study with planar bone scintigraphy, *J Nuclr Med Commun* 27(2006), P. 919.

[21] T. Kubo, S. Yamazo, N. Sugano, *et al.*, Initial MRI findings of non-traumatic osteonecrosis of the femoral head in renal allograft recipients. *J Magn Reson Imaging* 15(1997), P. 1017.

[22] S. B. Marston, K. Gillingham, R. F. Bailey, *et al.*, Osteonecrosis of the femoral head after solid organ transplantation: a prospective study. *J Bone Joint Surg Am* 84A (2002), P. 2145.

[23] R. Lopez-Ben, T. R. Mikuls, D. S. Moore, *et al.*, Incidence of hip osteonecrosis among renal transplantation recipients: a prospective study, *J Clin Radiol* 59(2004), P. 31.

[24] G. S. Lausten, T. Lemser, P. K. Jensen, *et al.*, Necrosis of the femoral head after kidney transplantation. *J Clin Transplant* 12(1998), P. 572.

[25] K. K. Kopecky, E. M. Braunstein, K. D. Brand, *et al.*, Apparent avascular necrosis of the hip: appearance and spontaneous resolution of MR findings in renal allograft recipients. *J Radiol* 179(1991), P. 523

[26] J. Brian. Lipworth, Systemic adverse effects of inhaled corticosteroid therapy: A systematic review and meta-analysis, *J Arch Intern Med.* 159(1999), P. 941

[27] T. Kubo. H. Tsuji H, T. Yamamoto T, *et al.*, Antithrombin III deficiency in a patient who has mulitifocal osteonecrosis. *J. Clin Orthop.* 378(2000), p. 306

14

Pediatric Kidney Transplant in Uropaties

Cristian Sager, Juan Carlos López, Víctor Durán,
Carol Burek, Juan Pablo Corbetta and Santiago Weller
Hospital Nacional de Pediatría Prof. Dr. J. P. Garrahan
Argentina

1. Introduction

It has been long reported that for children with end-stage renal disease (ESRD), renal transplant is the treatment of choice (Fine et al., 1978; Gradus & Ettenger, 1982). With this approach the lost renal function is reestablished and the pondo-stature, psycho-intellectual and social development is not affected (Ferraris & Rodriguez, 2008).

Hemodialysis or ambulatory peritoneal dialysis are modalities used in the treatment of children with ESRD when there is no living donor available or when patients are waiting for a cadaver donor (Galvez et al., 2005). However, these patients will eventually present growth and intellectual development alterations.

In 1954 Murray performed the first truly successful pediatric kidney transplant from one homozygous twin to another (Murray et al., 1958). In 1966 Kelly reported a kidney transplantation in a patient with dysfunctional bladder who had undergone ileal segment urinary diversion (Kelly et al., 1966). Until that time, patients with ESRD and untreatable dysfunctional urinary tract were excluded from renal transplant programs. At that time, it was believed that the renal allograft connected to a dysfunctional bladder would run the same risk as the native kidneys, that is, the result would be again renal insufficiency (Sheldon et al., 1994).

As a consequence, the focus began to be placed on the restoration of the dysfunctional lower urinary tract with the aim of creating urinary reservoirs of adequate volume and low pressure that could have complete voiding capacity (Mitchell & Piser, 1987). At present, children with ESRD can benefit from renal transplantation provided the lower urinary tract dysfunctions are corrected or reestablished by means of medical and/or surgical treatment (Broyer et al., 2004). Otherwise, the bladder dysfunction that is not corrected would have a negative effect on the allograft function (Salomon et al., 2000).

Several studies reporting long term encouraging results on patients that have received kidney transplantation with urinary tract reconstructions have been published. However, higher risks and incidence of complications related to the allograft and reconstruction have also been informed (Shekarris et al.,2000). Despite these risks, Luke obtained comparable and acceptable results in children with reconstructed urinary tract, similar to the renal transplanted subjects that had normal lower urinary tract function, following a careful pre-transplant evaluation and an appropriate post-transplant follow-up (Luke et al., 2003)

Nevertheless, there exists considerable controversy around the best approach to handle these types of patients, since there are no guidelines designed with defined reconstructive surgical criteria, optimal surgical procedures or recommendations as to when the best time to perform such interventions (Riley et al.,2010).

2. Etiologies for end stage renal disease – Uropathies

Among the most frequent etiologies for end stage renal disease are renal hypodysplasia (17%), obstructive uropathies (16.9%), focal segmental glomerulosclerosis (9%), vesicoureteral reflux (6.3%), renal polycystosis, uremic hemolitic syndrome, Prune belly, neurogenic bladder due to neural tube defects, among others (North American Pediatric Renal Transplant Cooperative Study (N.A.P.R.T.C.S.), 2007)

The predominance of one or other etiology is conditioned by the different geographical regions. The deterioration of the renal function is not the most common consequence of vesicoureteral reflux (VUR), with an estimated risk lower than 1%. There is a direct relationship between the degree of VUR and the incidence of the nephropathy (Skoog et al, 1987). Up to 35% of renal scarring is congenital, due to dysmorphic renal tissue from the gestational stage, especially in high degree VUR. When there is vesicoureteral reflux the patient is prone to develop pyelonephritis, and if this occurs during the first months of life or in repeated fashion, there are more chances of developing renal scars and aggravating the renal function. The incidence of chronic pyelonephritis is within 15 and 25% of ESRD.

The term 'obstructive uropathies' includes entities such as pyeloureteral stenosis, ureterovesical stenosis, obstructive megaureters and prior surgically corrected obstructive uropathy remnants. All these uropathies manifest as hydronephrosis or ureterohydronephrosis. The obstruction to the urine flow, if not corrected, eventually produces irreversible reduction of the function, depending on whether the obstruction is bilateral, affects only one kidney or an insufficient one (Podestá & Bertolotti, 2008).

Posterior urethral valve (PUV) remains the most frequent organic-anatomical obstruction in males and it is due to a congenital defect in the development of the membranous urethra. This condition can manifest along a spectrum of severity, ranging from disease incompatible with postnatal life to conditions that have minimal impact later in life. Chronic obstruction of the outlet urinary tract during the critical stage of organogenesis of the urinary system exerts a deep impact on the kidneys, ureters and vesical function. Approximately a third of the patients with PUV progress to ESRD (López & Durán, 2008).

In the case of Prune belly syndrome the kidneys may exhibit: ureterohydronephrosis, VUR, renal dysplasia, anatomical infravesical obstruction. This syndrome has a broad spectrum of affected anatomy with different levels of severity, from incompatibility with life to minimally compromised renal function (Woodward & Smith, 1998). Many patients require multiple urological surgeries with some cases of irreversible deterioration in the renal mass.

Patients with a neurogenic bladder caused by spinal dysraphism that do not receive appropriate treatment can progress to ESRD (De Jong et al., 2008). Spinal dysraphism abnormalities mainly include myelomeningocele, lipomeningocele and caudal regression syndrome. All of them generate different types of behavior of the neurogenic bladder and particularly affect the renal function (Torre et al., 2011).

The urodynamic variables that are more involved as risk factors are: detrusor hyperactivity, reduced compliance, detrusor-sphincter dyssinergia.

Medical therapies implemented during the first months of life and sustained by anticholinergic drugs and clean intermittent catheterization greatly help to avoid compromise or deterioration of the renal function.

3. Evaluation of the urinary tract

There is general consensus among the most prominent health care centers that assessment of the lower urinary tract before performing a renal transplant is of the utmost importance. If alterations are found, they must be corrected before the allograft is implanted. A dysfunctional lower urinary tract that has promoted the deterioration of the native kidneys represents a risk for the allograft.

In the first place, a history of baseline pathologies and a thorough physical examination are fundamental, since they determine which complementary studies will be needed. It is not necessary to have all patients undergo all possible urological studies. For that reason it is useful to define beforehand whether ESRD was caused by a nephropathy or by an uropathy. If the latter applies, it is necessary to classify patients into two groups: those who did not require urinary tract surgery and those who did.

Overall, for the group of patients who required lower urinary tract surgery most of the complementary studies described below will be needed. When the signs and symptoms reported by patients or parents are not clear enough, especially with respect to urinary incontinence or alterations of the voiding frequency, keeping a voiding diary and a record of urinary leakage becomes very useful.

On occasions, when the history or symptoms of urologic pathology are not defined, we must resort to other specialties for further evaluation, such as neurology-neurosurgery, in order to search for the etiological diagnosis of certain urinary dysfunctions.

The physical examination also includes the assessment of the abdominal and pelvic region for position of dialysis catheters, intestinal and urinary stomas, either for possible reconstructions of the urinary tract or to locate a future allograft implantation. In addition, it is necessary to analyze the status and mobility of lower and upper limbs, with the purpose of deciding whether intermittent catheterization could be used for bladder voiding, via the urethra or via continent stoma.

Ultrasound scanning is the initial technique of choice in order to detect morphological abnormalities. Although it is operator/observer-dependent, it does not present any contraindications and it can be repeated as many times as necessary without having damaging effects on the patient (Bibiloni, et al., 2008). In ESRD, ultrasound is used in order to characterize degree of ureterohydronephrosis, double ureter systems and characteristics of the vesical wall. If diuresis exists, ultrasound scanning with full and empty bladder is required in order to evaluate if there is post void residual or ureterohydronephrosis alterations.

Voiding cystourethrogram is mandatory, especially in the case of patients with a history of urinary infections and lower urinary tract surgeries. It is an irreplaceable method to detect vesicoureteral reflux, to show anatomical details of the bladder neck, of the male urethra, and to characterize other findings, such as bladder stones and irregularities of the bladder wall. This methodology also provides information on voiding pathophysiology. As it is an invasive procedure that uses fluoroscopy radiation, it must be carried out by trained professionals, so that the method can be optimized.

Urodynamic studies record the activity of the lower urinary tract in the filling and voiding phases of the bladder. The variables recorded, such as volume, bladder pressure, urinary leakage pressure, bladder compliance, detrusor muscle stability, coordination of the cycle, perineal surface electromyography activity, among others, determine the type of bladder dysfunction and help to indicate the most appropriate treatment and to control the evolution and therapeutic response (Burek & Sager, 2008). Urodynamic studies are required when there is a history of spinal dysraphism and other etiologies of neurogenic bladder, posterior urethra valves, lower urinary tract surgeries, urine incontinence, therapy with anticholinergic drugs, anatomical alterations as shown in the voiding cystourethrogram and high degree of vesicoureteral reflux.

In the latter case, a video urodynamic study is the preferred method, since it combines the benefits of voiding cystourethrography and urodynamic records. This results in a thorough anatomic and functional evaluation of the urinary tract. The video urodynamic study requires a certain degree of technical complexity and it must be performed by very well-trained professionals. In the case of some patients, in order to simplify and reduce manipulation, the following algorithm can be applied: renovesical ultrasound and video urodynamic study (Cerruto & Artibani, 2006).

4. Adequate bladder function

The urinary tract can be described as being "functional" if the storage and voiding phases of the bladder function in a coordinated way. In the first phase, the pelvis and ureters must void an adequate volume of urine into a bladder or neobladder of low pressure without leaks. Competent ureterovesical junctions stop urine from refluxing into the upper urinary tract. During the voiding phase, the bladder muscle (detrusor) contracts at regular intervals and in a sustained fashion, with relaxation of the outlet urinary tract (bladder neck and sphincter) with the purpose of eliminating urine. Many patients cannot achieve normal voiding and require clean intermittent catheterization.

After evaluation is completed we must define whether the lower urinary tract is in good condition to receive an implant. The parameters used to define "adequate bladder function" are:

- Absence of signs and symptoms of low urinary tract dysfunction.
- Absence or scant post void residual urine on renovesical ultrasound.
- Adequate volume capacity and bladder compliance, stability of the detrusor muscle, adequate voiding, no post void residual and no leaks as assessed by urodynamic/video urodynamic studies (Barry, 2004).

If assessment outcome shows that the lower urinary tract is not in adequate condition to receive a new kidney, therapy customized to the particular urologic condition should be indicated and a new evaluation should be carried out prior to transplantation. If reconstruction of the lower urinary tract is to be performed, the objective is to achieve a functional urinary tract.

5. Treatments for the lower urinary tract

5.1 Medical treatments

The objective of any treatment is to provide a safe mechanism of drainage for those patients who have voiding difficulties, by means of clean intermittent catheterization (CIC) and pharmacological reduction of storage pressure or non-inhibited contractions with the use of anticholinergic drugs.

CIC is the most significant advancement in the urological care of patients with neurogenic dysfunction of the lower urinary tract. This procedure provides adequate voiding and a reduced risk of urinary infections; it helps to avoid bladder overdistension; it facilitates resolution of the vesicoureteral reflux and favors urinary continence. CIC may be performed at any age, on both sexes and at any position and site. It can be indicated in the presence of high intravesical pressure, detrusor-sphincter dyssynergia, sphincter hypertonia, high residual urine volume and absence of spontaneous voiding. It is fundamental that instruction of the procedure be in charge of trained nurses, who will also supervise CIC management periodically.

CIC is a safe, easy and effective way of emptying the bladder with a low rate of complications. Although unusual, the most frequent complications are urethral bleeding and false passages, and epididymitis. Asymptomatic bacteriuria is observed in 70% of patients, but it is not associated to renal scarring; therefore, it is not treated. Antibiotic prophylaxis is indicated only at the beginning of CIC to patients with vesicoureteral reflux and those who have received a renal transplantation.

Anticholinergic drugs, mainly oxybutynin, are used for the treatment of hyperreflexia and bladder hypertonia. They are widely used in pediatric settings; they are of acceptable tolerance and they have proved to provide a beneficial therapeutic effect. For those patients who do not tolerate oxybutynin, tolterodine can be used. It is more selective; it has fewer adverse effects, but does not seem to have more efficacy. Other even more selective drugs, such as darifenacin, are also being used lately in the pediatric population.

The selective alpha-adrenergic blockade is a therapeutic alternative in cases of dysfunctional voiding of different etiologies. It facilitates the release of infravesical outflow obstruction. Doxazosin is one of the most commonly used drugs (Austin et al., 1999) Biofeedback therapy, mainly used with patients with non-neurogenic bladder dysfunction, contributes to educating, relaxing the perineum region and improving the dynamics of the detrusor-neck-sphincter unit.

5.2 Surgical treatment

5.2.1 Reconstruction of the urinary tract in children

The aim of the surgical intervention/s is to reestablish a new system that can protect the renal function and achieve adequate urine volume at low pressure, avoid urinary infections and lead to continence.

At present, most of the reconstructive procedures are performed in order to correct anomalies of the native urinary tract refractory to medical treatment. Children with bladder and sphincter dysfunction represent a big challenge and most patients who require reconstructive procedures have myelodysplasia as etiology for the neurogenic bladder.

The pathophysiological ways that lead to dysfunction of the excretory system are manifold; therefore, the evaluation of reconstruction should be meticulous and individualized. In addition to technical surgical matters, in questions of evolution and outcome it is important to consider the commitment of the patient and the family in the monitoring and post-surgery care. When a reconstruction of the lower urinary tract is considered, the aim is to achieve the characteristics of a functional urinary tract.

In general, vesicoureteral reflux is secondary to bladder dysfunction. In other etiologies, such as Prune belly syndrome and posterior urethra valves, the reflux can be primary and secondary. In the case of secondary reflux of low degree in patients that will undergo bladder augmentation, it is not necessary to correct the reflux, since after the augmentation, this type of reflux may resolve without the need for reimplantation. If the reservoir has adequate low pressure volume, reimplantation is not necessary. However, some surgeons prefer correction of the reflux, since they state that bacteiruria can unfold episodes of pyelonephritis.

Furthermore, when thinking of reimplanting dilated ureters, it should be taken into account that sometimes they have fibrous walls, and tunnelization and aggressive remodeling can lead to ureterovesical obstruction. For patients suffering from ESRD with vesicoureteral reflux and ureterohydronephrosis, pre-transplant nephroureterectomy can be beneficial. If ureteral dilation comes first and the patient requires bladder augmentation, ureteral segments can be used for the reconstruction.

The urothelium is exempt from complications that are inherent to intestinal segments (Nahas et al, 2004, Hitchcock, 1994). In this case, an extraperitoneal approach is taken: lumbotomy incision for the nephrectomy of the dysplastic kidney and mobilization of the dilated ureter and suprapubic incision for bladder augmentation. This approach is beneficial in that it avoids the risks of peritoneal adhesions, and it should be considered in the case of ventriculoperitoneal diversions and of patients who are still under ambulatory peritoneal dialysis (Bellinger, 1993; Dewan et al., 1994; Reinber et al., 1995; Wolf & Turzan, 1993).

Ureterocystoplasty that is laparoscopically assisted has been used since a few years ago. No serious complications have been reported with the use of this procedure, although the need for reaugmentation has been informed to a high degree in the case of native bladders with severely reduced compliance. It is thought that the best candidates to receive ureterocystoplasty have moderately reduced compliance (> 20 ml/cmh2o) and available ureter of a diameter greater than 15 mm to be used in the reconstruction (Husmann et al., 2004)

When it is not possible to obtain urothelial tissue for bladder augmentation, segments from the digestive tube are used: from the stomach, now hardly ever used, to bowel segments. The native bladder is preserved and, for a better anastomosis to the bowel segment, a sagittal incision is performed in order to divide it in two valves. The intestinal segment is open along its antimesenteric border in order to detubularize it and reconfigure it into spherical shape thus achieving maximum volume per given surface area, blunting of intestinal contraction, and improving overall compliance and distensibility.

In many health care centers, ileal segments are chosen to perform colocystoplasty (Nahas et al., 2007), whereas at Hospital de Pediatría Prof. Dr. J. P. Garrahan and since several years ago, sigmoid colon segments without specific bowel preparation have been the segments of choice. No significant infection complications have been observed postoperatively. We have adopted the colon because of its proximity to the native bladder; it has a low rate of metabolic complications and no technical complications.

It is necessary to train the patient and their family in the postoperative care of the colocystoplasty. This consists of clean intermittent catheterization, daily vesical washes and periodical visits to the urologist, because there is a certain risk of complications, such as symptomatic urinary infections, lithiasis, perforations and tumoral neoformations.

Once a bladder or reservoir with adequate volume and low pressure is obtained, it is essential to resolve the urinary incontinence. One of the greatest technical challenges that the urologist surgeon faces in the reconstruction of the vesical neck is to be able to provide adequate outlet resistance. Especially in the case of the neurogenic bladder due to spinal dysraphism, bladder outlet is generally incompetent. There are many surgical options that include adjustments of the neck and proximal urethra thanks to the aponeurosis slings, creation of valve mechanisms, endoscopic injection of artificial volume-formation agents and artificial urinary sphincter.

Several techniques that increase outlet resistance may also deteriorate the detrusor status, reducing its compliance or generating instability. These events will occur depending on the baseline pathology. Therefore, previous urodynamic evaluations carried out and a strict follow-up post-reconstruction and post-transplantation are the golden rule. The final option will undoubtedly be customized according to the baseline disease, the goals of the patients and technical limitations of medical nature.

It is reasonable to say that clean intermittent catheterization may have been the most significant contribution in terms of reconstruction of lower urinary tract functions. The potential need or absence of need for CIC in every reconstruction should always be considered, and both patients and family must be updated as to the objectives of reconstruction as well as the importance of adapting themselves to long term CIC regimens in a strict way. In most cases, the CIC procedure will be needed and patients must learn about it and accept CIC before reconstruction.

When the urethra is inaccessible, sensitive or carries irreparable obstructions, a tubular system with continence mechanism is built with the purpose of facilitating the access to the bladder or the reservoir. The Mitrofanoff principle (1980) solved this dilemma, thanks to the creation of a conduit, being the cecal appendix the most commonly used, reimplanted in the submucosal bladder tunnel at one extreme and converted into a catheterizable stoma at the other extreme, in the abdominal wall. When the bladder is full, optimal coaptation is achieved avoiding urine leakage. If it is not possible to use the cecal appendix, other tubular structures can be used, for instance the ureter, the Fallopian tubes or the reconfigured small intestine (Monti). It should be taken into account that complications that are not so infrequent, such as conduit stenosis, mucous prolapse and false passages, may occur.

5.3 Defunctionalized urinary tract: dry bladder

Anuric children who are awaiting for a kidney transplantation deserve special attention. Patients without a relevant history of urologic disorders, in general patients with nephropathies, have a high probability of recovering the normal functional bladder parameters after the renal transplant, since their bladder has simply defunctionalized due to lack of diuresis. Thus, this alteration is reversible.

On the other hand, patients with a history of neurogenic bladder or posterior urethra valves have a few chances of recovering, with the artificial bladder cycling or after the renal transplant, the adequate features of a functional urinary reservoir. In such cases, due to the chronic status of the baseline disease, the bladder walls suffer an important deposit of collagen connective tissue, with the subsequent reduction or lack of bladder compliance to accommodate increasing volumes of urine. Therefore, the urodynamic alterations are irreversible without an appropriate treatment after the renal transplant.

Pre-transplant augmentation cystoplasty in anuric children can represent a problem if it is not appropriately controlled. The cumulus of intestinal mucus is the main enemy to manage. The lack of regular cycles/washes leads to the appearance of urinary infections, mucus plugs, development of lithiasis and risk of intestinal perforations. Three to four daily washouts with distilled water are recommended with the aim of achieving augmentation distension and eliminating the mucus. It is important to emphasize that the washout liquid must not contain mineral salts in order to avoid precipitates with intestinal mucus, which is an important factor involved in the lithogenesis. Finally, the urodynamic evaluation must be repeated prior to renal transplantation.

5.4 Timing of reconstruction of the lower urinary tract

The reconstruction of the lower urinary tract may be performed before, during or after kidney transplantation. Many authors claim that reconstruction must be done before transplantation (Ali-El-Dei et al., 2004; Nahas et al., 2004) on the assumption that the uropathy is directly responsible for ESRD and must be corrected; furthermore, as post-transplant immunosuppression is far away in time from reconstruction, it will not affect the plastic procedures of the surgery (Fontaine et al., 1998).

In general the reconstruction of the lower urinary tract before the renal transplantation is preferred, since in this way the complications related to the reimplanted ureter that could lead to the loss of the graft are reduced (Taghizadeh et al., 2007). It is worth considering that in already augmented bladders the surgery of the renal transplant may become technically more complex because of the special care needed to avoid damaging the vascular pedicle of the cystoplasty during reimplantation, with the consequent risk of cystoplasty necrosis (MacInerny et al., 1995).

The lower urinary tract reconstruction performed simultaneously with renal transplantation has the main disadvantage of interference in the process of tissue remodeling after bladder augmentation, generated by steroid-based immunosuppression, which would increase tissue fragility. This would promote complications, such as perforations and urinary infections. The manipulation of bowel segments a short time prior to kidney implantation would lead to infection complications related to the allograft. Nevertheless, there exist specific situations in which some patients would benefit from such an approach. That is the case of patients who at the moment of the transplant surgery present important vesicoureteral reflux to the native kidneys and a bladder with low capacity and high pressure. Then it would be advisable to consider nephroureterectomy of the native kidneys and the use of urothelium segments of dilated ureters for ureterocystoplasty immediately before the placement of the graft. In this way, the reconstruction of the lower urinary tract is resolved with adequate tissues, with a low rate of infection complications for the graft.

The reconstruction of the lower urinary tract after the renal transplantation may be performed when the renal function is stable and immunosuppression has been reduced, in order not to interfere with the postoperative remodeling processes. The main advantage of this approach is that the lower urinary tract is reconstructed 'only' when the infection complications appear, which are related to the difficulties in urinary voiding. That is why it has been suggested that continent apendicovesicostomy of the Mitrofanoff type should be performed before renal transplantation, and augmentation cystoplasty, after the renal transplant, if necessary. Several reports describe acceptable outcomes in terms of complications, survival of the graft and the receptor, compared to the patients that have been operated on before renal transplantation (Sheldon et al., 1994; Thomalla, 1990; Nahas et al., 1997).

However, there is evidence that lower urinary tract reconstructions post renal transplant may trigger a high incidence of complications (Barisi et al., 2002), including episodes of pyelonephritis. Another disadvantage of this approach is that the time needed to reduce the immunosuppression doses exposes the graft and urinary tract to risky situations, where the patient requires a quick surgical solution to a transplant that may be deteriorating but it is not possible yet to reduce the immunosuppression drug doses.

Our team adheres to Taghizadeh, who concludes that augmentation cystoplasty 'before' the renal transplant is preferable, because the incidence of complications related to the transplanted ureter and loss of graft is reduced.

6. Renal transplant – Surgical technique – Anesthetic questions

A main part of the preparation of the living donor's kidney is done in situ by the surgical team of the donor. In general, the cadaveric donor's kidney requires major manipulation in order to be able to be implanted, in a procedure called bench surgery, where the dissections of perirenal tissues are performed, technical procedures are applied in order to prepare the blood vessels to be anastomosed and the kidney is irrigated with specific solutions.

By means of Gibson technique or paramedian cut, the incision extends from the costal border to the pubis and into the retroperitoneal space of the iliac fossa. The choice of one side, right or left, over the other is determined by the availability of the left or right kidney, localization of peritoneal dialysis catheter, stomas and available vascular access. Anastomosis between renal artery and vein is performed with primitive ileac artery and vein or hypogastric ones, and sometimes inferior vena cava and aorta, in a terminal-lateral fashion, with continuous polypropylene sutures 7/0. The procedure is performed by a cardiovascular surgeon.

In the case of small patients, weighing less than 15 kilograms, a transperitoneal approach is preferred, using midline incision, from the xyfoid appendix to the pubis, with release and dissection of aorta and inferior vena cava. Anastomosis is also done in these vessels using continuous polypropylene sutures 7/0 (Madeiros-Domingo et al., 2005).

Prior to declamping of the vessels for blood reperfusion of the graft, it is essential to maintain central venous pressure between 15 to 20 cmh2o, with the use of hematic, colloidal and crystalloid products. When reperfusion is done, the graft can sequester up to 300 ml of liquid volume; that is why it is important to keep substantial reposition of liquids post-clamping.

If the size of the organ is considerable in relation to the recipient, it may displace de liver and diaphragm upwards, making breathing and venous return difficult due to obstruction of the inferior vena cava (Madeiros-Domingo et al., 2005).

On the contrary, when the kidneys to be transplanted are small or shorter than 6 cm, they can be implanted in unit fashion, with anastomosis of the distal extreme to the aorta and inferior vena cava of the recipient vessels in a terminal-lateral way, as a segment interposed with proximal and distal anastomosis (Madeiros-Domingo et al., 2005).

Uretero-neo-cystostomy (ureterovesical reimplantation) is performed using extravesical Lich-Gregoire antireflux ureteroneocystostomy method (Lich Jr. et al., 1961). Some groups use intravesical reimplants, according to Politano-Leadbetter technique (Politano, 1958), and it is performed by a urologic surgeon. The former is preferred, since it is fast, does not require extra cystostomy or big ureteral length.

In most cases in our series, and when it was possible, the ureter was reimplanted into the native bladder. When the ureteric reimplantation wass difficult or the ureter caliber small, a double J (pig tail) catheter was used and it is removed 6 weeks following transplantation. For the rest of the patients, a K33-like catheter was used up to the renal pelvis of the graft, with an exit site other than the incision site and it was removed 5-7 days after the surgical procedure. The systematic use of a ureteral tutor for all recipients has reduced the incidence of ureteral complications (Pleass et al. 1995).

In the case of patients with bladder augmentation, the ureteroneocystostomy technique is the same, although special attention should be taken not to interfere in the continent diversion site (Mitrofanoff) in order to avoid urine leakage.

In all recipients, in order to guarantee a complete drainage of the bladder, vesical drainage through the urethra or by way of continent appendicovesicostomy (Mitrofanoff procedure) was established for 7 days, and drainage of the perirenal space was performed.

7. Modifications of the lower urinary tract after the renal transplantation

After re-evaluation during follow-up, there are cases in which for different reasons, such as course of the baseline pathology, alterations in the bladder behavior due to reconstructive procedures, inadequate management and care after reconstruction, among others, there appears a need for another reconstruction of the urinary tract in order to keep the features of a "functional urinary tract." Thus, on some occasions bladder re-augmentations, continent apendicovesicostomies of the Mitrofanoff type or procedures in the neck and/or proximal urethra must be performed so as to treat urinary incontinence. There is approximately 3% of cases described in the literature that needed procedures in the lower urinary tract after renal transplantation, although they had undergone evaluation and surgeries previously to the transplantation (Sager et al., 2011). This evidences that although we may think that everything that was done was enough, in surgical terms, the nephro-urologic follow-up show us that evaluation and follow-up are fundamental and many times it is necessary to do adjustments in order to protect the allograft.

8. Graft survival

Extensive bibliography shows that renal transplantation can be indicated safely in the case of patients with lower urinary tract reconstructions, achieving acceptable survival and function of the graft. The results are comparable to the ones obtained for patients with normal urinary tract (Franc-Guimond & Gonzalez, 2004; Capizzi et al., 2004).

At Hospital Nacional de Pediatría Prof. Dr. J. P. Garrahan, 156 renal transplants have been performed up to date on children with uropathies, 38 of which received reconstructions of the dysfunctional urinary tract. No significant differences have been found between the latter and those patients that had no lower urinary tract reconstructions regarding survival of the graft or levels of creatininemia at year 1 and 5 after transplantation (Sager et al., 2011). In general terms, the actuarial global functional survival rate after the first year postoperatively was higher than 93%, and at year 5 it was between 75% and 85% (Figure 1)

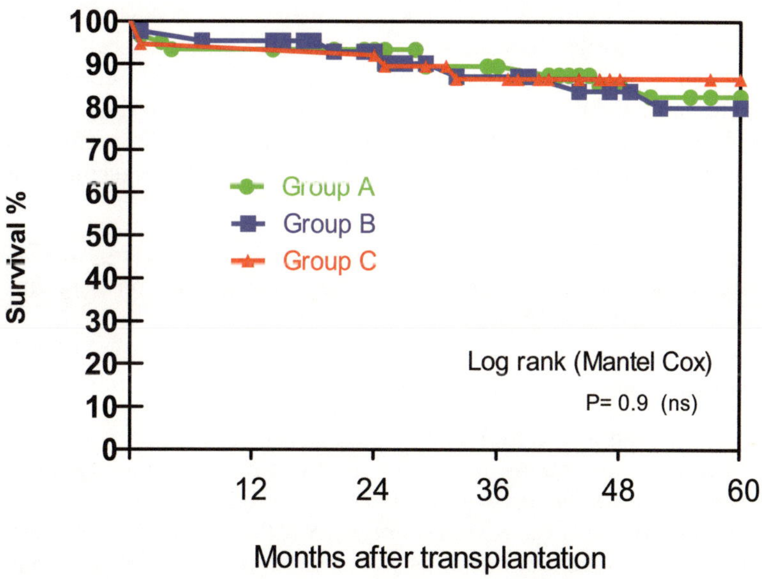

Fig. 1. Actuarial allograft survival in patients with uropathies. Group A: Patients without surgeries in lower urinary tract; Group B: Patients who underwent surgeries in lower urinary tract and preserved adequate bladder function; Group C: Patients who underwent surgeries in lower urinary tract due to inadequate bladder function.

Other authors have shown that patients with dysfunction in the urinary tract that required reconstructions had an increased risk of complications and loss of the graft (Mochon et al., 1992; Salomón et al., 1997). Such discrepancies can be explained because of the heterogeneity of the series published, the wide scope of the disease, the severity of the lower urinary tract and its different treatments (Riley et al., 2010)

9. Complications

9.1 Vascular complications

Vascular thrombosis is the third cause of loss of the graft in children according to the NAPRTCS (North American Pediatric Renal Transplant Cooperative Study), with an incidence of 11.6% (Benfield, 2003). When the receptor is very young and has a low weight, the risk increases because of the reduced diameter in the vascular structures.

Vascular thrombosis, especially venous thrombosis, may occur immediately and up to 90 days post-transplantation. It is a devastating complication, since besides the graft loss, it may unleash rupture of the graft capsule, major hematomas, massive hemorrhage, thromboembolic events and sepsis.

Arterial thrombosis is the most feared, since it invariably conditions the loss of the graft and subsequent nephrectomy. In children its incidence is 6% (Singh et al., 1997).

The causes of vascular thrombosis are intimal dissection, atherosclerosis, immunological factors and hypercoagulable state. Furthermore, high doses of cyclosporine or antilymphocyte globulin, systemic lupus erythematosus, antiphospholipid syndrome, and deficiency of protein C and S are involved.

Arterial stenosis, with an estimated frequency of occurrence between 2% and 10% can appear during the post-transplant period or many years later, and it is localized at the site of anastomosis or distal to it. Immunological and mechanical factors generate a hyperplasic response of the intima. Arterial stenosis manifests as out of control arterial hypertension and deterioration of the function of the graft. This entity forces physicians to perform procedures such as transluminal percutaneous angioplasty with or without endovascular prosthesis or vascular bypass.

Other vascular complications that are less frequent but not less severe are arteriovenous fistulas and perigraft hematomas or ureterovesical joint hematomas on the reimplantation site; the latter are also resolved surgically.

9.2 Urologic complications

Forced immunosuppression and complexity of the reconstructed urinary tract facilitate the appearance of different complications. By far, the most frequent bacteria infection in patients with a renal transplantation is the urinary tract infection (UTI) (Abbott et al., 2001; Karakayali et al., 2001). The incidence of UTI varies significantly across the literature: from 6% to 86% after renal transplantation. This variation responds to the different criteria in defining what UTI involves, the methods of urine collection and type of antibiotic prophylaxis, among others.

The possible impact of UTI increases mortality and morbidity rates due to infection itself, and the potential effects on the processes of acute and chronic rejection. UTI episodes occur especially in the first postoperative stage, when the patient is hospitalized. A great percentage of UTI occurs between 6-12 months after the implant.

Numerous risk factors for UTI are involved in renal transplantation; among the most important are the patients with a reconstructed lower urinary tract. The major causes are: anatomical conditions, characteristics of the intestinal mucus, vesicoureteral reflux and immunosuppression. Most of these patients who are under a clean intermittent catheterization program present with asymptomatic chronic bacteriuria. Reports have shown that this event has no effect on the survival of the graft (Warhom et al., 1999; Hatch et al., 2001). However, some authors believe that when pyelonephritis and recurrent episodes of asymptomatic UTI appear, the function of the graft is at risk, with the subsequent possibility of extirpation (Mendizabal et al., 2005; Alfrey et al., 1997). Other authors claim that recipients of the renal transplant with repeated UTI episodes show deterioration of the graft function, although its survival does not differ from the survival rate of the general population (Sullivan et al., 2003; Surange et al., 2003).

In some reports, instituting an aggressive treatment for UTI at an early stage post-transplant is recommended, since UTI may trigger acute rejection (Sullivan et al., 2003); other reports, however, suggest that intensive treatment in the case of asymptomatic UTI may favor the development of resistant bacteria strains. In our center, the approach followed consists of using as antibiotic prophylaxis trimetropin/sulfametoxazol even in the presence of positive urocultures in asymptomatic patients, without alteration of the function of the graft. Intensive antibiotic therapy is reserved for those patients with symptomatic UTI, worsening of the renal function or the presence of aggressive germs such as pseudomonas aeruginosa or those related with lithogenesis, like proteus mirabilis.

In our case report we showed that 25% of patients with renal transplantation and reconstructed urinary tract presented low UTI; 42.5% presented high UTI, and two patients developed sepsis of urologic cause; one of them with graft loss. Due to the detection of more episodes of UTI in this subgroup, vesicoureteral reflux was more frequently diagnosed (25%) compared to the subgroup of patients with uropathies without reconstructions, where reflux was observed in only 1% of the group (Sager et al., 2011).

Vesicoureteral reflux to the graft, especially of high grade, which is associated to symptomatic UTI, is generally treated first with endoscopic approach. Different materials are used as endoscopic bulking agents in ureterovesical junction: the most common one is dextranomer/hyaluronic acid. Many times the endoscopic technique becomes difficult because the bladder has undergone previous surgery or augmentation, and the opening of the urethral meatus may not always be located. In cases of neurogenic bladders with vesicoureteral reflux to the graft and failure of the bulking agents, as the urinary tract has already been reconstructed, open ureterovesical reimplantation is very frequently done.

If intermediate or low grade vesicoureteral reflux to the graft is detected under ureterohydronephrosis study and there are no UTI leaks nearby and the renal function is preserved, a vigilant attitude under antibiotic prophylaxis is taken before resorting to surgical techniques to resolve the reflux, provided the urodynamic studies do not show significant alterations.

Ureterovesical stenosis may have an incidence between 2% and 4%. Different procedures can be required in order to reestablish the adequate urinary flow, such as pig tail catheters via percutaneous nephrostomy and posterior ureterovesical reimplant. Ureteral fistulas are produced by ischemic necrosis of the distal ureter, as a consequence of vascular lesion during donor nephrectomy. Hematoma of the ureterovesical juncture, urinary fistulas and necrosis of the distal ureter (2 to 4%) are directly associated as causative agents of ureterovesical stenosis and require in all cases open exploration (Sager et al., 2011).

Perirenal collections are another frequent surgical complication with an incidence of approximately 49% (Pollak, et al., 1988). Lymphoceles cause several collections and are generated by the cumulus of lymphatic liquid in the retroperitoneum, due to the dissection and binding of lymphatic vessels at the moment of forming the vascular pouch. Their occurrence has been associated to the use of Sirolimus (Giessing & Budde, 2003). Some lymphoceles may grow until displacing or comprising the reimplanted ureter, generating ureterohydronephrosis extrinsic to the implant. If the lymphocele grows progressively or is persistent, it may be treated by means of external percutaneous drainage or with laparoscopic exploration and marsupialization.

Transplants	Group A	Group B	Group C
n	68	48	40
Complications *n(%)*			
Vascular:			
Arterial Stenosis	4(6)	2(4.2)	-
Arterial Thrombosis	2(3)	2(4.2)	-
Venous Thrombosis	1(1.5)	2(4.2)	1(2.5)
Arteriovenous Fistula	1(1.5)	-	-
Hematoma	1(1.5)	-	1(2.5)
Urologic:			
Ureterovesical Junction Hematoma	-	1(2)	-
Ureterovesical Stenosis	2(2.9)	2(4.2)	1(2.5)
Vesicoureteral Reflux (>grade II)	1(1.5)	1(2.1)	10(25)
Urinary Fistula - Ureteral Necrosis	2(2,9)	2(4.2)	1(2.5)
Renal Pelvis Necrosis	-	-	1(2.5)
Lymphocele	5(7.5)	2(4.2)	-
Vesical Lithiasis	-	-	2(5)
Retained drainage in surgical site	1(1.5)	-	-
Urinary Infections:		-	-
-Lower:	6(9)	3(6.2)	10(25)
-Upper:	8(12)	11(23.1)	17(42.5)
Sepsis of urologic origin	-	-	2(5)
Urinous Peritonitis	-	-	1(2.5)
Infection of surgical wound	1(1.5)	2(4.2)	6(15)
Abdominal wall abscess	-	-	2(5)
Urine Incontinence	-	-	1(2.5)
Total n(%)	35(51.5)	30(63)	53(132)

References: Group A: Patients without lower urinary tract; Group B: Patients that required surgery in lower urinary tract and preserved adequate bladder function; Group C: Patients that needed surgery in lower urinary tract due to inadequate function.

Table 1. Vascular and Urologic Post Renal Transplant Complications in Patients with Uropathies.

Other causes of perirenal collections include: hematomas, urinomas and sera cumuli, all of which are not resolved unless surgical intervention is performed.

Other urologic complications in decreasing order of presentation are: surgical wound infections, wall abscess, vesical lithiasis and urinous peritonitis due to colocystoplasty perforation.

Recently, colocystoplasty neoformations –infrequent but of poor prognosis- have been reported as appearing several years after bladder reconstruction-augmentation. The exact etiopathogenic mechanism for these neoformations is unknown, but the possible explanations include: increased nitrosamines at the vesicointestinal anastomosis site; influence of disguised and chronic urinary infections, among others. At a histological level, the neoformations may be adenocarcynomas, urothelial tumors located in the native bladder, in the bowel segment or at the vesicointestinal anastomosis site, and in general they exert a very aggressive effect (Bono Ariño, et al., 2001). This poses a serious ethical-medical dilemma, since so far the established modality widely embraced has been the re-functionalization of the lower urinary tract by means of intestinal segments in patients that will surely be put under immunosuppression regimens. Up to date, the only weapon to protect this complex subgroup of patients is a strict clinical, ultrasound and endoscopic follow-up, especially when hematuria is present.

In our case report we describe the following complications and interventions post renal transplant (Tables 1 and 2).

10. Vascular and urologic post renal transplant interventions

Transplants	Group A	Group B	Group C
n	68	48	40
Vascular Interventions			
Angioplasty	2	-	-
Bypass	1	2	-
Fistula embolization	1	-	-
Urologic Interventions			
Sigmoid vesical augmentation	1	-	2
Mitrofanoff	1	1	1
Mitrofanoff reoperation	-	1	2
Aponeurotic sling	-	-	1
Closure of bladder neck	-	-	1
Ureterovesical reimplant due to:			
- vesicoureteral reflux	1	-	-
-Stenosis	2	1	1
-Fistula	2	2	1

Transplants	Group A	Group B	Group C
n	68	48	40
Nephroureterectomy of native kidney	3	-	2
Drainage-punction of lymphocele	4	1	-
Drainage-punction of abscess-hematoma	2	-	2
Nephrostomy	3	1	3
Cystoscopy	2	-	-
Placement of pig tail catheter	2	1	3
Injection of substances due to vesicoureteral reflux	-	-	1
Injection of substances due to urine incontinence	-	-	1
Nephrectomy of the graft	5	2	4
Parcial Ureterectomy	-	2	
Ureterostomy	-	-	2
Endoscopic Cystolitotomy	-	-	1
Open Cystolitotomy	-	-	1

References: Group A: Patients without lower urinary tract; Group B: Patients that required surgery in lower urinary tract and preserved adequate bladder function; Group C: Patients that needed surgery in lower urinary tract due to inadequate function.

Table 2. Vascular and Urologic Post Renal Transplant Interventions.

11. Graft loss

There are different causes of graft dysfunction, such as renal rejection and nephrotoxicity due to cyclosporine, tacrolimus and vascular problems. The vascular thromboses that are more associated to graft loss are venous thromboses. Urologic causes have infrequent relation to the renal graft loss, but recurrent urinary infections, such as pyelonephritis generate lymphocyte and intratubular neutrophilus deposits. As a consequence, but not exclusively due to pyelonephritis, the normal functional renal tissue is replaced by interstitial fibrosis and tubular atrophy (IF/TA).

Even though the patients who have received a kidney transplantation and have corrected or reconstructed urinary tracts are subjected to an important incidence of urologic complications, the main cause for graft loss in our series was the presence of vascular events (Sager, et al., 2011).

12. Survival and quality of life

Survival rates at years 1 and 5 post-transplantation are 98.8% and 94.2%, respectively. In our series, 8 out of 150 patients died due to cardiovascular causes, lymphoproliferative disease and non urologic sepsis (Sager et al., 2011).

In other studies, 100% of transplanted patients with over 10 years of follow-up reported that they feel they have good or excellent health status; 94% stated that their health status does not interfere with their family and social life; 90% of them study or work; 70% have an active sexual life, and absence from their work or study places was in general minimal (Ferraris & Rodriguez, 2008).

The success of this type of therapy also depends on "the patients's adherence to treatment." Lack of adherence is the most important risk factor for the development of chronic allograft nephropathy (CAN) and sub-clinical rejection. The critical period is when the adolescent goes from dialysis to the post-transplant phase, when the responsibilities as to being alert, managing care and decision-making increase.

13. Follow-up

Strict follow-up is essential in order to carry out a continuous assessment of the following aspects: function of the graft and drainage to the lower tract; function of the lower urinary tract; record of the urinary volume and frequency voided by means of voiding records; need for contrasting studies, such as cystourethrography and urodynamic studies.

It is necessary to monitor compliance with medication therapy, for instance, anticholinergic drugs; compliance with daily bladder washes in the case of those who have undergone bladder augmentation, and the correct use of catheters for those who need catheterization via Mitrofanoff or urethra.

It is likewise important to bear in mind that many patients and parents gradually lose interest in the urologic follow-up after the renal transplant. Thus, physicians should emphasize how essential monitoring is since the first consultation, so that parents, patients and medical caregivers become committed to a thorough and long-term follow-up program.

14. Conclusions

Along the time, it has been demonstrated that the renal transplant is the best option for children with end stage renal disease. At present these children can benefit from this type of therapy provided the functions of the dysfunctional lower urinary tract are corrected, either by means of medical and/or surgical treatment. Otherwise, the bladder dysfunction that is not corrected will negatively affect the function of the graft.

Among the most frequent etiologies for ESRD we can find renal dysplasia, obstructive uropathies, focal and segment glomerulosclerosis, nephropathy due to vesicoureteral reflux, renal polycystosis, hemolytic uremic syndrome, Prune belly, neurogenic bladder due to neural tube defects, and other conditions. All of them must be exhaustively evaluated so that it can be determined whether the lower urinary tract is in optimal condition to receive a renal implant, following the principle of "functional urinary tract." This term refers to the condition that a lower urinary tract should be a reservoir with adequate volume, low intravesical pressure and continence, and correct and complete urine voiding.

For those cases that do not meet these criteria, different treatments are offered in order to provide a safe mechanism of drainage when voiding difficulties are present, via clean intermittent catheterization and pharmacologic reduction of filling pressure or contractions that are not inhibited, with the use of anticholinergic drugs.

When the objectives cannot be reached in spite of applying medical treatments, the option is surgical intervention for reconstruction of the urinary tract. Here the possibility of using urothelial tissues should be considered, since these patients usually have high grades of vesicoureteral reflux or obstructive ureterohydronephrosis. When it is not possible to obtain urothelial tissue to perform bladder augmentation, segments of the digestive tube can be used, either from the small or the large bowel, according to the criterion of each health care center.

Favorable long term outcomes have been reported on patients who underwent renal transplantations with reconstruction of the urinary tract; however, there is considerable controversy around which is the best way to manage these patients, since there are no guidelines with defined criteria for reconstructive surgeries, optimal surgical procedures, or even recommendations as to when is the best time to do them.

Our team adheres to Taghizadeh, whose report claims that augmentation cystoplasty before renal transplant is preferable, as the incidence of complications and graft loss is reduced, especially in relation to lesions of the transplanted ureter.

It has also been agreed that renal transplantation can be indicated in a safe way to patients with lower urinary tract reconstructions, with acceptable survival and function of the graft. Results are comparable to those obtained in the case of patients with normal urinary tract. Nevertheless, it is undeniable that forced immunosuppression and the complexity of the reconstructed urinary tract favor the appearance of complications, especially infections related to the urinary tract. Potentially, this would promote the increase of morbidity and mortality rates and it would attempt against the implant. However, urologic causes have an infrequent relationship with the loss of the renal graft.

In the case of these complex and heterogeneous patients, it is essential to provide a careful and individualized evaluation of the lower urinary tract prior to transplantation and a strict postoperative follow-up in order to diminish and control possible urological complications. Since at present there are no sound guidelines or protocols for the management of pediatric patients with dysfunctional lower urinary tract and end stage renal disease, it is necessary to design randomized multicenter studies in order to achieve better results on morbidity.

15. Acknowledgments

The authors thank all the members of the Nephrology Department at Hospital de Pediatría Dr. Juan P. Garrahan for their collaboration.

16. References

Abbott KC, Oliver JD III, Hypolite I, et al. (2001). Hospitalization for bacterial septisemia after renal transplantation in the United State. *Am J Nephrol;* 21:120-127.

Alfrey EJ, Salvatierra O Jr, Tanney DC et al. (1997). Bladder augmentation can be problematic with renal failure and transplantation. *Pediatric Nephrol;* 11:672-5.

Ali-El-Dei B, Abdol-Eneim H, El-Husseini A, et al. (2004). Renal transplantation in children with abnormal lower urinary tract. *Transplant Proc;* 36:2968.

Austin PF, Homsy YL, Masel JL, et al. (1999). Alfa-adrenergic blockade in children with neuropathic and nonneuropathic voiding dysfunction. *J Urol;* 162:1064-1067.

Barisi A, Hosseini Moghaddam S, Khoddam R. (2002). Augmentation cystoplasty before and after renal transplantation: Long-term results. *Transplant Proc;* 34:2106.

Barry J. (2004). Kidney transplantation into patients with anormal bladders. *Transplantation;* 77:1120-23.

Bellinger MF. (1993). Ureterocystoplasty: a unique method for vesical augmentation in children. *J Urol;* 149:811-13.

Benfield MR. (2003). Current status of kidney transplant: update 2003. *Pediatr Clin North Am;* 50: 1301-34.

Bibiloni N., Bertolotti J., Ferrari C. M. (2008). Diagnóstico por imágenes del riñón y del tracto urinário, In: *Nefrología Pediátrica,* Ferraris JR, Briones LM. 75-89. Fundación Sociedad Argentina de Pediatría-FUNDASAP, ISBN 978-987-1279-16-6, Buenos Aires, Argentina.

Bono Ariño A, Sanz Vélez JI, Esclarin Duny MA, et al. (2001). Adenocarcinoma de células en anillo de sello en colocistoplastia. *Actas Urol Esp;* 25 (4): 312-314.

Broyer M, LeBihan C, Charbit M; Guest G, et al. (2004). Long-term social outcome of children after kidney transplantation. *Transplantation;* 77: 1033-1037.

Burek C & Sager C (2008). Vejiga neurogénica, In: *Nefrología Pediátrica,* Ferraris JR, Briones LM. 480-493. Fundación Sociedad Argentina de Pediatría-FUNDASAP, ISBN 978-987-1279-16-6, Buenos Aires, Argentina.

Capizzi A. Et al. (2004). Kidney transplantation in children with reconstructed bladder. *Transplantation;* 77:1113-16.

Cerruto MA & Artibani W (2006). Urodynamics, In: Pediatric neurogenic bladder dysfunction. Diagnosis, treatment, long-Term Follow-up. Esposito C, Guys JM, Gough D, Savanelli A. 133-146, Springer, ISBN-10 3-540-30866-0, Berlin, German.

De Jong TP, Chrzan R, Klijn AJ, Dik P. (2008). Treatment of the neurogenic bladder in spina bifida. *Pediatr Nephrol;* 23:889-96.

Dewan PA, Nicholls EA, Goh DW. (1994). Ureterocystoplasty: an extraperitoneal, urothelial bladder augmentation technique. *Eur Urol;* 26:85-89.

Ferraris JR & Rodriguez L (2008). Transplante renal In: *Nefrología Pediátrica,* Ferraris JR, Briones LM. 682-699. Fundación Sociedad Argentina de Pediatría-FUNDASAP, ISBN 978-987-1279-16-6, Buenos Aires, Argentina.

Fine RN, Malekkadek MH et al.(1978). Long term results of renal transplantation in children. *Pediatrics,* 61: 641.

Fontaine E, Gagnadoux MF, Niaudet P, et al. (1998). Renal transplantation in children with augmentation cystoplasty: long-term results. *J Urol;* 159:2110.

Franc-Guimond J, Gonzalez R. (2004). Renal transplantation in children with recontructed bladders. *Transplantation;* 77:1116-20.

Galvez MP, Cusi MP, Corral Molina JM. (2005). Generalidades del trasplante renal pediátrico. *Arch Esp Urol;* 58, 6: 553-562.

Giessing M, Budde K. (2003). Sirolimus and lymphocele formation after kidney transplantation: an immunosuppressive medication as co-factor for a surgical problem? *Nephrol Dial Transplant;* 18: 448-9.

Gradus D, Ettenger RB. (1982). Renal Transplantation in children. *Pediatr Clin North Am,* 29: 1013.

Hatch DA, Koyle MA, Baskin LS et al. (2001). Kidney transplantation in children with urinary diversion or bladder augmentation. *J Urol;* 165:2265-8.

Hatch DA. (1994). Kidney transplantation in patients with an abnormal lower urinary tract. *Urol clin North Am;* 21:311.

Hitchcock RJ, Duffy PG and Malone PS. (1994). Ureterocistoplasty: The bladder augmentation of choice. *Br J Urol;* 73:575.

Husmann DA, Snodgrass WT, Koyle MA et al. (2004). Ureterocystoplasty: indications for a successful augmentation. *J Urol;* 171:376-380.

Karakayali H, Emiroglu R, Arslan G, et al. (2001). Mayor infectious complications after kidney transplantation. *Transplant Proc;* 33:1816-17.

Kelly WD, Merkel FK, Markland C. (1966). Ileal urinary diversion in conjunction with renal homotransplantations. *Lancet;* 1:22.

Lich R Jr., Howerton LW, Davis LA. (1961). Vesicourethrography. *J Urol;* 85: 396-7.

López JC & Durán V (2008). Obstrucción de la vía urinaria Baja, In: *Nefrología Pediátrica,* Ferraris JR, Briones LM. 432-437. Fundación Sociedad Argentina de Pediatría-FUNDASAP, ISBN 978-987-1279-16-6, Buenos Aires, Argentina.

Luke P, Herz D, Bellinger M, et al. (2003). Long term results of pediatric renal transplantation into a disfuntional lower urinary tract. *Transplantation;* 76:1578-82.

Mac Inerny PD, Picramenos D, Koffman CG, et al. (1995). Is cystoplasty a safe alternative to urinary diversion in patients requiring renal transplantation? *Eur Urol;* 27:117.

Madeiros-Domingo M, Romero-Navarro B, Valverde-Rosas S, et al. (2005). Trasplante renal en pediatria. *Rev Inv Clin;* 57,2:230-36.

Martz k. (2007). NAPRTCS 2007 Annual Report, In: North American Pediatric Renal Trials and Collaborative Studies, 2007, available from: <www.emmes.com/study/ped/annlrept/annlrept2007.pdf>

Mendizabal S, Estornell F, Zamora I, et al. (2005). Renal transplantation in children with severe bladder dysfunction. *J Urol;* 173:226-9.

Mitchell ME, Piser JA. (1987). Intestinocystoplasty and total bladder replacement in children and young adult: follow up in 129 cases. *J Urol;* 138: 579.

Mochon M, Kaiser BA, Dunn S, et al. (1992). Urinary tract infections in children with posterior urethral valves after kidney transplantation. *J Urol;* 148:1874.

Murray JE, Merril JP. Harrison JH. (1958). Kideney transplantation between seven pairs of identical twins. Ann Surg; 48: 343.

Nahas C. et al. (2007). Comparision of transplantation outcomes in children with and without bladder dysfunction. A customized approach equals the diference. *J Urol;* 179:712.

Nahas WC, Lucon M, Mazzucchi E, et al. (2004). Clinical and urodinamyc evaluation after ureterocystoplasty and kidney transplantation. *J Urol;* 171:1428.

Nahas WC, Lucon M, Mazzucchi E, et al. (2004). Clinical and urodynamic evaluation after ureterocystoplasty and kidney transplantation. *J urol;* 171:1428.

Nahas WC, Mazzucchi E, Antonopoulos I, et al. (1997). Kidney transplantation in patients with bladder augmentation: Surgical outcome and urodynamic follow-up. *Transplant proc;* 29:157.

Podestá M & Bertolotti G (2008). Uropatías obstructivas del tracto urinario superior: diagnóstico y tratamiento, In: *Nefrología Pediátrica,* Ferraris JR, Briones LM. 424-31. Fundación Sociedad Argentina de Pediatría-FUNDASAP, ISBN 978-987-1279-16-6, Buenos Aires, Argentina.

Politano VA, Leadbetter WF. (1958). An operative technique for the correction of vesicoureteral reflux. *J Urol;* 79: 932-41.

Pollak R, Veremis SA, Maddux MS, et al. (1988). The natural history of and therapy for perirenal fluid collections following renal transplantation. *J Urol;* 140: 716-20.

Reinber Y, Allen RC, Vaughn M et al. (1995). Nephrectomy combined with lower abdominal extraperitoneal ureteral bladder augmentation in the treatment of children with vesicoureteral reflux dysplasia syndrome. *J Urol;* 153:777-779.

Riley P, Marks S,Desai D, et al. (2010). Challenges facing renal transplantation in pediatric patients with lower urinary tract dysfunction. *Transplantation;* 89:1299-1307.

Sager C, Burek C, Duran V, et al. (2011). Outcome of renal transplant in patients with abnormal urinary tract. *Pediatr Surg Int;* 27:423–430.

Salomón L, Fontaine E, Gagnadoux MF, et al. (1997). Posterior urethral valves: Long-term renal function consequences after transplantation. *J Urol;* 157:992.

Salomon L, Fontaine E, Guest G, et al. (2000). Role of the bladder in delayed failure of kidney transplants in boys with posterior urethral valves. *J Urol;* 163: 1282.

Shekarris B, Upadhyay J, Demirbilek S, et al. (2000). Surgical complications of bladder augmentation: comparicion between enterocystoplasties in 133 patients. *Urology;* 55.123.

Sheldon C A, Gonzalez R, Burn MW, et al. (1994). Renal transplantation into the dysfunctional bladder. The rol of adjunctive bladder reconstruction. *J Urol;* 152: 972.

Singh A, Stablein D, Tejani A. (1997). Risk factors for vascular thrombosis in pediatric renal transplantation: a special report of the North American Pediatric Renal Transplant Cooperative Study. *Transplantation;* 63: 1263-7.

Sullivan ME, Reynard JM, Cranston DW. (2003). Renal transplantation into the abnormal lower urinary tract. *BJU int;* 92:510-15.

Surange RS, Johnson RW, Tabakoli A, et al. (2003). Kidney transplantation into an ileal conduit: a single center experience of 59 cases. *J Urol;* 170:1727-30.

Taghizadeh AK, Desai D, Ledermann SE, et al. (2007). Renal transplantation or bladder augmentation first? A comparision of complications and outcomes in children. *BJU Int;* 100:1365.

Thomalla JV. (1990). Augmentation of the bladder in preparation for renal transplantation. Surg *Gynecol Obstet;* 170:349.

Torre M, Guida E, Bisio G, et al. (2011). Risk factors for renal function impairment in a series of 502 patients born with spinal dysraphisms. *J Pediatr Urol;* 7:39-43.

Warhom C, Berglund J, Andersson J, Tyden G. (1999). Renal transplantation in patients with urinary diversion: a case-control study. *Nephrol Dial transplant;* 14:2937-40.

Wolf JS, Turzan CW. (1993). Augmentation ureterocystoplasty. *J Urol;* 149:1095-98.

Woodward J.R. & Smith E.A. (1998). Prune-Belly Syndrome, In: *Campbell´s Urology*, Walsh PC, Retik AB, Vaughan ED, Jr, Wein AJ. 7 edition, Vol 2: 1917-36, WB Saunders, ISBN 0-7216-44-63-5, United States of America.